Practical Homoeopathy

A COMPLETE GUIDE TO HOME TREATMENT

Beth MacEoin

BLITZ EDITIONS

For Denis with fondest love

The information in this book is intended to be advisory in nature and should not be regarded as a replacement for professional medical treatment and advice. If in doubt, always consult your GP or homoeopathic practitioner.

Neither the publishers nor the author of this book can be held liable for any errors, omissions, or actions that may be taken as a consequence of using it.

This edition published in 1997

Published by Blitz Editions
an imprint of Bookmart Limited
Registered Number 2372865
Trading as Bookmart Limited
Desford Road, Enderby
Leicester, LE9 5AD

ISBN 1 85605 388 1

10 9 8 7 6 5 4 3 2 1

Designed by Neysa Moss
Typeset by Hewer Text Composition Services, Edinburgh
Printed in Great Britain by Clays Ltd, St Ives plc

Contents

Introduction   1

Chapter 1   Understanding Homoeopathy   3

Chapter 2   Homoeopathy In The Home: How To Use This Book   10

Chapter 3   Homoeopathic First Aid   23

Chapter 4   A–Z Of Common Ailments   46

Chapter 5   Homoeopathy And Sports Injuries   91

Chapter 6   Homoeopathy For Babies And Children   106

Chapter 7   Homoeopathy For Women   144

Chapter 8   The Stresses Of Modern Living: How To Cope   187

Chapter 9   Homoeopathy For The Over Fifties   211

Chapter 10 Remedy Information: Essential Aspects   236

Homoeopathic Remedies And Their Abbreviations   336

Useful Addresses   338

Recommended Reading   340

Index   343

Acknowledgements

Many thanks are due to the following, who have helped in various ways during the writing and production of this book: Rowena Gaunt, Teresa Chris, Dr Mike Whiteside, Kathy Rooney, Kate Bouverie, Isabelle Rickard, and Kate Morris. In addition, special thanks must also be extended to my husband Denis and my mother Nancy for providing vital emotional and practical support at stressful times during the writing process. Last, but not least, my special thanks go to Samantha for being an endless source of amusement and pleasure when the pressures of work got too tough.

Introduction

H omoeopathic medicine provides us with an exciting approach to health and healing, which is eminently suitable for those of us who are interested in tackling ill health at its most fundamental level. Instead of temporarily dampening down or suppressing symptoms, the homoeopathic approach to treatment stimulates the body's capacity for self-healing and self-renewal. As a result, symptoms depart when the underlying disorder has been efficiently dealt with, and not before.

The homoeopathic interpretation of cure is also extremely ambitious, since it encompasses much more than the mere removal or temporary absence of symptoms. From the homoeopathic perspective, genuine freedom from illness is a positive state which results in enhanced energy levels, an improved sense of well-being and vitality, and clearer thought processes, as well as a true sense of emotional balance and harmony. In other words, cure can be understood to have been established when the mind, emotions and body function in a state of optimum harmony, which is unfettered by pain, distress, exhaustion or trauma.

Although this may initially sound a little daunting, it is important to bear in mind that the homoeopathic approach is also extremely practical, offering effective treatment for a wide range of problems. Patients regularly consult homoeopaths for treatment of a variety of conditions, which may include any of the following: eczema, asthma, hayfever, irritable bowel syndrome, depression, migraines, anxiety, psoriasis, bronchitis, arthritis, sinusitis and pre-menstrual syndrome.

However, there are also conditions that can be effectively treated at home, provided enough clear, practical information is made available to the home prescriber. It is the aim of this book to give the newcomer to homoeopathy the basic information they need in order to treat straightforward conditions with confidence and security.

With this in mind, the structure of this book has been deliberately set out to guide the home prescriber, initially identifying the conditions they should and should not treat, and giving clear instructions about how to obtain the essential information they need to choose the most appropriate homoeopathic prescrip-

1

tion. In addition, general, practical self-help advice is given regarding changes in diet or lifestyle that will support a move towards cure. Most important of all, clear indications are also provided which suggest when the home prescriber may be getting out of his or her depth, and that professional medical advice (homoeopathic or otherwise) is needed.

As a result, it is to be hoped that users of this book will be empowered to treat simple conditions at home, discovering the exciting potential of using an extremely safe, gentle and effective system of restoring the body to optimum health.

■1■

Understanding Homoeopathy

These days it is common practice in medical circles to make casual references to the useful role of complementary or holistic therapies in medical treatment. As a result, we may often be led to believe that homoeopathy, in common with other alternative therapies, should be limited to an adjunctive capacity, being 'tacked on' to more vigorous, conventional treatment.

Although advocates of complementary approaches are frequently well-meaning in striving for better treatment for patients, this limited interpretation of the potential of alternative therapies can seriously distort the facts. As a result, we may be unable to grasp the radical contrasts between the basic theories underlying alternative and orthodox medical systems.

Before we can appreciate this fundamental difference, we must explore the basic concepts of health and disease, in order to demonstrate how alternative and conventional medicine are radically different from each other.

The Conventional Medical View Of Disease

Conventional medicine takes a broadly mechanistic view of disease, regarding the human body as a highly sophisticated and specialized machine which can succumb to injury, infection or degenerative processes. As a result, a great deal of effort is put into finding ways of combating these problems by refining and perfecting surgical techniques, identifying and developing 'magic bullet' drugs, and replacing worn out or damaged parts such as knee or hip joints.

As a rule, orthodox drugs work by opposing symptoms so that the discomfort is diminished as long as the drug is effective. Good examples of this process would include the use of analgesics for acute pain, antacids for acidity, anti-inflammatories for inflammation, tranquillizers for anxiety and laxatives for constipation. However, if the underlying problem that has led to the initial development of the symptoms has not been dealt with, many patients may find that they need to take drugs on a long-term or permanent basis in order to keep their symptoms suppressed. Unfortunately long-term drug treatment of this kind can lead to undesirable side effects, which can further undermine our overall quality of health.

In many ways we can regard this approach to disease as an aggressive one, with the analogy of 'waging war on illness' commonly being used within this context. As a result, some orthodox measures may be violent or highly toxic, such as the use of radical surgery, chemotherapy or radiotherapy in cancer treatments. It has been said in defence of such procedures that, within the context of a crisis, drastic problems require equally drastic solutions if the illness is to be overcome. However, although this approach may achieve results, it is sometimes at the expense of great trauma and distress to the system as a whole.

Before the appropriate orthodox treatment can be selected and given, the most accurate diagnosis must be made and the range of tests to which a patient may be exposed can be astonishingly detailed and wide-ranging. While this can play a vitally important role in identifying the nature of the illness, it can also have the undesirable effect of distancing the physician from his or her patient as sophisticated and potentially invasive technology is increasingly being relied upon.

Conventional medical theory also encourages a high degree of specialization, with remarkably detailed information being gathered regarding individual organs such as the liver, brain and heart, or systems of the body such as the endocrine or immune system. As a result, the higher one rises in the medical hierarchy, the more specialized one's knowledge is likely to become.

In addition, treatments tend to be focused on the specific organs that may be affected, so that we may be given one course of tablets for one disorder, such as acidity of the stomach, a different drug for constipation, and yet another for the diarrhoea that may result from over-vigorous action of the laxative.

If we take this argument further, and consider that we may suffer from conditions affecting more than one organ at a time, this can create a scenario where each separate part of the body needs treatment from a different consultant. Consequently, we and our consultants are likely to lose sight of our bodies as an integrated whole.

The Alternative View Of Disease

Alternative therapists generally adopt what is termed a 'holistic' perspective when discussing the issues of health and disease. Unlike conventional doctors, who may equate health with the absence of disease, alternative therapists will refer to good health as a positive, dynamic state which is much more than the mere absence of illness. From the alternative perspective, good health involves an ideal sense of balance and harmony of mind, emotion and body. In other words, temporary absence of physical symptoms is not considered indicative of optimum health if, say, depression or anxiety remain. It is only when a change for the better has taken place on all levels that a genuine improvement can be assumed to have occurred.

In contrast to the conventional approach, which puts its greatest efforts into suppressing symptoms, alternative healing systems such as homoeopathy or acupuncture seek to stimulate the in-built capacity of the body to heal itself. Treatment is given which is designed to mobilize the self-healing of the body as a whole, rather than seeking to eliminate symptoms on a piecemeal basis.

From this perspective we can see that the alternative approach seeks to deal with the underlying reasons for illness developing, rather than concentrating on suppression of the signs and symptoms of disease. When symptoms retreat as a result of successful alternative treatment, it is because the body has dealt with the problem at a fundamental level as a result of its own defences being strengthened. It is this fundamental difference between the conventional and alternative approach which leaves the patient of successful alternative therapy liberated from permanent drug treatment once his or her body is capable of functioning at its peak performance once again.

It is also worth stressing that apart from the prescription of medication, many alternative therapists will also be very well-versed in additional measures that may be taken by the patient to stimulate a generally improved state of health. This usually includes practical advice on nutrition, relaxation and exercise techniques, while many therapists will also employ basic counselling skills to enable their patient to explore emotional problems. This holistic approach to treatment usually leads to a greater sense of empowerment in the patient, who can make vital changes in lifestyle that will support a much-improved experience of health and vitality.

This ideal may be achieved through the responsible prescription of herbal or homoeopathic remedies, use of acupuncture in combination with Chinese herbs, hypnotherapy, osteopathy or chiropractic treatment. The major systems of healing such as homoeopathy are capable of dealing with a broad spectrum of health problems, including acute illnesses such as coughs, colds and food poisoning, as well as more established disorders such as hayfever, asthma, eczema, migraines, arthritis and recurrent digestive problems. As we can see, the potential use of alternative medicine for a wide range of health problems is very exciting indeed.

Although extremely effective, alternative treatments such as homoeopathy do not have the toxic or stressful side effects of some conventional drugs. This is because a well-indicated remedy stimulates self-healing, therefore it is working in harmony with the body's efforts, rather than against them. In the case of homoeopathy, it is also worth noting that the extremely dilute nature of the remedies themselves is also a guarantee against toxic side effects.

Homoeopathy And The Alternative Approach

Homoeopathic medicine provides a genuine alternative to the conventional approach to the treatment of illness. It fits very appropriately within a holistic framework, since it is a perspective on healing which emphasizes the vital importance of establishing a state of balance and harmony at the most profound level. As a result, homoeopathic treatment is capable of dealing with a broad spectrum of disorders affecting the mind and body.

Treating With Similar Medicines

While orthodox drugs work by opposing or combating symptoms as described in the previous section, the appropriate homoeopathic remedy is chosen on the basis of its similarity to the symptoms being experienced by the patient. By giving a sick person a remedy that would produce similar symptoms if repeatedly given to someone in good health, the body's capacity for self-healing is given a boost. Because the symptoms of illness are resolved by the body's own efforts, once this process is well under way additional treatment is unnecessary. As a result, permanent or extended reliance on homoeopathic remedies should not be necessary.

The Gentlest Way To Cure: The Minimum Dose

Unlike conventional drugs, homoeopathic medicines are given in the smallest dose possible in order to avoid the risk of toxic build-up in the system. This preoccupation with using the gentlest possible medicinal stimulation in order to induce a cure originated with the German physician Samuel Hahnemann (1755–1843) who developed the theory and practice of homoeopathy.

Although we may consider some current orthodox medical treatments to have undesirable side effects, these are minimal when compared with the horrific results of medical treatments in frequent use in Hahnemann's day. Bleeding and purging were popular measures that left the patient weakened and exhausted to an extreme degree, while the administration of highly toxic substances such as mercury for the treatment of venereal disease, gave rise to side effects that were often worse than the symptoms of the disease itself.

When Hahnemann witnessed the trauma and distress that conventional medical treatments caused in pursuit of a cure, he abandoned his career as a physician. He began to conduct experiments, investigating gentler ways of restoring patients to good health. Once he adopted the principle of using similar rather than opposite medicines, he began to work with increasingly smaller doses in an effort to avoid distressing side effects During his experiments he observed that the more dilute a substance became, the stronger its action would be, provided it had gone through a process of succussion (vigorous shaking) at each stage of dilution, and provided the symptoms of the patient were sufficiently well matched to the symptoms that could be produced by the remedy in a healthy person.

Single Doses

Although some homoeopathic preparations are available in combination form (more than one remedy combined together), homoeopaths generally prescribe only one remedy at a time. This is done in order to observe how effective the action of the remedy has been. If a number of remedies are given at the same time, it can be very difficult to establish which one has been instrumental in promoting an improvement.

It is also important to stress that the extremely detailed information outlined in the *Materia Medica* (a comprehensive textbook which lists in great detail the sphere of action of each homoeopathic remedy) has been gathered using single rather than multiple substances at a time. As a result, we have no reliable information on what the action of combination remedies may be.

However, there are special circumstances where the use of combination formulas may be appropriate. These are mainly situations where it is extremely difficult to obtain enough guiding symptoms from the patient, so that differentiating between one remedy and another may be almost impossible. If we take the example of travel sickness, it can be an extremely arduous job to decide which of the main indicated remedies may fit the symptoms most closely. This is likely to be especially hard for the beginner to homoeopathic prescribing, who is less familiar with the remedies themselves. It can be helpful, therefore, to select a travel sickness combination which may include up to half a dozen appropriate remedies. However, if an individually-selected remedy is obviously indicated after considering the main symptoms of the patient, it is always worth trying the single remedy first.

Treating The Whole Person

A homoeopath works very differently from an orthodox doctor when gathering information on which to base the selection of an appropriate homoeopathic remedy. While a conventional physician will be interested in symptoms that can be classified in an appropriate disease category, a homoeopath is much more interested in symptoms that convey something of the individual person.

For example, a homoeopath may see two patients who have been given a diagnosis of arthritis. Although both may have received the same broad diagnosis, one patient might complain of joint pains that are very severe on waking, which improve progressively as the limbs are loosened up. They may also be extremely restless and depressed when lying still in bed at night, and made much more comfortable after a hot bath. The second patient, however, might feel that their joint pains are much improved when resting in bed, or keeping the limbs as still as possible. Becoming overheated may result in great discomfort and distress, while cool surroundings may give general relief.

As we can see, although both patients are suffering from the same general problem, each experiences their illness in their own individual way. It is the uncommon or unusual symptoms which convey a sense of the individual person that the homoeopath is searching for, rather than the common or general features of illness such as inflammation, pain or swelling. Although these common symptoms give the homoeopath a basic framework within which to work, they begin to take on more significance once it is possible to obtain additional information about them.

It is essential for a homoeopath to understand the detailed nature of a symptom in order to grasp how the individual is affected by it. If we take the example of pain, a homoeopath will question the patient very closely in order to establish the specific nature of the sensation. They are likely to be asked how long it has been present, what makes it better or worse, whether it shifts from place to place, how it affects them emotionally, and to try to find a way of describing the nature of the pain (stabbing, cutting, stinging, throbbing, aching or dull). The general effect on the mind and body of suffering chronic pain is also likely to be explored, with some time being devoted to exploring the possible triggers which may have contributed to the onset of the problem.

In this way, the practitioner is able to build up a rounded picture of the problem, within the context of the overall health of the patient on mental, emotional and physical levels. Once this information has been gathered and analysed, it is then possible for the homoeopath to select the most appropriate homoeopathic remedy which will fit the symptoms of the patient as a whole.

The Homoeopathic 'Symptom Picture'

Because it is the overall condition of the individual patient that is being prescribed for, rather than specific symptoms in isolation, it is misleading to speak of a specific homoeopathic remedy that is used to treat migraine, heartburn, eczema, flu, and so on. It is more appropriate to regard homoeopathic remedies as multi-faceted medicines that can be used to treat a range of disorders, depending on the specific match between the symptoms of the patient and the chosen remedy.

For example, the homoeopathic remedy **Arsenicum alb** can be used effectively in cases of anxiety, insomnia, heartburn, food poisoning, hayfever, eczema, diarrhoea, painful periods or flu. However, it will only be effective in treating any of these conditions if the specific symptoms of the patient match the chief characteristics of the remedy.

Therefore, regardless of their condition, someone who responds well to this remedy must have the characteristic nightly intensification of symptoms, extreme mental and physical restlessness, chilliness, burning pains relieved by warmth, and scanty, clear, burning discharges. If they are chilly, but respond very badly to heat, feel much better for cool surroundings, have discharges that are thick, bland and yellowish-green in colour, and feel very weepy, an alternative remedy must be chosen which covers these leading symptoms such as **Pulsatilla**. The symptoms of the patient must match the characteristics of the homoeopathic remedy as closely as possible for improvement to take place.

■2■

Homoeopathy In The Home: How To Use This Book

The information contained within this chapter has been written with a view to answering most of the practical questions that arise when using homoeopathy in the home. It assumes that no previous knowledge of practical homoeopathy exists, and identifies the main areas of concern or confusion that arise when working with homoeopathic remedies.

It also provides important information on additional basic issues, such as where to obtain homoeopathic remedies, how to store them, how long they retain their shelf-life, and how to expand on a basic knowledge of homoeopathy. More importantly, it also gives very firm guidelines on how to spot situations that need professional help, and how to avoid getting out of your depth.

Becoming familiar with the information contained within this chapter should leave the user feeling confident about resolving problems that are within their grasp, and totally at ease about calling on further help when appropriate.

Identifying Conditions That Are Appropriate For Home Prescribing

Before we learn to select and administer the most appropriate homoeopathic remedy, it is essential to first establish the situations in which homoeopathic self-help is appropriate.

Broadly speaking, conditions which respond well to homoeopathic self-help are classed as *acute*. These tend to be of short duration, are self-limiting, and have a clear beginning, middle and end. Simple examples of this kind of condition would include:

■ Infectious illnesses such as colds, influenza and chickenpox.
■ Food poisoning that results from eating or drinking contaminated food or water.

■ Cuts, bruises and grazes that occur as a result of accidents and injuries.

■ Immediate symptoms of emotional distress following bad news or shock.

Although conditions of this kind can become complicated by secondary developments that make recovery more prolonged, such as recurrent catarrh or sinusitis that remain after a bout of cold or flu, an uncomplicated episode should respond well to homoeopathic prescribing, especially when combined with practical self-help measures.

However, many conditions fall into another category which is regarded as *chronic*. These are long-term problems which do not clear up of their own accord, and are subject to repeated flare-ups of symptoms that are likely to gather in intensity and severity with the passage of time. Good examples of these conditions would include the following:

■ Asthma

■ Hayfever

■ Eczema

■ Migraines

■ Irritable bowel syndrome

■ Recurrent depression and anxiety

■ Arthritis

■ Pre-menstrual syndrome

■ Psoriasis

Because these conditions arise from a fundamental weakness in the system, often referred to by homoeopaths as a 'constitutional' problem, they are best treated by a trained practitioner who will strive to address the problem at this fundamental level. As a result, a homoeopath will prescribe an appropriate homoeopathic remedy which is selected after an analysis of the patient's symptoms as a whole – mental, emotional and physical.

By matching the 'totality' of the symptoms with the most appropriate homoeopathic remedy in this way, it becomes possible to stimulate the whole system of the patient into an improved state of balance and harmony. When this happens, symptoms recede because the body's own self-regulating mechanism has been stimulated into action. Because this is not done on the basis of selecting a remedy that fits the immediate symptoms of an acute flare-up alone, it is a task that is beyond the scope of the home prescriber who would soon get out of their depth when dealing with a complex situation of this kind.

This advice is reiterated in the individual sections that deal with chronic conditions in this book. Although general self-help measures are suggested that may aid the condition on a basic level (such as dietary changes, exercise and relaxation), clear advice is given on the need for professional help when dealing with long-term conditions of the kind mentioned above.

How To Begin: Obtaining The Relevant Information

In order to achieve the best results, it is very important to be clear about the information that needs to be obtained before beginning the process of home prescribing. By being confident about the relevant information at this point, it is possible to avoid confusion later on.

■ First of all, identify any factors that may have contributed to the development of illness. These triggers may be very wide-ranging, and may include anything from exposure to chill or hearing bad news, to suffering the consequences of too little sleep or too much alcohol.

■ Note the main symptoms, remembering that you are interested in any changes that have occurred since illness began. In other words, if someone normally has a high colour, or if they are irritable by nature, this information is not helpful in acute prescribing. However, if this person has become noticeably pale and weepy since the onset of illness, these are relevant symptoms that can lead you to the choice of an appropriate remedy.

■ Begin this process by asking questions that relate to the most obvious symptoms such as fever, pain or nausea. In other words, if a headache is the main problem, ask where the pain is lodged, how it feels, and what makes it better or worse (movement, eating, cool compresses, etc.).

■ Once you have obtained all the information that relates to the specific problem, broaden it out by asking more general questions about any other changes that have taken place since the onset of illness. It is often most helpful to ask questions that relate to different parts of the body, starting at the head and moving downwards. For example, is there any light sensitivity or discomfort in the eyes, nasal discharge, earache, toothache, mouth ulcers, more or less saliva, bad taste in the mouth, cold sores, swollen glands, sore throats or difficulty swallowing? Continue in this way, asking questions as you mentally move down the parts of the body, always bearing in mind that you are looking for any changes that have occurred since illness set in.

■ Once a symptom picture has been obtained by putting together this specific information, do not forget to ask more general questions about sensations affecting the system as a whole. For example, is the patient more chilly, hot, restless, weary, sweaty or dry since illness began? This is also the appropriate point to discover the factors that make the patient feel generally better or worse. These may be varied in nature and may include any of the following: fresh air, movement, resting, warmth, cool, eating, drinking, company, light, dark, sympathy, weeping, peace and quiet or distraction.

■ Most important of all, try to establish whether there have been emotional changes since illness set in. Remember that anxiety in an already anxious person is not as valid as irritability, or short temper in a normally placid individual, or weepiness in someone who usually keeps a stiff upper lip.

Using The Information: Selecting The Most Appropriate Remedy

■ Sift through the symptoms you have written down, initially looking for a characteristic feature that runs through them or a factor that has brought illness on. The latter could be exposure to stress or chill, while the former could be anything that is a marked, characteristic, or unusual feature of the symptoms. Whatever you have selected should be placed under the heading of *Typical features* on your list.

■ Work through the bulk of the symptoms you have obtained, organizing them in order of importance (severity of symptoms or amount of distress caused to the patient). It can be helpful to underline the most central symptoms with three lines, those that are slightly less severe or characteristic with two, and those that are least pressing with one line. Once the bulk of the symptoms have been arranged in this way, they should be listed under the heading of *General symptoms*.

■ Remember, the most valuable symptoms are those that are classed as strange, rare or peculiar. In other words, these are symptoms that are unexpected or unusual (dry mouth without thirst, indigestion or nausea that is better for eating, or hot, burning pains that are relieved by warmth). If a symptom of this kind is present, it should be regarded as especially important since it can often clinch the choice of a remedy.

■ Finally, establish the factors that make the patient feel better or worse. Above all, remember that you have to take into account the features that improve or aggravate the patient in general, as well as the factors that improve or intensify individual symptoms (e.g. a headache may be improved by contact with cool, fresh air while the person generally wants to be kept warm). This information should be organized into *Worse from* and *Better for* columns.

Using The Remedy Tables

■ You are now ready to turn to the relevant remedy table, in order to establish the homoeopathic remedy that will match the symptoms of the patient most closely. In order to do this, consider the information you have included under the heading *Typical features* and see how closely it matches the entries under the left hand column entitled *Type*.

■ Once you have identified a general approximation to the symptoms you have isolated, move on to the second column entitled *General symptoms*. Check that there is a broad correspondence between this information and the symptoms that you have included under this heading in your list. Remember that it doesn't matter if not all the symptoms in this section correspond with your list, provided that those you have underlined twice or three times are present (see page 13). In other words, the most characteristic or severe symptoms must correspond with the information under this heading, even if others do not.

■ If you are satisfied that there is a good match between your list of symptoms and the information given under the heading *General symptoms* in the table, move on to the *Worse from* and *Better for* columns in order to check that these also correspond to the information you have gathered from the patient. If so, there is every chance that the remedy which appears under the heading *Remedy name* is the most appropriate for the patient.

■ If there is any doubt, turn to the remedy information in **Chapter 10** in order to confirm your choice.

■ Always bear in mind that the information in the remedy tables can be used as creatively as required. For example, if someone is suffering from a cold and cough, or vomiting and diarrhoea at the same time, it is possible to combine the information given in both tables in order to establish whether one remedy covers the characteristic symptoms of both problems. Again, if there is any doubt about the suitability of the remedy selected, or if there is a need to choose between two potentially appropriate remedies, turn to **Chapter 10** in order to confirm your choice.

■ Once you become familiar with using the remedy tables, you will discover that certain homoeopathic remedies appear regularly under different headings. For example, the homoeopathic remedy **Belladonna** may be used to treat a wide variety of conditions including the following: earache, high temperatures, sore throats, chickenpox, cystitis, and sunburn, while **Arsenicum alb** may be helpful in treating insomnia, anxiety, vomiting, diarrhoea, coughs, flu, and heartburn.

Selecting The Appropriate Potency (Strength) Of Remedy

■ Before deciding on the appropriate potency of a selected remedy, it is important to establish the intensity of the symptoms. In other words, if an illness has set in slowly and insidiously over a few days, leading to low-grade symptoms, it is best to give a low potency remedy two or three times daily for a few days in order to provide gentle, cumulative stimulation towards cure.

■ On the other hand, if illness has set in rapidly with marked severity of symptoms, it is more appropriate to match the potency of the remedy with the strength of the symptoms. Therefore, in fast-developing, strong symptoms a higher (stronger) potency is indicated which should be repeated frequently (every half or three-quarters of an hour for up to three doses) in the early stages of illness until improvement sets in.

■ When we talk about the lowest potency of homoeopathic remedy, this generally means a 6c strength (the 'c' stands for centessimal dilution, i.e. the remedy has been diluted in a proportion of 1:99 drops of water and alcohol). It is the most easily obtainable over-the-counter homoeopathic potency from pharmacies or health shops. Generally speaking, this is the most appropriate potency for the beginner to buy when putting together a home remedy kit, since it should meet the needs of most first-aid or home-prescribing situations.

■ Alternatively, if a higher potency is required, this means that a 12c or 30c will be called for. Generally speaking, a 30c can be obtained from health shops, while a 12c potency needs to be ordered from a homoeopathic pharmacy. Always remember that the higher potencies should be used less frequently than the lower in order to avoid over-stimulation and too energetic a response.

■ It is helpful to bear in mind that there is no need to agonize over the choice of potency as long as there is sufficient confidence about the selected remedy. Provided the homoeopathic remedy chosen matches the symptoms of the patient as closely as possible, it should stimulate a positive response. Therefore, if all that is available is a 6c potency, but you feel a higher potency would meet the situation more appropriately, do not hold back from using the 6c since it may just need more frequent repetition than a higher potency.

How To Administer The Appropriate Remedy

■ Once the most appropriate remedy and potency has been selected, tip a tablet (this constitutes a single dose) on to a clean spoon or the cap of the remedy bottle. This is done in order to avoid touching the tablets, since this may contaminate them.

■ Suck or chew the tablet, allowing it to be absorbed by the mucus membranes of the mouth. Above all, avoid taking the tablets when there are any strong flavours around which may interfere with the effective action of the remedy. Offending substances may include any of the following: strong tea or coffee, peppermint, spearmint, eucalyptus or strongly-flavoured mouthwashes. Other substances which may counteract the action of homoeopathic remedies include aromatic oils or rubs such as Olbas Oil (brand name), inhalations, and some essential oils such as lavender, rosemary or eucalyptus.

■ When giving remedies to small children or babies, it is more practical to use granules rather than tablets. Remedies in granule form may be ordered by telephone or post from a homoeopathic pharmacy (addresses and telephone numbers are given at the back of the book).

■ If a remedy needs to be given urgently, it is possible to crush the tablets into a fine powder. In order to do this, place the tablets between two clean teaspoons and press hard with the back of one against the bowl of the other until a fine powder is formed. Alternatively, place two tablets in a clean fold of paper and use a heavy object such as a rolling pin to grind them into a powder.

■ Place a pinch of powder or granules inside your child's cheek, or rub it along the gums. This allows the remedy to be absorbed by the membranes of the mouth without requiring your child to suck or chew a hard tablet.

■ If you accidentally spill too many tablets or granules out of the bottle, throw them away rather than putting them back, since they may have been contaminated.

Evaluating The Response

■ Once the first dose has been given, wait for thirty minutes, observing any changes that have occurred in the condition of the patient. This might involve any of the following:

- ■ Easing of discomfort or pain.
- ■ Reduction of fever.
- ■ Improved appetite.
- ■ Enhanced energy levels and/or sense of well-being.
- ■ Improved ability to rest, or reduction in physical and/or mental restlessness.
- ■ Reduction in distress, anxiety or despondency.

This list is not presented in order to give an exhaustive account of all the symptoms that might respond favourably to a remedy; its function is merely to outline the wide scope of sensations and symptoms that need to be taken into account when assessing the response to a well-selected homoeopathic medicine.

■ In cases of marked, acute, rapidly-developing symptoms, if there is no improvement within thirty minutes, and you still are confident about your choice of remedy, another dose should be given. This is also the case if there has been a brief improvement that has failed to hold.

■ Remember when evaluating the response of the patient that a positive response may consist of a **general** sensation of relief, even though specific symptoms may remain. For example, someone may respond by feeling an increased sense of vitality and energy after taking a remedy, even though their headache, sore throat or indigestion has not yet improved. In this situation, it is the degree of distress that is caused by the symptom that improves before the symptom itself is diminished. If this occurs, it should be considered a positive reaction, and the remedy should **not** be repeated unless and until a relapse occurs.

■ If after repeating a remedy three times as suggested above (at intervals of thirty to forty-five minutes for rapidly-developing or severe symptoms) there is no improvement, go back to the remedy tables in order to check if another remedy is better indicated.

■ This should also be done if the remedy has helped the initial symptoms but they have changed in nature. For example, after giving a well-selected remedy a dry, tickly cough may change into a loose, productive one, or a scanty, clear, burning nasal discharge may change to a thick, greenish-yellow, bland discharge. In such a situation, it is essential that the new symptoms are matched by the most appropriate remedy.

■ If a low potency (6c) remedy has helped a great deal initially, and the symptoms are unchanged but it stops working, a higher potency (12c or 30c) should be considered. However, it must always be borne in mind that higher potency remedies should not be repeated as frequently as low potencies. Use the same guidelines as above in deciding when, and when not to give a remedy, leaving two-hour gaps (depending on the reaction) in between doses than would be expected when using a 6c remedy.

■ In cases of insidious, slow-developing problems that emerge over a few days, it is appropriate to regulate dosage so that slower, more extended stimulation can be given. In such a situation, the remedy can be given two or three times daily over the course of three or four days. However, once improvement sets in, the same principles apply as outlined above.

■ If symptoms get more intense after taking a well-indicated remedy too frequently, this can be rectified by stopping the dosage. This potential problem can occur if the system is over-stimulated in its fight against illness, resulting in symptoms briefly becoming stronger. This reaction can be easily identified, in contrast to a general deterioration of the original condition being treated, since the intensification of symptoms should be speedily followed by an improvement once the remedy is withheld and the body has a chance to return to a state of equilibrium. The best way of avoiding this problem arising is to always refrain from routinely taking a homoeopathic remedy once improvement has set in.

Problems That Suggest Professional Help Is Needed

■ In each section dealing with a medical condition guidelines are given that indicate when a professional opinion should be consulted. Symptoms that suggest a medical emergency may be developing are also given so that the home prescriber may become fully aware that, even though a condition may have begun as a problem that can be appropriately treated at home, complications may develop later that require professional help. In such a situation, it is essential to spot these indications as quickly as possible in order to ensure the best outcome.

■ Seeking professional or medical help should be interpreted within this context as consulting a GP or alternative health practitioner in less pressing circumstances; calling an ambulance or taking the patient to the casualty department of a local hospital in more urgent situations. If there is severe concern about the condition of a patient, or a sense that the situation is deteriorating rapidly, lose no time in sending for medical help.

■ If the situation is not as severe as the one outlined above, but there is a general sense that self-help measures and home prescribing are not resolving the problem, or there is a general feeling of being out of one's depth, never be afraid to call on professional advice. This can be obtained from your alternative health practitioner, GP or homoeopath.

■ Always be extra careful when looking after babies, small children and the elderly, since they share the characteristic of becoming ill with alarming rapidity and severity. With children in particular, it is always best to err on the cautious side if you sense that there are any indications that your child may be seriously ill. These may be no more than an altered cry or feeding pattern in a listless baby, or a marked, uncharacteristic change in behaviour or energy levels in your child.

■ Apart from specific symptoms that are peculiar to each condition, there are some indications that generally suggest that the situation requires professional help. These may include the following:

   ■ Symptoms that do not respond to self-help measures or become more severe.

   ■ Signs of drowsiness, confusion or disorientation.

   ■ Persistent high temperature that reaches or rises above 103°F. (39°– 40°C)

   ■ Persistent or severe pains anywhere in the body.

   ■ Muscular tension and/or stiffness combined with light sensitivity and/or severe headache.

   ■ Loss of consciousness.

   ■ Severe or protracted loss of fluid as a result of sweating, vomiting and/or diarrhoea. This can be especially serious in the very young or the elderly.

   ■ General debility and difficulty in recovering.

   ■ Signs of infection including fever, redness, pain and/or pus formation.

   ■ Any severe illness in babies, young children and the elderly.

   ■ If there is any cause for concern about the condition of the patient.

Buying Homoeopathic Remedies

As homocopathy has grown in popularity and profile over the past ten years or so, it has become proportionally easier to obtain homoeopathic remedies from over-the-counter outlets. A major high street chemist recently launched a range of homoeopathic remedies in 6c strength, making them even easier to obtain. In addition, health food stores will usually carry a wide range of remedies, often in 6c and 30c potencies, while homoeopathic pharmacies stock a full range of potencies, from the highest to the lowest.

However, the needs of the newcomer to homoeopathic prescribing should be very adequately met by the range of remedies offered by retail outlets of the kind mentioned above. It should only be necessary to order from a homoeopathic pharmacy when potencies are required which cannot be obtained easily (such as a 12c), or when a less well-known remedy is needed. In such a situation, orders can be easily placed by telephone or in writing. It is also worth considering that staff who work in homoeopathic pharmacies can be very helpful in giving general advice about prescribing.

Advice is given in **Chapter 3** on how to put together a basic home-prescribing kit, as well as combinations of remedies that meet more specific needs such as the *Accident and Emergency/Sports Injury* or the *Mother and Baby* kits. It is best to initially acquire remedies in 6c potency, adding to these with 12c or 30c as expertise and confidence in home prescribing develops.

Remedies can also be obtained in decimal potency (these have an 'x' or 'd' after the name), which means that the original substance is made into a liquid and diluted with alcohol. One drop of this tincture is added to nine drops of alcohol or distilled water and shaken in order to obtain the first potency of 1x. The same process is repeated, adding one drop of the previous potency to nine drops of dilutant before shaking at regular intervals in order to obtain remedies in an ascending scale of 2x, 3x, 4x, and so on. The centessimal scale of dilution operates in exactly the same way, the only difference being that 1 drop of tincture is added to ninety-nine drops of distilled water or alcohol each time.

Storing Homoeopathic Remedies

Provided they are kept in appropriate conditions, homoeopathic remedies appear to have an indefinite shelf-life. In order to preserve the quality of the remedies, avoid storing homoeopathic medicines where they may come into contact with the following:

■ Aromatic substances such as essential oils, Olbas Oil, or camphorated items.
■ Sunlight may also damage remedies, and so it is best to keep remedy bottles in a darkened place.

■ Exposure to extremely hot or cold conditions. They are best kept in moderately cool but not cold surroundings.

■ Continued exposure to air. The tops of remedy bottles should always be screwed back on very tightly after use.

■ X-ray equipment at airports may also adversely affect the quality of homoeopathic remedies. It is best to ask that the remedies should be examined by staff, rather than leaving them in luggage which will be X-rayed.

The Practicalities Of Home Prescribing When Conventional Medication Is Being Taken

Generally speaking, there are no obvious problems of adverse interaction between homoeopathic and conventional medicines such as a toxic reaction occurring, because of the extremely dilute nature of homoeopathic medication. However, if drugs such as antibiotics are taken, there is the strong possibility that they may interfere with the medicinal action of a well-indicated homoeopathic remedy.

In reality, most acute conditions covered in this book are likely to be appropriate for initial treatment with homoeopathic prescribing, which can make resorting to antibiotics or decongestants less necessary. In this way, it becomes possible to use gentle but effective measures in order to deal with an acute problem, leaving the more toxic conventional measures as a later resort if the condition is escalating in seriousness, or refusing to respond to holistic measures.

On the other hand, it is important to stress that when conventional drugs are being given for a chronic condition such as asthma, high blood-pressure or anxiety, they should **never** be withdrawn abruptly or without medical supervision, since they can have a rebound effect when stopped. As a result, the original condition can return with renewed severity, leaving the patient extremely vulnerable. It is always best to seek alternative or conventional medical advice if there are any queries about long-term management of a chronic condition.

For more information about how to differentiate between an acute and chronic condition, see the section entitled *Identifying Conditions That Are Appropriate For Home Prescribing* at the beginning of this chapter.

How To Expand Your Knowledge Of Homoeopathy

If using this book stimulates a basic interest in homoeopathy, there are practical steps that can be taken to deepen your knowledge and expand your horizons with regard to this fascinating subject.

If you want to learn more about the theory behind homoeopathy, you will benefit greatly from reading some of the excellent books on the subject which are listed in the *Recommended Reading* section. These have been especially selected for the newcomer to homoeopathy, who has gained some practical experience with regard to acute prescribing, but who wants to learn much more about the context within which homoeopathy exists. The books that have been selected for inclusion in this list explain how homoeopathy developed as a medical science out of conventional medicine in the nineteenth century, as well as giving more technical advice on how homoeopathic remedies are prepared, and how this radically different approach to healing fits in with current research.

At the same time, this developing knowledge can be expanded by attending one of the many homoeopathic self-help classes that are held at regular intervals throughout the country. These usually last for six weeks or so, and are geared to the needs of the newcomer to homoeopathic prescribing. Much of the ground covered will be similar to the material dealt with in this book, with great emphasis being laid on the practicalities of identifying and treating acute problems in the home. However, attending such a class gives the new prescriber a vital opportunity to ask practical questions which can be answered on the spot: this is something that, unfortunately, even the most comprehensive book cannot do.

Details of courses such as these can usually be obtained from your local homoeopathic college (look in the Yellow Pages for details), local homoeopathic group, public library or local education authority (extra-mural studies).

How To Contact A Homoeopathic Practitioner

Since at many stages in this book it is suggested that help and advice should be sought from a professional homoeopath, it would seem an oversight not to give advice on the easiest and most reliable way in which to make contact with a local practitioner.

Generally speaking, registers can be obtained from two main sources. These are the Society of Homoeopaths, which provides a list of professional homoeopaths who have undergone a minimum of four years' training at an approved college, and the British Homoeopathic Association, which provides a register of conventionally-trained doctors who have done an additional course in homoeopathy. The former can be identified in the Yellow Pages by the initials RS Hom, while the latter may use MF Hom.

Although the presence of these letters gives a guide to the basic level of training, which in itself provides a degree of reassurance, the best way of finding a competent, experienced practitioner tends to be by word of mouth. If a family member, friend or colleague has been favourably impressed by the treatment offered by a homoeopath, and you discover that they also possess a qualification of the calibre mentioned above, it is certainly worth contacting the practitioner in order to obtain further details.

Most practitioners will be happy to answer any questions a prospective patient may have over the telephone. These may include queries about the length of the first consultation and follow-up visits, obtaining a rough guide to the costs that may be involved, and establishing the degree of experience the practitioner may have in treating patients with similar problems.

Always bear in mind that the rapport and relationship that develop between a patient and homoeopath is unique, and that the practitioner who answers the needs of one patient may not be as appropriate for another. However, an enthusiastic recommendation from someone whose opinion you trust may be the best way of pointing you in the right direction as you begin to make enquiries.

■3■

Homoeopathic First Aid

n this chapter you will find a range of common problems that require first aid measures. Within this context, homoeopathic prescribing has a tremendously important role to play. When used side by side with basic first aid techniques, homoeopathic prescribing for common accidents and injuries can be immensely valuable in aiding the casualty to deal with physical and emotional shock and to ease the trauma and pain of cuts and bruises. It also encourages the speedy knitting of fractured bones and the re-absorption of blood from injured tissue.

By using homoeopathic medicines for first aid, the essential practicality of this system of healing becomes apparent. We may be amazed at how effective **Calendula** or **Hypericum** cream is in speeding up the healing of wounds, or at the efficiency with which **Arnica** diminishes the pain and tenderness of deep bruising. In other words, this chapter shows how homoeopathy can be effectively used for conditions that we may have previously thought could only be treated by orthodox medical measures.

This is not to suggest that we abandon sensible conventional medical first aid techniques; on the contrary, knowledge of these practical measures can save lives. However, the information contained within this chapter will add a range of effective complementary medical resources that may prove of invaluable help in an accident or emergency situation.

Putting Together A Homoeopathic First Aid Kit

In addition to the items included in a standard first aid kit, such as adhesive tapes, bandages and dressings, the following are essential homoeopathic remedies.

Topical Preparations (For Application To The Skin)

■ **Calendula** or **Hypercal** (brand name – a mixture of Calendula and Hypericum) tincture. It is important to note that tinctures must *always* be diluted before use.
■ **Urtica urens** tincture.

■ **Calendula** or **Hypercal** cream and ointment. Creams are best for cut or lacerated wounds, while ointment is most suited to treating grazed or roughened skin. However, ointment should be avoided by those with sensitive skin because of the possibility of a reaction to the lanolin base.

■ **Arnica** cream.

Homoeopathic Remedies For Internal Use

When putting together an initial selection of homoeopathic remedies, it is best to start with a basic kit that can be expanded to accommodate individual needs at a later stage.

The Accident and Emergency/Sports Injury Kit

Apis
Arnica
Bryonia
Cantharis
Carbo veg
Hypericum
Ipecac
Ledum
Phosphorus
Rhus tox
Ruta
Symphytum
Urtica urens

The Comprehensive Kit

The following remedies, added to the above, should meet most requirements of the newcomer to homoeopathic prescribing:

Aconite
Argentum nit
Arsenicum alb
Belladonna
Calc carb
Gelsemium
Hepar sulph
Ignatia
Lachesis
Lycopodium

Mercurius
Natrum mur
Nux vomica
Pulsatilla
Sepia
Staphysagria
Sulphur

Mother and Baby Kit

The following are valuable additions to the above list:
Bellis perennis
Caulophyllum
Chamomilla
Colocynthis
Dioscorea
Ferrum phos
Kali bich
Kali carb
Kreosotum
Mag phos

Any other conditions, including menopausal symptoms, men's problems and stress-related disorders, are likely to be covered by the remedies mentioned in the above lists. By referring to the relevant remedy tables for each condition, it will be clear which remedies are likely to be indicated.

Bites And Stings

The severity of symptoms associated with a sting or bite can vary enormously. Some of us may experience extreme distress and discomfort, while others feel minimal unpleasantness. The range of bites and stings may come from any of the following sources:

Bites:

Dogs or cats
Snakes
Midges
Fleas
Spiders

Stings:

Bees
Wasps
Scorpions
Horseflies
Nettles or other stinging plants

Symptoms

■ Pain, redness and swelling around the site of entry of a sting, or itching and swelling if the skin has been bitten.
■ General symptoms of distress or mild shock.

Basic First Aid

■ Bathe the affected area with *diluted* **Hypericum** tincture. One part of tincture should be added to ten parts of boiled, cooled water.
■ After bathing, **Hypercal** (a blend of Hypericum and Calendula) cream may applied directly to the damaged skin. Alternatively, **Hypercal** or **Calendula** cream may be applied to a sterile dressing which can be used to cover the wound.
■ In the case of stings, bear in mind that a wasp does not leave a sting behind, but a bee does. After being stung by a bee, remove the sting carefully with a pair of tweezers, ensuring that the venom sac is not ruptured.
■ If itching is troublesome after coming into contact with a stinging plant such as a nettle, bathe the affected area with *diluted* **Urtica urens** tincture. Additional relief may also be obtained from applying **Urtica urens** cream to the inflamed skin after bathing.

Homoeopathic Help

Type of injury	General symptoms	Worse from	Better for	Remedy name
Stings and bites that look water-logged, pink and swollen.	Extreme puffiness around the site of the bite or sting. Stinging pains that cause great fidgetiness and agitation. Contact with any form of heat is intolerable.	Warm bathing. Warm air. Touch. Keeping still.	Cool bathing. Cool air. Uncovering. Moving about.	**Apis**

Type of injury	General symptoms	Worse from	Better for	Remedy name
Bites and stings with pains that radiate along the affected limb.	Wounds are extremely sensitive to touch. Pains are intermittent, sharp and stitching. Soreness and tenderness are aggravated by cold in any form.	Cold. Touch. Movement.	Keeping still.	**Hypericum**
Stings and bites that result in violent, burning sensations.	Terrible burning in affected areas: feels as though skin is on fire. Hypersensitivity of the skin to touch with extreme restlessness.	Movement. Touch.	Warmth.	**Cantharis**
Bites and stings that feel cold or numb.	Stabbing, tearing pains that feel much better for contact with cool air, or cold bathing. Wound may be swollen and taut.	Heat. Movement. Touch.	Bathing in cool water. Contact with cool air, or cold compresses. Resting.	**Ledum**
Skin problems that develop after a sting, such as hiving.	Itching, burning pains that are very much worse when touched. Skin looks swollen, blotchy and raised in patches.	Contact with cool air. Cold bathing. Touch. Lying on painful area.		**Urtica urens**
Severely itchy midge bites.	Driven to desperation by the severity and extensive nature of insect bites. Skin is extremely sensitive with stinging, smarting, sharp pains. The least touch causes great distress.	The least contact with the skin. At night. Being irritated.	Resting. Warmth.	**Staphysagria**

Seek Prompt Medical Help In Any Of The Following Situations:

■ **If the person who has been stung has a history of allergic reactions to bee or wasp stings, professional medical help should be sought as soon as possible. This is done in order to prevent a condition called Anaphylactic Shock developing. Signs of this potentially life-threatening problem include the following:**

■ **Pale, bluish-tinged, clammy skin.**
■ **Irregular, shallow or laboured breathing.**
■ **Prostration or collapse.**
■ **Drowsiness that leads to unconsciousness.**

If any of these symptoms appear, get medical help immediately.
■ **Any indication of rapid swelling advancing around the face, mouth or throat.**
■ **Signs of infection developing around the bite or sting. These might include redness, heat or pus at the site of entry.**
■ **Check that the casualty is up-to-date with protection against tetanus if there is a possibility that dirt has entered the wound.**

Bleeding

The severity of blood loss determines whether it is appropriate to treat accidents where bleeding occurs at home, or whether professional medical help is required. Episodes of bleeding can vary from a very minor wound or nosebleed to severe haemorrhage which may be life-threatening. However, even in the latter situation, knowledge of simple first aid techniques can save lives while waiting for emergency medical help to arrive.

Basic First Aid

■ The first priorities should be to slow down or stop the bleeding. In minor wounds, all that may be needed is to cover the wound with a clean dressing, securing it with adhesive bandages. If this is sufficient, see *Cuts, Abrasions and Bruises* for advice on how to ensure that the wound is clean before it is covered by a bandage.
■ Where bleeding is severe and difficult to stop, emergency help should be obtained as quickly as possible. While waiting for help to arrive, gently remove clothing where appropriate and apply pressure to the wound in an effort to slow down blood loss. In the case of a puncture wound, never apply

direct pressure because of the danger of pushing an embedded object further into the wound.

■ If bleeding is severe as a result of a wound in the arm or leg, raise the injured limb in an effort to slow down the blood flow. Apply pressure to the appropriate pressure point for five to fifteen minutes. Cuts to the chest should be treated with the casualty sitting propped-up, leaning in the direction of the injured side. Wounds affecting the back, stomach or legs should be treated with the patient lying down.

■ Once bleeding has stopped, or considerably slowed down, cover the wound with a clean, absorbent dressing, and bandage firmly in place with a clean cloth or scarf.

■ If there are any signs of drowsiness, do not give food or drinks.

■ Monitor the casualty's breathing and pulse, checking for any indications of shock.

■ If bleeding occurs from the ear, nose or mouth after a blow to the head or chest, let the blood drain on to a clean dressing after sending for emergency medical help.

■ Never remove an object which is deeply embedded in a wound since it may be operating as a plug. If it is dislodged without expert help, blood flow may rapidly accelerate.

■ If blood is seeping through a bandage, do not remove the dressing but cover it with an extra layer of clean fabric.

■ If a simple, uncomplicated nosebleed occurs with no attendant injuries, pinch the bridge of the nose between forefinger and thumb, and keep applying the pressure for roughly five minutes. If any blood enters the mouth, spit it out rather than swallowing it in an effort to prevent vomiting occurring.

Homoeopathic Help

Type of bleeding	General symptoms	Worse from	Better for	Remedy name
General trauma associated with blood loss and bruising.	Disorientation as a result of an accident. Rejects help and maintains that nothing is the matter as a reaction to shock. General state of blood loss and bruising following an accident.	Touch. Being approached. Movement.	Lying with head low.	**Arnica**

Type of bleeding	General symptoms	Worse from	Better for	Remedy name
Pallor and prostration with blood loss.	Skin is clammy, pale and bluish-tinged. Cold and sweaty with a craving for fresh air: feels better for being fanned. Faint, dizzy and nauseated with loss of blood. Bleeding is dark and oozing.	Stuffy, airless rooms. Pressure of clothes.	Cool, fresh surroundings. Being fanned. Raising feet slightly higher than the body.	**Carbo Veg**
Bright, gushing bleeding with terrible nausea.	Breathlessness, faintness and sick feeling accompany loss of blood. Generally feels much worse from the slightest movement.	Movement. Warmth. Being over-heated or chilled.	Resting. Keeping as still as possible. Keeping the eyes closed. Fresh air.	**Ipecac**
Small wounds that bleed excessively.	Indicated where blood loss exceeds expectation for the size of the wound. Also suitable for frequent or exceptionally heavy nosebleeds.	Cold, open air. Being alone. Anxiety.	Reassurance. Physical contact. Bathing the face in cool water.	**Phosphorus**
Bright red bleeding with flushed, hot face.	General picture of congestion and excitability. Pulse is rapid, pounding and laboured. Muscles may go into spasm or become twitchy.	Touch. Company. Movement. Sensory stimulation.	Sitting propped-up. Light covering. Resting.	**Belladonna**

Seek Prompt Medical Help In Any Of The Following Situations:

■ **Where there are multiple injuries with such severe bleeding that it cannot be stopped in any one area.**

■ **If the pulse rate increases and external bleeding has been controlled, it is likely that there may be internal haemorrhaging. If this is the case, emergency help should be sought immediately.**

■ **Difficulty in breathing.**

■ **If symptoms of shock develop. These include:**

■ Confusion, drowsiness or unconsciousness.
■ Nausea and vomiting.
■ Pale, grey or blue-tinged skin.
■ Weak or rapid pulse.
■ Increased thirst.

■ **Bear in mind that the consequences of severe blood loss in a child are more serious than in an adult. If your child is losing blood rapidly, get professional help immediately.**

Burns And Scalds

Burns and scalds can happen readily as minor or much more serious accidents in the home. While minor or first-degree burns may be treated with simple first aid measures at home, severe second or third-degree burns demand expert medical treatment in hospital.

The following will give an idea of how we differentiate between the main categories of severity:

■ *First-degree burns*: These are minor burns that involve painful reddening or inflammation of the affected skin, without blister formation.
■ *Second-degree burns*: May be characterized by severe pain, blistering and fluid retention beneath the affected skin.
■ *Third-degree burns*: This is the most serious category of burn, involving deep or widespread destruction of tissue, loss of fluid, and severe shock.

If a burn or scald affects an area larger than the palm of the hand, emergency medical help must be obtained immediately.

Burns may be caused by any of the following:

■ Contact with hot oven doors, hotplates or over-heated radiators.
■ Fire.
■ Friction.
■ Over-exposure to direct sunlight.
■ Electrical burns from faulty or inadequately-maintained electrical equipment.
■ Chemical burns may occur from contact with caustic household cleaning agents.

Scalds are often caused by the following:

■ Contact with very hot liquids, e.g. mugs of boiling beverages or soups that may be accidentally spilt.

■ Steaming saucepans or kettles can cause a nasty scald if the lid is lifted without taking adequate measures to protect hands, e.g. using a cloth or oven glove.

■ Bathwater that is excessively hot. Always check the temperature of bathwater before stepping in. Small children, babies and the elderly are especially vulnerable to this kind of scald.

Basic First Aid

■ If the casualty has been injured in a fire, the first priority is to get them away from the flames. If their clothing is alight, cover them with any heavy fabric that is available such as overcoats, curtains or blankets. Once the flames have been quenched treat them as described below.

■ If the accident involves an electrical burn, the most essential priority is to switch the electricity supply off at the mains, or to get the casualty away from contact with the electric current. In doing so, it is essential to bear in mind that the victim may still be 'live'. If this is the case, touching them could be extremely hazardous since the current would pass through the person trying to help. As a result, a non-conductive material must be used to break the contact between the casualty and the electrical appliance. Appropriate items that may be used include a wooden chair, broom or mop handle. Once the electricity supply has been safely dealt with, treat as for **Shock**, checking pulse and breathing, while also following the advice given below if necessary.

■ Bathe or immerse damaged areas in cool water for roughly ten minutes. If you have **Hypericum** or **Calendula** tinctures to hand, ten drops of either should be added to each pint or half litre of water.

■ Remove any jewellery that is near to damaged areas of skin, since these may become very difficult to take off once the skin swells.

■ Cover burnt areas lightly with clean, non-fluffy, non-adhesive dressings in an effort to prevent infection. If burnt clothing is stuck to the skin, on no account try to remove it, but cover the area with a dressing.

■ Where a large area of skin is affected, do not use a large dressing; instead use small amounts of clean coverings that may be removed more easily once the casualty has reached hospital.

■ Treat burnt areas extremely gently, trying to have as little contact with the skin as possible. **Never** break blisters deliberately, since these form a barrier to the entry of infection.

■ If a third-degree burn has occurred, and fluid loss has been severe, ensure that the casualty is given regular sips of water in an effort to prevent dehydration (excessive fluid loss). If the patient is very drowsy or unconscious, do not attempt to give fluid by mouth.

■ If you suspect that the casualty is approaching unconsciousness, see section entitled *Shock*. Treat accordingly after having sent for emergency medical help.

■ If a chemical burn has occurred, wash the affected area in water only in order to remove any residue of the chemical, and treat the damaged skin as described above.

■ In cases of first, or very minor second-degree burns, bathe the affected area with cool water in which **Urtica urens** tincture has been diluted (see above for suggested proportions). Alternatively, a cool compress that has been soaked in diluted **Urtica urens** tincture may be applied to minor burns.

■ Cover the affected area with a clean, non-fluffy dressing on which **Calendula** or **Hypercal** cream or ointment has been applied.

■ These instructions apply to any burn except for severe second-degree or third degree burns which require immediate medical treatment and attention.

Homoeopathic Help

Type of burn or scald	General symptoms	Worse from	Better for	Remedy name
Minor burns and scalds without blistering.	Painful, sensitive skin with redness and burning. Burnt area stings and smarts. The remedy may be taken internally in tablet form, or the tincture may be diluted as a solution for external application.	Touch. Cool bathing.		**Urtica urens**
Minor second-degree burns with minimal blistering.	Stinging, inflamed skin with slight blistering. Diluted **Urtica urens** tincture may be used initially, for external application, switching to **Calendula** if the blisters should break.	Touch. Cool bathing.		**Urtica urens**

Type of burn or scald	General symptoms	Worse from	Better for	Remedy name
Severe second-degree burns.	Violent burning of skin with severe smarting pains. Raw sensations in burnt skin with rapidly-developing blisters Burning pains are more intense when skin is touched.	Touch.	Bathing with cool water.	**Cantharis**
Lingering pains after deep burns.	Sore, drawing pains that persist after burns have superficially healed. Indicated for emotional trauma that follows a severe, deep burn or scald.	Exposure to dry, cold winds or draughts. Exertion. Extreme changes of temperature.	Becoming warm in bed.	**Causticum**
General symptoms of shock that accompany a minor burn or scald.	Denies there is anything wrong and wants to send offered help away. Give initial dose of **Arnica**, and then move on to one of the more specific remedies listed above for burns or scalds.	Touch. Exertion. Being approached. Jarring movements.	Lying with head lower than the body.	**Arnica**

Seek Prompt Medical Help In Any Of The Following Situations:

■ **A severe second or third-degree burn, or any scald or burn that covers an area larger than the palm of the hand.**

■ **If a blister breaks, always check for any signs of developing infection. These may include increased heat or redness around the edges of the damaged skin, or any hint of pus formation. In the case of severe blistering, always seek medical opinion if the surface breaks.**

■ **Check the pulse and breathing rate of anyone who has suffered severe burns, while waiting for emergency help to arrive. Check for any signs and symptoms of shock. These include:**

■ **Pale or blue-tinged skin.**
■ **Drowsiness, confusion or unconsciousness.**
■ **Shallow or laboured breathing.**

- Feeble, fast pulse.
- Thirst.
- Nausea or possible vomiting.
- Yawning, panting or gasping.

Cuts, Grazes and Bruises

Any accident tends to result in bruises and cuts, but the severity of the damage will depend on the seriousness of the trauma. As a result, cuts and bruises can span the range from extremely minor problems which can be easily dealt with by home first aid measures to medical emergencies which need urgent hospital admission. The latter may be especially the case if internal injuries are suspected.

Basic First Aid

- With minor cuts or grazes, the first priority is to clean the wound of any foreign matter or debris. This is most easily and gently done by bathing or soaking the injured area until the wound looks clean. Use boiled, cooled water to which **Calendula**, **Hypericum** or **Hypercal** tincture has been added. One part of tincture should be dissolved in ten parts of water.
- Once they are clean, minor cuts and grazes should be covered with a sterile dressing. **Calendula** or **Hypercal** cream or ointment can either be applied directly to the wound or squeezed on to the dressing which covers the cut or graze. Ideally, the cream is best suited to cuts with lacerated edges, while the ointment is most appropriate for grazes and roughened skin.
- If skin is bruised and not broken, apply ice packs to the injured area for roughly half an hour in an effort to reduce swelling. Provided the skin is intact, **Arnica** cream may be rubbed into bruised tissue in order to ease pain. However, *never* use Arnica cream on broken or cut skin.
- If a cut looks very wide or severe, bear in mind that it will need stitches if the edges of the wound will not come together easily.

Homoeopathic Help

Type of cut, graze or bruise	General symptoms	Worse from	Better for	Remedy name
General trauma and bruising after an accident.	Mild shock following an accident or injury. Reacts as though nothing has happened and may reject help. Pains are sore and aching, with sensitivity of skin to touch and extreme restlessness.	Movement. Touch. Being approached.	Lying with head lower than the body.	**Arnica**
Minor cuts and grazes.	While the suggested remedy should be taken internally in order to help with physical and emotional shock, **Calendula** cream may be applied to clean cuts, and **Calendula** ointment to bathed, grazed skin.	Touch. Movement.	Resting	**Arnica**
Bruised or crushed fingers and toes or deep cuts with nerve involvement.	Indicated for damage to areas that are rich in nerve supply, e.g. fingers, toes and base of the spine. Pains are intermittent and sharp, and shoot along the injured limb.	Jarring movements. Touch. Contact with cold or damp.	Rubbing injured part. Keeping still.	**Hypericum**
Bruises or black eyes that are soothed by cool compresses.	May be needed after **Arnica** has ceased to be helpful. Eases pain and helps speed up the healing process in the bony socket of the eye.	Warmth. Moving.	Cool bathing. Cool compresses. Resting.	**Ledum**
Black eyes or injuries to the soft tissue of the eye.	Often needed after the eyeball has been hit by a blunt object such as a tennis ball. Indicated after **Arnica** if the initial swelling has subsided but the pain remains.	Touch.	Moving the head.	**Symphytum**

Type of cut, graze or bruise	General symptoms	Worse from	Better for	Remedy name
Bruising of areas where bones are thinly-covered, e.g. shin or elbow.	Deep bruising to the periosteum (the membraneous sheath that covers bones). Pains may initially improve with **Arnica**, but deep aching remains in areas thinly-covered with skin.	Exertion. Cold or damp conditions. Stooping. Going up or down stairs.	Warmth. Lying down.	**Ruta**
Bruising to deeply-located tissues, e.g. the breasts.	Bruises that are sustained as a result of a heavy blow, e.g. a knock to the breasts. It may also be needed after surgery which involves bruising to deeply-located tissues.	Touch. Becoming chilled. Warmth.	Cold locally applied.	**Bellis perennis**
Incised wounds as a result of surgery.	Indicated for lacerated wounds that cause stitching, sharp pains. Often needed after surgery involving the genital areas, e.g. hysterectomy or episiotomy in childbirth.	Touch. Stretching the affected area. Emotional stress.	Warmth. Resting.	**Staphysagria**

Seek Prompt Medical Help In Any Of The Following Situations:

■ In the case of deep or wide wounds that require stitches. If a wound cannot be held together by adhesive dressings, professional help is needed.

■ If bleeding from a wound cannot be stopped.

■ Deep cuts to the chest, abdomen or face.

■ Where signs of infection develop around a wound. This may involve symptoms of redness, heat, high temperature or pus formation.

■ If there is a risk of tetanus developing, professional medical help should be consulted. Tetanus is a very serious condition which can advance rapidly and severely. Possible symptoms include:

■ Rapidly advancing rigidity and muscle spasm of the neck, spine and abdomen.

■ **Stiffness and rigidity of the jaw muscles.**
■ **Red streaks radiating from the wound along the injured limb.**

■ **If dirt is deeply embedded and cannot be removed from a wound.**
■ **Wounds to the fingers or underside of the palm of the hands. Bear in mind that these areas may become rapidly infected.**
■ **If someone shows signs of repeated or easy bruising.**
■ **Bruising or injury to the head, especially if there is any bleeding from the nose, ears or mouth.**
■ **Numbness, tingling or loss of strength in an injured limb.**

Fractures

Those who are especially at risk of suffering broken bones include the very young, sports enthusiasts and the elderly. Children as a rule often sustain fractures because of the rough and tumble nature of their games, while vigorous sports carry their own associated problems of sprains, strains, and bruised or broken bones. However, women occupy the most vulnerable category when they reach the post-menopausal years. This is because of the risk of osteoporosis: a condition which results in brittle or porous bones which break under the least stress or strain. The joints that are especially affected include the small bones of the wrist, the spine and the hip.

Symptoms

■ Difficulty in moving or putting weight on the injured limb.
■ Extreme pain or obvious distortion of the injured area.
■ In cases of spinal injury there may be numbness, tingling or loss of control of the limbs, as well as severe pain in the neck or spine. In such a situation, it is vital that the casualty should *on no account be moved*, unless there is a risk of the patient choking on their vomit. In the latter situation, they should only be moved the absolute minimum amount in order to ensure that their airways are kept open.

Basic First Aid

■ If you suspect a fracture has occurred as a result of an accident, keep the casualty as still as possible and make them as comfortable as you can, while waiting for professional medical help to arrive.

■ If any signs of unconsciousness, drowsiness or confusion occur, treat for **Shock**, making sure that emergency medical help is on its way.

■ If swelling is severe and the skin has not been broken, apply ice packs to the swollen area.

■ If there is severe bleeding in addition to a fracture or dislocated joint, efforts should be made to stop the bleeding while waiting for emergency medical attention.

Homoeopathic Help

Type of injury	General symptoms	Worse from	Better for	Remedy name
General pain and trauma following an accident.	The first remedy to be given after an injury of any kind in order to promote re-absorption of blood and ease pain. It also helps symptoms of emotional shock.	Touch. Being approached.	Lying with head low.	**Arnica**
Fractures that have been set in place.	Only to be used once bones have been set in alignment since knitting of fractures is likely to be considerably speeded up. Most useful when initial pain and swelling have subsided.	Touch.		**Symphytum**
Fractures with little swelling but severe pain.	Weakness from extreme pain in fractures. Violent, aching pains in bones. Generalized muscle aching leading to nausea, restlessness and chill.	Movement. Lying on painful area. Coughing. Contact with cold air.	Lying on the stomach. Being spoken to.	**Eupatorium**
Fractured ribs that cause immense pain on movements.	Terrible sensitivity and distress on the slightest movement. More comfortable for firm pressure, or lying on the painful part. Wants to take a deep breath in, but is prevented because of the severity of pain.	Movement. Coughing. Heat in general. Stooping. Taking a deep breath. Light touch.	Keeping as still as possible. Firm pressure. Cool, fresh air. Being left in peace.	**Bryonia**

Type of injury	General symptoms	Worse from	Better for	Remedy name
Stubborn fractures that take ages to heal.	Indicated if bones are slow to knit, even after the use of **Symphytum**. Painful stiffness and numbness in injured areas. Poor quality bones that are soft, thin or brittle.	Cold, draughty conditions. Exertion. Movement. Lifting.	Lying down. Warm, dry conditions.	**Calc phos**

Seek Prompt Medical Help In Any Of The Following Situations:

■ **Where multiple injuries have occurred involving severe bleeding.**
■ **If symptoms of shock develop.**
■ **Any suspicion of fracture to the spine. Symptoms may include severe pain in the neck or back, numbness, tingling, or loss of strength in any limbs. Additional problems may include loss of bladder or bowel control.**
■ **Coldness, numbness or blueness affecting the area beyond the injury.**
■ **If the injured area looks distorted.**
■ **Where there is severe bruising or bleeding beneath the skin around the damaged area.**
■ **If the injured limb cannot be used within twelve hours of the accident occurring.**
■ **If women experience repeated easy fractures after the menopause. Joints that may be especially weak include the small bones of the hand and wrist or the hip joint.**

Puncture Wounds

Puncture wounds generally occur as a result of sharp, pointed objects entering the skin. Because of the nature of this kind of injury, it carries with it certain specific problems that may not apply as much to simple cuts (lacerations) or grazes (abrasions). These include an increased chance of dirt entering the wound, with a higher attendant risk of tetanus developing. There are also additional problems associated with the removal of the foreign object if it is deeply embedded in the skin.

Basic First Aid

■ Where a piece of glass or other sharp material is deeply embedded in a wound, do not attempt to remove it if you suspect that it is acting as a plug. If it is removed there is a danger that bleeding may become extremely severe, thus causing further complications. In a situation such as this, it is best to call on professional medical help so that the foreign body can be removed under appropriate conditions of safety.

■ If bandaging is needed in order to stop bleeding while waiting for medical help, use a raised dressing so that pressure is not applied directly over the point of entry of the foreign body.

■ If blood loss is severe and must be slowed down, never apply pressure directly over the wound if a pointed object remains in it. This is to prevent the foreign body being pushed further into the injured area. Instead apply pressure a short distance away from the puncture wound.

■ If the sharp object has not remained in the injured area, make sure that all dirt or debris is removed from the wound. This is often most efficiently and easily achieved by soaking the damaged skin in a solution of ten parts of boiled, cooled water to one part of **Calendula** or **Hypercal** tincture. Bathing serves the dual function of ensuring that the wound is kept open, which encourages removal of debris and foreign bodies, while also improving circulation which enhances the healing process.

■ Once satisfied that the wound is clean, apply **Calendula** or **Hypercal** cream to the dressing which is being used to cover the punctured area

■ If the edges of the wound need help in order to be held together, apply 'butterfly strips' across the damaged area.

■ If the wound cannot be effectively cleaned, or if it is very large or deep, medical advice should be obtained.

■ If the casualty is at risk of developing tetanus, professional medical advice should be sought.

Homoeopathic Help

Type of wound	General symptoms	Worse from	Better For	Remedy name
Puncture wounds that fell cold and numb.	Tense swelling around wound with tearing pains. Affected limb may feel weak and numb. Although injured area feels cold to the touch, pains are soothed by cool bathing.	Warmth. Moving injured limb.	Cool bathing. Cold compresses. Resting.	**Ledum**

Type of wound	General symptoms	Worse from	Better For	Remedy name
Puncture wounds with puffy, water-logged swelling.	Stinging, prickling pains with rosy-red puffiness surrounding the wound. Extreme sensitivity to touch and heat in any form.	Contact with warm air. Warm bathing. Touch. After sleep.	Contact with cool air. Cool bathing. Cold compresses. Uncovering. Sitting propped-up.	**Apis**
Puncture wounds that are very sensitive.	Pains shoot intermittently along injured limb from the site of wounds. Indicated where injury affects areas that are rich in nerve supply.	Jarring movements. Touch.	Keeping as still as possible.	**Hypericum**
Puncture wounds that refuse to heal well.	Often needed by those who have poor-healing skin. Watery, thin, clear discharge from wound. Injury may leave a painful scar behind. Aids in the expulsion of foreign bodies.	Cold air. Uncovering. Jarring movements. Touch.	Warmth. Dry, warm conditions.	**Silica**

Seek Prompt Medical Help In Any Of The Following Situations:

■ If a foreign body is firmly embedded in the wound and cannot be removed easily and without great distress.

■ If you suspect that the sharp object is acting as a seal, preventing severe blood loss. In this situation, ensure that the casualty receives medical attention before removal is attempted.

■ Always seek medical attention if dirt remains deeply embedded in the wound.

■ If the casualty is at risk of developing tetanus, seek a professional opinion as soon as possible. Tetanus is a potentially life-threatening disease which is characterized by the following symptoms: tension, rigidity or severe muscle spasms in the affected limb spreading to the neck, jaw, abdomen, or spine; red streaks radiating from the wound along the injured limb.

■ If a puncture wound is still extremely tender and sensitive after a couple of days.

■ If any signs of infection develop. These may include heat, redness, excessive swelling or pus formation around the wound. More general indications of infection include a raised temperature or feeling of unwellness or malaise.

■ If the puncture wound affects the thin covering of skin over a joint, especially if any symptoms of infection are present.

■ Where a very deep puncture wound has occurred or if it affects any area apart from the extremities.

■ Wounds which affect the palms or backs of the hands rather than the fingers.

■ If the casualty complains of any numbness, tingling or weakness in the affected limb.

Shock

Symptoms of severe shock constitute a medical emergency and must be dealt with as quickly as possible by seeking professional medical help. Indications that someone is suffering from shock may include any of the following:

■ Pale, clammy or bluish-tinged skin.
■ Collapse.
■ Drowsiness or confusion.
■ Unconsciousness.
■ Laboured or irregular breathing.
■ Feeble or irregular pulse.
■ Nausea.

Shock may be associated with any of the following situations:

■ A severe allergic reaction to bites or stings.
■ Loss of blood.
■ Heatstroke.
■ Severe burns.
■ As a result of dehydration if vomiting and diarrhoea are protracted.
■ Blood poisoning or septicaemia.
■ Internal bleeding.

Basic First Aid

■ If someone appears to be entering a state of shock, the first priority must be to send for medical help immediately.

■ While help is on its way, loosen clothing at any points that may be causing constriction, e.g. around the neck.

■ If the patient is conscious, elevate the legs slightly.

■ If there are any signs of impending unconsciousness, place the casualty in the recovery position with their head facing downwards and forwards in order to enable them to breathe freely. To place someone in the recovery position, roll them on to their front, with the leg nearest to you placed at right angles to their body. The arms should also be bent at the elbows so that the body weight is supported in a secure and comfortable position. Also ensure that the head is slightly tilted, with the chin jutting forwards. Monitor their pulse and breathing rate at regular intervals while help is on its way.

■ If someone has gone into shock as a result of a spinal injury, they should not be moved into the recovery position unless there is a risk of their choking on vomit. In the latter situation, movement should be restricted to the absolute minimum in order to avoid flexing the spine.

■ Make sure that the casualty is not exposed to extreme temperatures, either of heat or cold.

■ Reassure the patient as much as possible while waiting for help to arrive.

Homeopathic Help

Type of shock	General symptoms	Worse from	Better for	Remedy name
General trauma as a result of an accident.	Gets up from an accident and claims that nothing is wrong, and refuses medical help. Lapses in and out of drowsiness and confusion. Indicated where injuries have occured to the head and neck.	Being approached. Jarring movements. Touch.	Lying with head outstretched.	**Arnica**
Emotional shock and panic.	Terror-stricken and restless as a result of emotional or physical trauma. Panic leads to a conviction that death is imminent. Collapse from sudden loss of strength. Shock may develop after surgery or injury.	Becoming chilled. Noise. Bright light. Touch.	Resting. Fresh air.	**Aconite.**

Type of shock	General symptoms	Worse from	Better for	Remedy name
Shock resulting from a severe allergic reaction.	Indicated where there is a severe reaction to wasp or bee stings. Puffy swellings of the face, eyes, lips or throat leading to breathing problems.	Warmth. Touch. Pressure. Lying down.	Cool air. Cool bathing. Sitting propped-up. Moving.	**Apis**
Faintness with pale, clammy skin.	State of collapse with 'air hunger': needs to be fanned in order to feel more comfortable. In severe stages of shock, skin is sweaty, cold, grey or bluish-tinged.	Warm, stuffy surroundings. Becoming chilled. Weight or pressure of clothes.	Fresh air. Being fanned. Raising feet slightly higher than the body.	**Carbo veg**

Shock is a medical emergency that requires swift professional attention. If the following symptoms occur, lose no time in sending for medical help:

- **Confusion or drowsiness**.
- **Unconsciousness**.
- **Weak or rapid pulse**.
- **Shallow panting or laboured breathing**.
- **Grey or bluish-tinged skin, especially around the lips**.
- **Sweating**.

■4■
A–Z Of Common Ailments

T he conditions discussed in this chapter are broad-ranging problems that are generally not specific to age or gender. Many of these can be defined as 'acute' disorders. This means that they usually follow the pattern of an abrupt onset, a short life-span, and they generally clear up of their own accord given appropriate conditions for recovery. The latter may include a light diet, increasing fluid intake where appropriate, resting and avoiding extreme fluctuations of temperature. For a more detailed discussion of acute prescribing, see **Chapter 2: *Homoeopathy In The Home: How To Use This Book*.**

In many ways, the majority of the conditions discussed in this chapter are the most appropriate for the newcomer to homoeopathy to deal with. This is because of the limited nature of acute problems, and the fact that many of them can be helped by the simple practical measures that are included in each section. In this way, the new prescriber can ease themselves gradually into using homoeopathic remedies for acute conditions, only taking on cases that they feel comfortable with. Most important of all, this guards against the danger of the novice getting into situations where they feel out of their depth. However, where more complicated 'chronic' problems are discussed (such as asthma), it is made clear why home prescribing is not appropriate.

Asthma

Asthma is a condition that may vary in severity from symptoms of mild breathlessness and constriction of the chest to extreme distress, wheezing and inability to breathe. It is a problem that often emerges in childhood, with a good chance of spontaneous recovery occurring during the teenage years. However, the general incidence of asthma is growing, probably as a result of increasing levels of atmospheric pollution and correspondingly poor air quality.

Although homoeopathy has a great deal to offer asthma sufferers of all ages, this is a condition that should be dealt with by an experienced homoeopathic practitioner rather than the home prescriber. This is because a homoeopath will be well-versed in the care that needs to be taken regarding the role of conventional asthma medication, and the importance of *never* withdrawing medication abruptly. As a result, the professional judgement of a homoeopath is of paramount importance in assessing the progress of an asthma case and advising on when and how to adjust conventional medication, ideally in consultation with the patient's GP.

The professional opinion of a homoeopathic practitioner is also invaluable in taking all the information of a patient's case into consideration when selecting the appropriate homoeopathic prescription. For instance, if someone is suffering from asthma as well as eczema and/or hayfever, a homoeopathic strategy will be selected on the basis of improving all of these conditions as a whole. The potential complications involved in case management of this kind can be considerable, since one condition may briefly become more active as another improves. The experienced homoeopathic practitioner, however, has the necessary perspective to manage the situation, knowing when it is best to take action and when it is crucial to wait.

If a homoeopath is consulted by someone suffering from asthma, they are likely to be treated on a 'constitutional' level. This involves a holistic approach to treatment, with mental, emotional and physical symptoms being taken into account, as well as a full family medical history. When this approach to treatment is successful, the patient's general experience of health and well-being improves, as established patterns of ill health recede into the background. As a result, homoeopathy is a system of healing that is not concerned with haphazard removal or suppression of symptoms, since it is aiming to restore a much more ambitious experience of improved health.

Since asthma sufferers are best treated along the lines outlined above for the most positive outcome to ensue, home-prescribing for this condition is not recommended. Even if a well-indicated homoeopathic remedy were selected for an acute asthmatic episode, it would be likely to alleviate the immediate symptoms in the short term but would probably do nothing to discourage further episodes from occurring in the future.

The following self-help measures may be of practical use in addition to professional homoeopathic help.

Practical Self-Help

■ Avoid contact where possible with substances that may aggravate the condition. The potential range of problematic factors that can trigger a reaction is very wide, and may include the following:

■ Animal fur or bird feathers.
■ Certain drugs.

- Chest infections.
- Dust.
- Exercise in frosty, dry air.
- Fungal spores.
- Household sprays and cleaners.
- Pollen.
- Some foods such as eggs, shellfish or milk.
- Stress or emotional strain.

Practical measures for limiting exposure to some of these items include: ensuring that surroundings are as free of dust as possible, using pillows that are filled with man-made fibres rather than feathers or duck down, and staying indoors as much as possible while keeping doors and windows shut during the hayfever season.

- If stress is a contributing factor, explore relaxation and breathing techniques. See **Chapter 8: *The Stresses of Modern Living: How to Cope*** for advice on general management of this distressing problem.
- Sipping a warm drink in relaxed surroundings may help alleviate a mild bout of wheezing, especially if the attack has been sparked off by inhaling very cold air.
- If breathing is difficult, avoid lying down since this tends to make things worse. For maximum relief, sit leaning slightly forwards with elbows resting on the back of a chair. Relax as much as possible while doing this, breathing as evenly and gently as you can while concentrating on slowly expanding the chest.
- Avoid dairy products as much as possible such as milk, cream, and cheese. Apart from being possible *allergens* (substances that may trigger an allergic reaction), they also contribute towards the production of mucus, thus making any chest problem worse. Other potential allergens include chocolate, convenience foods that contain colourings and preservatives, shellfish and peanuts.

Seek Immediate Medical Help If The Following Occur:

- **A severe asthma attack with any of these symptoms:**

  - **Loud wheezing.**
  - **Pallor and clamminess of the skin.**
  - **Any tinge of blue to the skin or lips.**
  - **Rapid, shallow breathing.**
  - **Increased pulse rate.**
  - **Anxiety or panic.**

- **A severe chest infection in an asthma sufferer.**
- **If asthma attacks are becoming increasingly severe, or frequent, or if they are accompanied by hayfever or eczema.**

Colds

Very few of us are likely to be strangers to the miseries of the common cold. Although in itself a minor health problem, the attendant complications, such as residual catarrh or sinus involvement, can lead to weeks of discomfort long after the original cold has gone. For those of us who suffer repeated bouts of cold through the winter, the problems can become even more severe, leaving us with a general feeling of being below par for most of the winter months.

Within this context, homoeopathic prescribing has an enormous amount to offer. Although using the appropriate homoeopathic remedy is unlikely to stop a cold in its tracks (especially if it is already into the well-established stage), it can do a great deal to make us feel better able to cope with the symptoms. It also has the added bonus of speeding us through the stages of a cold more rapidly and easily, leading to a lessened risk of residual complications of the kind mentioned above.

Generally speaking, a cold goes through three stages. The first stage may include initial symptoms of sneezing, irritation in the throat and a general sensation of being unwell. The second stage is likely to result in what we refer to as a 'head cold', including a streaming or obstructed nose, and possible irritating cough. By the third stage of a cold, if a cough is present, it is likely to have become more productive, or it may alternate between dry and loose. Mucus discharges from the nose and chest may have turned a yellowish green colour, and the ears and nose often feel blocked.

Although these are the common stages experienced by cold sufferers, many us may find that we go through stages one and two without the complications of the third stage, while others may find that the initial phases of a cold are not too troublesome, while the third stage seems to drag on for ages. However, for those of us who are unlucky enough to have little resistance to infection, the boundaries between stages of a cold are difficult to identify, since one cold seems to merge into another, creating the impression of one interminable illness that seems to last for weeks or months.

Practical Self-Help

■ At the first sign of a cold, take a gram of vitamin C daily for a few days. The supplement may be obtained in single, one gram tablets, or doses of 500mgs (half a gram) or 250 mgs (quarter of a gram). In the case of the latter, four doses may be spaced through the day by taking one tablet in the morning, lunchtime, mid-afternoon and evening. Taking a vitamin C supplement appears to aid the body in fighting infection. As a result, it is often useful to take a short course of vitamin C as quickly as possible if you know you have been exposed to a cold virus and want to avoid developing symptoms. Those who suffer from kidney stones should avoid taking high doses of vitamin C over a lengthy period of time.

■ Rest as much as possible in the earliest stages of a cold in order to assist your body in fighting infection. By making other demands on energy that is required to fight a cold, you are likely to take longer to get over the illness. By taking it easy when needed, time spent off work is generally reduced overall. You will also find that you are better able cope with work effectively when you return, rather than if you force yourself back too early. There is also the added practical bonus with this approach of not spreading the cold to colleagues during the infectious stage.

■ Drink as much water as possible in order to support your body in flushing toxins out of the system more effectively. Avoid drinks that have a fluid-reducing or dehydrating effect such as coffee, strong tea and caffeinated, cola-type drinks. Instead choose water as a cold drink, and opt for some of the more refreshing fruit teas as warm beverages.

■ Keep in as stable a temperature as possible in order to avoid getting over-heated or chilled. Either extreme will put extra strain on the body, requiring adjustments that put additional demands on energy levels. The situation becomes even more taxing where the system has to cope with the body's own rapid or extreme temperature changes.

■ If you have a history of chest or sinus problems that develop after a cold, consider using a garlic supplement as a natural anti-bacterial agent. It also has a beneficial effect in breaking down thickened or discoloured mucus.

■ Avoid foods or drinks that put an extra strain on the liver. The latter is one of the main organs responsible for de-toxifying the body, and it needs to be supported as much as possible in this role during acute illness. Avoid foods that are high in fat, and concentrate instead on easily-digested soups, salads and lightly-cooked fish or chicken. If you aren't hungry, don't feel that you have to eat but make sure that you drink as much as possible. On the other hand, avoid alcohol since the liver has to work very hard in order to deal with its toxic effects.

Homoeopathic Help

Type of cold	General symptoms	Worse from	Better for	Remedy name
Early stage of a cold that develops after exposure to cold winds.	Sudden onset of severe symptoms which primarily affect the nose, eyes and throat. Feverishness with dry throat and marked thirst.	Chill. Touch. At night. Noise.	Resting. Fresh air.	**Aconite**

Type of cold	General symptoms	Worse from	Better for	Remedy name
Early stage with rapid onset of feverishness.	Hot, dry and flushed with raised temperature. Skin, nose and throat look bright red and inflamed. Liquids are difficult to swallow because of sore throat: sips drinks. Symptoms are likely to affect the right side.	Jarring movements. Light. Noise. Lying flat. Touch.	Sitting propped-up in bed. Light covering. Resting.	Belladonna
Early stage with earache and sore throat.	Looks alternately flushed and pale in the first stages of a cold. Sore, swollen throat which is worse for swallowing saliva. Loss of hearing with earache.	At night. Movement. Jarring. Chill. Cold drinks.	Lying down. Cold compresses.	Ferrum phos
Severe head cold with streaming eyes and nose.	Burning, smarting eyes that constantly water bland tears. Streaming nose with sore nostrils and upper lip. Constant violent sneezing bouts with burning nasal discharge.	Over heated rooms. In the evening. Damp conditions.	Bathing. Movement. Cool, fresh air.	Allium cepa
Violent head cold with profuse, burning discharge from eyes.	Streaming eyes and nose with loose cough. Nasal discharge is abundant and bland, while watering eyes are burning and smarting.	Sunlight. Warm rooms. Walking in the wind. In the evening.	Blinking or wiping eyes. Fresh air.	Euphrasia
Cold symptoms that get much worse as the night progresses.	Chilly, restless and anxious with illness. Burning sensations in eyes, nose and throat that are eased by contact with warmth. Chest becomes tight and wheezy with irritating dry cough: has to sit propped-up on pillows to get comfortable.	Exposure to cold or chill. As the night progresses. Lying on the painful side. Making an effort.	Warmth. Sips of warm drinks. Hot water bottle. Movement. Sitting propped-up. Company.	Arsenicum alb

Type of cold	General symptoms	Worse from	Better for	Remedy name
Head cold with generally 'hungover', headachy feeling.	Tired, irritable and grouchy with a cold. Terribly sensitive to cold draughts, and generally much better for peace and quiet. Stuffed-up nose is most severe at night. Nose runs in warm surroundings and during the day.	Being disturbed. Cold conditions. Loud noise. Relying on sedatives or stimulants. First thing in the morning.	Peaceful surroundings. Warmth. Sound sleep. As the day goes on. Hot drinks.	**Nux vomica**
Colds with clear, streaming nasal discharge that runs like a tap.	Dry, cracked lips with cold sores. Discharge from nose is either clear and extremely runny, or like the white of an egg. Difficulty breathing from stuffed-up sensation high in nose.	Sunlight. Sympathy. Making an effort. Noise. Touch.	Being left alone. Cool surroundings. Cool compresses. Skipping meals. Fresh air.	**Nat mur**

Seek Prompt Medical Help In Any Of The Following Situations:

■ **Severe cold symptoms in the very young or the elderly.**

■ **Sore throats in anyone who has previously suffered from rheumatic fever.**

■ **If breathing becomes laboured, wheezy or difficult, especially in those who do not have a history of asthma.**

■ **Severe earache in a young child.**

■ **Feverishness that does not respond to self-help measures, especially in the very young or the elderly.**

Constipation

Although the misery of constipation is something that can affect us at any time, there are certain periods in our lives when we may be more likely to suffer from this frustrating condition. These include the teenage years when scant attention may be paid to the quality of our diets and when eating disorders can be a problem, during the later months of pregnancy, or as we become elderly. Certain features of our daily routine can also compound the situation, such as a sedentary lifestyle (especially if working hours are spent behind a desk), poor-quality diet that is lacking in essential fibre, dependence on painkillers, or living in an over-stressed environment with little space for relaxation and reflection.

However, there are a range of practical steps that can be taken which should render constipation a problem of the past. By dealing with it in this way rather than masking the symptom temporarily by relying on laxatives, the outcome is far more likely to be successful in the long term.

Practical Self-Help

■ It is very easy to forget the role that drinking sufficient water plays in protecting against constipation. Many of us may feel we drink enough fluid because we take regular cups of tea or coffee through the day. However, this will do little to provide the necessary lubrication that is needed for an easy bowel movement since both tea and coffee have diuretic properties: in other words, they encourage the body to eliminate liquid rather than conserving it. Drinking between six to eight large glasses of water each day facilitates the movement of bowel contents. This also helps to guard against the formation of small, dry or hard stools that result in straining and distress.

■ Dietary fibre also plays a vital role in protecting against constipation by encouraging regular, easy bowel movements. The best source of fibre comes from fresh fruit, vegetables (ideally eaten raw or lightly steamed), whole grains (such as wholemeal bread), pulses and beans. Foods that encourage constipation because of their low fibre content include convenience foods, refined carbohydrates such as white sugar and flour, and items that are high in fat. By keeping foods in the latter category to a minimum, and increasing our intake of high fibre foods and the amount of water we drink, constipation should cease to be a problem. Easy ways of increasing fibre intake include ensuring that a large salad is eaten with each main meal, always eating a healthy portion of fresh vegetables with lunch and dinner, and regularly having fresh fruit as a pudding.

■ Eating frequent or large helpings of red meat can also cause particular health problems. These include a high risk of suffering from constipation because of the extended period of time that red meat takes to be broken down and digested. As a result, meat tends to sit for a long time in the gut, unlike more fibrous foods which pass through more speedily. Those who eat regular quantities of red meat and little fibre may be at more risk of developing constipation, and attendant problems such as diverticulosis or cancer of the bowel.

■ Achieving a regular, easy bowel movement is also dependent to a large extent on becoming conscious of the signals that our bodies give out, alerting us to the need to pass a stool. If these signals are persistently ignored because we are too preoccupied to act on them, constipation is usually the result. On the other hand, if we develop the ability of making time to act on the impulse to pass a stool when appropriate, regularity is usually established without a problem.

■ It is always best to avoid using laxatives where possible, especially on a long-term basis. If dependence on taking laxatives occurs, it eventually becomes impossible to achieve a bowel movement without them. This is because laxatives have the long-term effect of making the bowel increasingly 'lax', with the result that once they are withdrawn, the chances of resuming normal bowel action are diminished rather than increased. When taken over a long period of time, they can also result in an unhappy alternation between diarrhoea and constipation with an attendant risk of nutritional deficiency developing.

■ Regular, rhythmic exercise also has an important role to play in guarding against constipation. Aerobic activity such as running or cycling can do a great deal to improve bowel action, as well as improving the condition of the heart and lungs. If we sit behind a desk all day, drive home and sit on the sofa all night after eating dinner, we are doing nothing to improve the tone and condition of our muscles or digestive system.

■ Constipation is a common by-product of an overly-stressed lifestyle. 'Living in the fast lane' usually involves a poor-quality diet of fast foods, reliance on stimulants to keep going and sedatives to relax, too high a consumption of alcohol, over-consumption of painkillers, and very little quality time in which to relax and unwind. Generally speaking, feeling uptight and overstressed are very common factors in those who develop a condition called Irritable Bowel Syndrome. This diagnostic definition embraces a host of digestive problems, including a distressing alternation between constipation and diarrhoea. Within this context, learning to relax can play an essential role in helping the overall problem, especially with regard to chronic constipation. One of the best ways of learning to relax is to attend a yoga class. This should incorporate a lengthy relaxation session and advice on breathing techniques for stress-reduction. Other options include using audio or video tapes which provide a guided relaxation exercise, or exploring meditation techniques. The main thing is to give priority to the time spent relaxing each day so that it becomes an essential part of the daily routine. Once this happens it will feel like second nature and the general benefits to mind and body will become obvious.

■ Avoid cooking with aluminium pots and pans. Traces of the metal may enter food as it is being cooked, leading to potential problems with constipation, osteoporosis, learning problems in the young, and senile dementia. If you are concerned about unwittingly being exposed to aluminium, also avoid tea bags and aluminium-based antacids.

Homoeopathic Help

Type of constipation	General symptoms	Worse from	Better for	Remedy name
Constipation with constant, fruitless urging.	Overall picture of hyper-stress and tension with resulting headaches, indigestion, nausea, muscle tension and constipation. Persistent sensation of needing to pass a stool.	Over-use of painkillers. Coffee. Alcohol. Stress. Noise. Lack of sleep. On waking.	Being left in peace. Sound sleep. Warmth. As the day goes on.	**Nux vomica**
Constipation with no urge to pass a stool.	Irritable and headachy with constipation. Throbbing headache that is much worse for the least movement. Stools are large, dark, hard, very dry and extremely difficult to pass. Marked thirst for long, cold drinks.	Movement. Warm, stuffy surroundings. Being disturbed. Muscular effort.	Keeping still. Cool surroundings. Cold drinks.	**Bryonia**
Constipation with extreme difficulty in passing even a very soft stool.	Slow-developing constipation, especially in the elderly. Severe straining and bleeding when attempting a bowel movement. Stools are knotted, dry and hard.	Starchy foods. Cold conditions. Every other day. Sitting still.	Warmth. Eating. Warm foods. Warm drink.	**Alumina**
Constipation when routine is upset away from home.	Lots of bloating with rumbling, gurgling wind: has to loosen waistband in order to feel relief. Constipation from overuse of laxatives that alternates with a constant need to go.	Emotional strain. Anxiety. Pressure of clothes. Cool food or drinks. 4–8 p.m.	Gentle exercise in the open air. Loosening clothes. Keeping occupied. Warm food and drinks.	**Lycopodium**

Type of constipation	General symptoms	Worse from	Better for	Remedy name
Constipation with abundant, offensive-smelling wind.	Bloated abdomen with constant wind that moves upwards and downwards. Discomfort is not relieved by belching. Hard, dry, knotted stools covered in mucus. Anal fissure with constipation.	Becoming over-heated. Cold food and drinks. Before or after a period.	Fresh air. Resting.	**Graphites**

Seek Medical Advice If Any Of The Following Occur:

■ **Any change in bowel habits that cannot be accounted for, e.g. onset of constipation or diarrhoea for no apparent reason.**
■ **If stools become persistently dark or light in colour.**
■ **Difficult stools that cause straining and bright bleeding.**
■ **Severe constipation in pregnancy.**

Coughs

A persistent cough can be one of the most irritating and exhausting symptoms left behind after a heavy cold or flu. Although many of us are tempted to reach for a cough suppressant in an effort to obtain short-term relief from a hacking cough, it is important to understand why the problem is there, and what the coughing reflex is attempting to do for us.

Coughing is the basic mechanism used by the body to loosen and rid itself of mucus that is lying in the air passages. When this reflex acts successfully, we cough up phlegm and breathe more easily afterwards as a result. If we consider how important this process is to easing a congested chest, suppressing the cough is unlikely to have a long-term beneficial effect.

However, very often a coughing cycle is set up which becomes unproductive. In other words, spasmodic coughing happens at regular intervals, but it is unable to resolve the situation. When things have reached this stage, the appropriate homoeopathic remedy can give the body the necessary boost to get on with the job more efficiently. As a result, the cough may quickly become productive, releasing the necessary mucus and easing the chest. An appropriately-chosen remedy can also do a great deal to soothe the aching chest muscles that often result from persistent, violent coughing spasms.

Practical Self-Help

■ Use a humidifier to prevent the atmosphere becoming too dry. This is especially important in centrally-heated or air-conditioned surroundings. Custom-made machines can be purchased, or a home-made version can be created by placing bowls of water near radiators or heaters. Refill the containers at regular intervals as the contents evaporate.

■ Use a garlic supplement in order to encourage the breakdown of mucus and to discourage bacterial growth. Two capsules should be taken three times a day until the cough improves. A vitamin C supplement may also be helpful. See the self-help section on *Colds* for the recommended dosage.

■ If a cough is troublesome at night, a great deal of relief may be obtained by sleeping propped-up on two or three pillows. Lying flat tends to compress the chest area, making breathing more difficult.

■ Avoid taking a milky drink at night since it may increase mucus production. Also cut down on dairy products such as cheese, milk, and cream since these can also contribute to congestion in the chest from excess phlegm.

■ Steam may do a great deal to soothe dry, croupy-sounding coughs. Steam inhalations may be helpful, or spending some time in a steam-filled bathroom if coughing bouts are made worse by a dry, cold atmosphere.

Homoeopathic Help

Type of cough	General symptoms	Worse from	Better for	Remedy name
Dry, wheezy coughs that are better for sitting up.	Cough gets worse at night and in the early hours of the morning. Tight, wheezy chest with restlessness and anxiety. Cold air makes chest problems worse, while warmth helps. Burning in chest with coughing bouts.	Cold air. Cold drinks. At night. Early hours of the morning. Lying down.	Warmth. Sitting propped-up in bed. Company. Gentle movement.	**Arsenicum alb**
Persistent, tickly cough with sore chest.	Dry cough from irritation in the throat pit. Presses hand to chest in an effort to ease muscular pain caused by repeated coughing spasms. Wants to take a deep breath, but it makes the cough worse.	Entering a warm room. Movement. Breathing deeply. Dry cold or heat. Touch.	Cool fresh air. Pressing on chest. Keeping as still as possible. Sitting up.	**Bryonia**

Type of cough	General symptoms	Worse from	Better for	Remedy name
Tight, constricted chest with hoarseness and yellow expectoration.	Cough is brought on or aggravated by marked changes of temperature. Exhausting cough that strains the abdominal muscles. Burning sensations in chest with alternation between dry and loose cough.	Lying on the left side. Talking. Strong smells. Morning and evening.	After sleep. Sitting still. Massage. Reassurance.	**Phosphorus**
Brassy-sounding cough with mucus that is difficult to move.	Cough begins with tickling in the throat, followed by difficulty in raising stringy, ropy phlegm. Often required in the final stages of a cold that has led to congestion in the chest and sinuses.	Fresh air. Cold and damp. Eating. Sleep.	Dislodging mucus. Warmth.	**Kali bich**
Severe coughing spasms that end in vomiting.	Coughing starts as soon as the head touches the pillow. Exhausting bouts of coughing that follow each other in close succession. Coughing is brought on by talking. Irritating sensation of a crumb or feather in the throat.	Lying down. Warmth. Speaking. After midnight. Laughing. Stooping.	Fresh air. Pressure.	**Drosera**
Hoarse, rasping throat with croupy-sounding cough.	Sense of frightening suffocation: feels as though breathing through a sponge. Burning in chest and throat which gets worse from cold food or drinks. Wakes from sleep with a distressing sense of a foreign body in the throat.	Dry, cold winds. Waking from sleep. Physical exertion. Talking.	Warm food or drinks.	**Spongia**

Type of cough	General symptoms	Worse from	Better for	Remedy name
Choking cough set off by least draught of cold air.	Barking cough with thick, yellow phlegm that rattles in the chest. Loose cough with difficulty in raising phlegm. Coughing bouts are much worse in the evening and at night.	Uncovering. Contact with dry, cold air. Touch. Exertion. At night.	Warm surroundings. Wrapping up warmly. Moist heat. Humidity.	**Hepar sulph**
Coughing spasms that are brought on by touching the throat.	Insomnia from persistent coughing. Choking spasms with breathlessness. Raw, burning sensations in chest that feel worse for taking a deep breath. Phlegm is thin, frothy and abundant.	Cold air. Taking a deep breath. Changing temperatures. Movement. Pressure on throat. Eating.	Wrapping up well. Covering mouth.	**Rumex**
Well-established, loose cough with thick, yellowy-green phlegm.	Most symptoms are aggravated by a stuffy, over-heated environment. Lying or sitting still also feels very uncomfortable. Dry cough in the evening alternates with loose cough in the morning. Phlegm tastes sweet, salty or bitter.	Stuffy, airless rooms. Morning and evening. In bed at night. Resting. After eating.	Cool, fresh air. Gentle movement. Uncovering. Sympathy. Attention.	**Pulsatilla**

Seek Prompt Medical Help In Any Of The Following Situations:

■ **Where pronounced wheezing occurs without a history of asthma.**
■ **If a persistent cough does not clear up after using sensible self-help measures, especially if it is accompanied by a declining sense of well-being and energy.**
■ **A severe cough in the very young or the elderly.**
■ **Severe chest pain.**
■ **Breathing difficulties or marked distress in young children.**
■ **If a foreign body has been inhaled.**
■ **Where there is any suggestion of drowsiness or confusion.**

Diarrhoea

Diarrhoea is a distressing condition that can occur on either a short-lived acute basis, or it may become a more long-term chronic problem. If diarrhoea occurs as a temporary disorder it is usually the result of having eaten something that has not agreed with the digestive system. In this situation the body usually responds by expelling the contents of the stomach and bowel as quickly as possible in the form of vomit or diarrhoea. Other short-lived episodes of diarrhoea may result from anticipatory anxiety such as exam nerves, or tension before an interview. However, long-term anxiety or emotional strain can cause an extended problem with diarrhoea and other digestive disorders which may come under the diagnostic heading of *Irritable Bowel Syndrome*. Additional chronic problems that may result in frequent bouts of diarrhoea include *Ulcerative Colitis*, *Crohn's Disease*, or *Coeliac Disease*.

The homoeopathic remedies listed below are intended for use in occasional, acute bouts of diarrhoea in an otherwise healthy person. If the situation involves a more long-term digestive problem, professional help should be sought rather than attempting treatment with home prescribing.

Practical Self-Help

■ If the body is attempting to expel something disagreeable from the digestive tract, it is best not to go on eating since this is likely to irritate the situation further. However, it is essential to ensure that enough fluid is drunk in order to prevent dehydration. This becomes especially vital if vomiting and diarrhoea happen at the same time, since the risk of becoming dehydrated in this situation is very marked. Babies, small children and the elderly are especially vulnerable to serious fluid loss. Avoid drinks that irritate the stomach lining such as tea or coffee, orange juice, or sugary, carbonated drinks. Opt instead for still mineral water or soothing herbal teas such as peppermint or fennel. However, do remember that peppermint or spearmint may interfere with the action of homoeopathic remedies.

■ Since the body also loses salt during excessive fluid loss, a very weak saline solution can be made up as follows. Add a quarter of a teaspoon of salt and four level teaspoons of sugar to a pint of water, stir well until completely dissolved and drink as often as possible.

■ If hunger pangs occur, ensure that whatever is eaten is as light and easy to digest as possible. Suitable choices include clear broth and rice made from a vegetable base, home-made soups or puréed vegetables and lightly-steamed fish. Foods to avoid when digestion is sensitive include: cheese or meat that is high in fat such as salami or sausages, beans, fried foods and creamy puddings. If fruit or vegetables seem appealing, steam them lightly in order to make them more easily digestible.

■ Bear in mind that although conventional, anti-diarrhoea formulations may provide temporary relief, they also hinder the spasmodic, expulsive mechanism that the body is employing in order to rid itself of irritant material. By obstructing this process before the underlying problem has been resolved, we may feel nauseated and unwell, even though diarrhoea has stopped.

■ Rest as much as possible if feeling generally unwell with diarrhoea. By making demands on the body, energy that could be used to fight infection is diverted elsewhere and the process of getting well may take longer.

Homoeopathic Help

Type of diarrhoea	General symptoms	Worse from	Better for	Remedy name
Chilly, anxious, and restless with diarrhoea.	Diarrhoea may occur with vomiting as a result of eating spoiled meat or fruit. Burning sensations are relieved by sips of warm drinks or warm applications. Fearful, fussy and very difficult to please when ill.	Cold surroundings. Being alone. Cold drinks. During the night.	Warmth. Sips of warm drinks. Company. Sitting propped-up in bed.	**Arsenicum alb**
Diarrhoea with severe thirst for cold water.	Cold, pale, clammy and exhausted during and after a bout of diarrhoea. Vomiting may occur at the same time from food poisoning. Diarrhoea results in severe straining, prostration and muscle cramps. Appetite may be present between bouts of diarrhoea.	Movement. During muscle spasms. Pressure. After drinking.	Being snuggly covered up. Warmth. Resting.	**Veratrum alb**
Diarrhoea with excessive production of wind.	Cramping diarrhoea with faintness and clammy, pale skin. Involuntary bowel movements occur with violent passage of wind. Severe discomfort from tight clothing around the waist.	Overheated, stuffy, rooms. Tight waistbands. Becoming chilled. Spoiled chicken. Extreme changes of temperature.	Belching or passing wind. Being fanned. Fresh, cool air. Resting with feet elevated.	**Carbo veg**

Type of diarrhoea	General symptoms	Worse from	Better for	Remedy name
Profuse, watery, painless diarrhoea.	Nauseated, weak feeling after diarrhoea. Bouts of diarrhoea alternate with headache. Noisy gurgling before urgent need to empty bowels. Fruit and milk aggravate the condition.	Early hours of the morning. After eating. Movement. Before, during and after a bout of diarrhoea.	Lying on abdomen. Massage or stroking.	**Podophyllum**
Involuntary, gushing painless diarrhoea with extreme anxiety.	Very little control over passage of diarrhoea: feels as though anus is constantly open. Exhausting diarrhoea may occur after a fright or shock. Very thirsty for cold drinks that are expelled as soon as they become warm in the digestive tract.	Shock. Cold air. Exhaustion. Strong smells. Morning and evening.	Reassurance. Sound sleep. Bathing face with cold water. Eating a little. Cold drinks, until they are warmed in the stomach. Massage.	**Phosphorus**
Painless, 'nervous' diarrhoea before an important event.	Withdrawn, morose, and lethargic before a stressful event such as an interview or examination. Heavy, aching sensations in arms and legs with exhaustion. Headachy and dizzy with diarrhoea.	Anticipating a stressful event. Making an effort. Anxiety.	Resting. Bending forwards. Passing urine.	**Gelsemium**
Severe diarrhoea that comes on immediately after eating or drinking.	Diarrhoea from anticipatory anxiety. Talkative, excitable and nervous. Bloated abdomen with severe wind and loud belching. Noisy diarrhoea worse for sugary foods. Shivering and trembling with diarrhoea.	Anxiety. Confined spaces. Sweets. Cold or iced foods. Crowds.	Fresh cool air. Pressure. Movement. Belching. Bending double.	**Argentum nit**

Type of diarrhoea	General symptoms	Worse from	Better for	Remedy name
Watery, painless diarrhoea that is especially urgent on waking.	Has to hurry to pass violent, frothy diarrhoea in the morning. Frequency and severity of bowel movements leave the anus sore, burning, red and itchy. As a result of discomfort, puts off passing a stool until the last moment.	Warm bathing. In bed. Over-exertion. Sweets. Milk. Standing.	Fresh, open air. Drawing knees up. Moderate temperatures. Perspiring.	**Sulphur**

Seek Prompt Medical Help In Any Of The Following Situations:

■ **Severe or persistent diarrhoea in babies, small children, pregnant women or the elderly.**

■ **If any signs of dehydration occur. These may include:**

   ■ **Dry skin that does not spring readily back into place when pinched.**
   ■ **Reduced urine output and/or strong-smelling urine.**
   ■ **Sunken eyes.**
   ■ **Sunken fontanelle (the soft spot at the crown of the head) in young babies.**
   ■ **Lack of saliva or tears.**

■ **If severe abdominal pain and vomiting accompany diarrhoea.**
■ **Signs of mucus, pus or blood in stool.**
■ **Alternating diarrhoea and constipation.**
■ **Any marked change in bowel habit for no obvious reason, which does not resolve itself within a reasonable period of time.**

Eczema

Eczema is a similar condition to asthma with regard to severity of flare-ups. In other words, one eczema sufferer may experience very mild, limited episodes of irritation, while another may find that large surfaces of the body are regularly covered with severe, dry, itchy eruptions. There are strong links between eczema, asthma and hayfever, since many people who suffer from one of these conditions will often have espisodes of one or both of the others. Alternatively, an eczema sufferer may have a strong family history of asthma or hayfever.

Homoeopaths regard a skin disorder such as eczema or psoriasis as a superficial indication of a more deep-seated disorder. As a result, treatment is aimed at rectifying this established imbalance from inside by prescribing appropriately-selected homoeopathic remedies which treat the problem at the deepest level. Consequently, symptoms tend to improve from within outwards, with problems such as headaches, indigestion, asthma or joint pains clearing up before the skin condition. As improvement sets in, there is also an established pattern by which a homoeopath can determine whether the condition is moving in a positive direction. The most desirable outcome occurs when a skin eruption initially improves on the head, face and upper limbs, moving gradually and steadily downwards until the condition disappears. If symptoms also disappear in reverse order of their initial appearance, the indications suggest strongly that the problem has been dealt with at a profound level.

Because of the deep-seated nature of skin problems, eczema, psoriasis, urticaria (hives), warts, and impetigo should not be treated by the home prescriber. The newcomer to homoeopathy is unlikely have the required clinical knowledge and experience to correctly interpret the reactions of the patient and may rapidly get out of their depth. Professional help should be sought from a homoeopathic practitioner who will be able to evaluate and treat the case according to the principles outlined above. In addition, the following hints may be of help.

Practical Self-Help

■ See the self-help section for **Asthma**. Some of the advice given about substances that may cause an overly-sensitive reaction may also be helpful for eczema sufferers.

■ Wear thin cotton gloves when doing household chores that may involve contact with potential problem substances. This applies to chopping citrus fruit, tomatoes or potatoes, or using cleaning agents that may result in burning, itching or stinging skin. If you have an allergy to rubber, do not use rubber gloves to protect your hands.

■ Use detergents that have been specially formulated for those with sensitive or allergic problems. Always rinse washing twice over to ensure that the maximum residue of detergent has been removed from clothes, bed linen and towels.

■ If patches of eczema affect the face or neck, use cosmetics and skin care products that are hypo-allergenic. It may still be necessary to experiment in order to find a brand that is suitable for your individual situation. Also take care with perfumes and perfumed products such as soaps, body lotion or foam bath. Always patch test a new product on a small area of skin for a few days before use.

■ Limited and **moderate** exposure to sunlight may help a reasonable proportion of eczema and psoriasis sufferers. However, always ensure that exposure is for short periods only, during the times of day when the sun is not at its strongest. Avoid exposure in the late morning, lunch time and early afternoon. Also experiment until you find a sun screen that is suitable for those with sensitive or allergic skins. As before, never apply a new product over a large area of skin without carefully patch testing it first. It is important to bear in mind that some eczema sufferers find that sunlight makes their problems worse, and that they need to take extra care during hot, sunny weather.

■ Keep dry, itchy patches of skin well moisturized. Use emulsifying cream or ointment liberally, especially after a bath and during cold, winter weather. If changing to a new moisturizing cream, check if it contains lanolin. Although frequently used in skin creams and ointments, the latter can cause severe skin reactions in those who are allergic to it.

■ Certain foods may aggravate skin conditions such as eczema. These include dairy products such as cheese, milk or eggs, sugar, tomatoes, citrus fruit, potatoes, convenience foods including colourings and preservatives, and wheat in the form of bread, sauces and thickening agents.

■ Oil of Evening Primrose has a reputation for easing the irritability of eczema for some sufferers. It may be taken internally in capsule form or applied to irritable patches in oil or cream form. As before, always patch test on a small area of skin if you are using the cream or oil for the first time.

Professional Help Should Be Consulted In The Following Situations:

■ **If the skin has broken as a result of continued scratching and there are any signs of infection. These may include severe inflammation, pus formation or swelling.**

■ **If bouts of eczema are becoming increasingly widespread, severe, frequent or are complicated by associated problems such as hayfever or asthma.**

■ **Eczema in young babies or the elderly.**

Hayfever

Hayfever is classed as a chronic problem by homoeopaths (a long-term disorder subject to regular flare-ups), and should be treated by a homoeopathic practitioner for the most positive outcome to be obtained. However, because the acute symptoms of a bout of hayfever closely resemble the common cold, it is possible to obtain short-term relief by taking the appropriate homoeopathic remedy. This may be very positive in the short term, providing an alternative to taking antihistamines without any attendant side effects such as drowsiness. On the other hand, it must be stressed that this is unlikely to deal with the underlying disorder that leads to the problem. Therefore, if success is obtained with home prescribing for acute symptoms of hayfever, it is well worth consulting a homoeopath with a view to dealing with the problem at a deeper level.

Practical Self-Help

■ Increase water intake, avoiding beverages that act as diuretics (eliminating fluid) such as coffee or tea.
■ Bathe eyes and nasal passages with cool water as frequently as required.
■ If airways feel inflamed and sensitive, inhaling steam may be soothing.
■ Stay indoors as much as possible when pollen counts are known to be high.
■ Try to avoid exposure to additional irritants which may make symptoms more severe. These include perfumes, animal fur and dust.
■ Sunglasses may make your eyes more comfortable but avoid using contact lenses which may irritate the eyes, making them more sensitive.
■ Where possible, try to avoid rubbing your eyes. This will only give very temporary relief, and rapidly makes puffiness, swelling and itching around the eyes worse.

Homoeopathic Help

Type of hayfever	General symptoms	Worse from	Better for	Remedy name
Rapidly developing puffiness and swelling of eyes and throat.	Puffy, rosy-red swelling of eyes: 'water bag' puffiness of lids. Itching, stinging sensations in eyes and throat. Terrific sensitivity to heat which makes symptoms much worse.	Warmth in any form. Keeping still. Touch.	Cool air. Cool bathing. Cool compresses. Movement.	**Apis**
Hayfever with burning sensations relieved by warmth.	Puffiness and swelling around eyes with burning tears and light sensitivity. Lots of sneezing with scanty, clear, burning nasal discharge. Irritation and tightness in the chest that is especially marked at night.	Cold. At night. Out of doors.	Warmth. Indoors. Resting.	**Arsenicum alb**

Type of hayfever	General symptoms	Worse from	Better for	Remedy name
Hayfever with profuse, watery nasal discharge that drips constantly like a tap.	Severe light sensitivity with itching and burning of eyes. Sneezes constantly in bright sunlight. Alternating thin, watery nasal discharge and thicker, gelatinous consistency like egg white. Dry, cracked lips and cold sores after exposure to sun.	Heat. Sunlight. Sympathy or fussing. Making an effort.	Cool air. Cold bathing of irritated parts. Being left alone.	**Nat mur**
Hayfever with bland tears and burning nasal discharge.	Constant violent sneezing with acrid discharge from nostrils that burns the upper lip. Sensitive to smell of flowers and fruit. Profuse, bland watering of the eyes.	Warmth. Damp, humid weather. Evening.	Bathing. Cool, fresh air. Movement.	**Allium cepa**
Hayfever with bland nasal discharge and burning tears from eyes.	Eyes feel as though they are swimming in tears due to constant watering. Discharge from eyes is hot and burning, making the rims of the lids red and sore. Profuse, bland discharge from nose.	Warmth. Indoors. Windy weather. Evening.	Fresh, open air. Wiping eyes. Blinking.	**Euphrasia**
Hayfever with violent reaction to the smell or thought of flowers.	Dry, tickling sensation in nose spreads over the whole body. Sensitive to smells with profuse discharge from nose. Abortive sneezing bouts leaving one nostril blocked at a time.	Cool air. Cold drinks. Strong smells. Mental effort.	Warmth. Fresh air. Swallowing.	**Sabadilla**
Hayfever with thick, yellowish-green nasal discharge.	Although chilly, feels much worse in warm surroundings. Craves fresh, cool air. Blocked nasal passages at night, with fluent discharge during the day. Despondent and weepy with symptoms.	Warmth. Stuffy rooms. Lying down. In the evening or night.	Cool, fresh air. Cool compresses. Cool bathing. Gentle movement. Sympathy.	**Pulsatilla**

Type of hayfever	General symptoms	Worse from	Better for	Remedy name
Hayfever with symptoms that are at their worst on waking.	Irritable and bad-tempered with symptoms. Terrific sensitivity to the least draught of cold air and strong smells. Bloodshot eyes with itching in ears and throat. Feels generally hungover with symptoms.	Interrupted sleep. First waking. Cold draughts. Stress.	Warmth. Humidity. Sound sleep. Peace and quiet. As the day goes on.	**Nux vomica**

Professional Help Should Be Consulted In The Following Situations:

■ **If mild attacks of hayfever increase in severity, especially if they are associated with breathing difficulties or wheezing of the chest.**
■ **If acute prescribing of the appropriate homoeopathic remedy helps temporarily, help should be sought from a homoeopathic practitioner in order to deal more effectively with the problem. This is especially important where hayfever is linked to asthma and/or eczema.**

Headaches

There are many factors which can contribute to the onset of a headache. These include stress, high temperature, irregular or poor eating and drinking patterns, and poor posture. By identifying the elements in our lifestyle that trigger a headache, we are in the best position to rectify the situation.

A headache can vary considerably in nature and severity. The following are the main categories of headache that we are likely to encounter:

■ *Tension Headaches* are caused by muscle tension in the neck, shoulders, scalp and face.
■ *Vascular Headaches* are the result of swelling within the blood vessels that supply the head and neck.
■ *'Morning After' Headaches* are the result of drinking an excessive amount of alcohol. Because alcohol relaxes and widens the blood vessels, this type of headache is related to the vascular type.
■ *Migraines* are a more broad-ranging disorder, resulting in severe headaches, visual disturbance, nausea, vomiting, disorientation and a general feeling of unwellness.

■ *Cluster Headaches* consist of sporadic episodes of pain that affect one side of the head. The degree of pain may be severe, often waking the sufferer from sleep. The eye and nostril on the affected side may water profusely while the pain lasts. These headaches may recur over the period of a few hours or days, and may not then recur for months.

Practical Self-Help

■ If tension headaches are a problem, investigate ways of learning how to relax and unwind. Possibilities include taking up yoga, learning how to meditate or having a regular massage. For more detailed information on ways of relaxing and dealing with tension, see **Chapter 8: *The Stresses of Modern Living: How to Cope*.**

■ Ensure that conditions at work aren't contributing to the problem. Many headaches are caused by working hunched over a desk in poorly-lit or badly-ventilated surroundings. In order to combat this potential problem make sure that rooms are well-ventilated, providing adequate amounts of fresh air; check that chairs fit well under desks, allowing feet to reach the floor comfortably, and give adequate back support. Office lighting should be bright but not harsh; fluorescent lighting may be especially problematic for migraine sufferers.

■ Avoid, or cut down on, foods and drinks that may contribute to the problem. These include alcohol, coffee, chocolate and cheese. Since some headaches may be caused by lack of fluid, ensure that plenty of water, fruit juices or herbal teas are drunk at regular intervals through the day.

■ Avoid over-reliance on painkillers as a way of managing pain. Although the occasional dose of analgesic may be appropriate or necessary for a severe headache, always avoid reaching for the painkillers as a first resort. Potential problems associated with regular analgesic use include constipation, nausea, dizziness, rebound pain as the drug is withdrawn, and possible addiction. Also remember that especial care is needed when using paracetamol formulations: it is essential that the maximum dose should not be exceeded or liver damage may occur.

■ If eye strain is a potential contributing factor, have your eyes tested. This may be especially important if you are in your forties, since this is a time when long-sightedness begins to affect people who may not previously have needed spectacles.

■ Ensure that you are getting the right amount of good quality, restful sleep. This is especially important in a stressful lifestyle. Make sure curtains block out light adequately, that the room is neither too chilly nor too hot, that it is well ventilated and reasonably soundproofed. Avoid stimulating work before bed-time, and do not have caffeinated drinks as a bedtime drink. Opt instead for soothing herbal teas such as chamomile, or a milky drink, provided catarrh or excess mucus production isn't a problem.

Homoeopathic Help

Type of headache	General symptoms	Worse from	Better for	Remedy name
Left-sided headaches that are brought on by sleep.	Dizziness with headache that is aggravated by shutting eyes. Bursting pains that extend from left eye to the same side of the nose. Headaches may be brought on by sunlight or becoming overheated.	Morning. On waking. Warmth. Before or after a period. Alcohol. Movement. Closing eyes.	Cool compresses. Fresh air. Onset of a discharge.	**Lachesis**
Headache with band-like sensation over the eyes.	Unpleasant, dizzy feeling with headache. Pains extend from back of head over the eyes. Sore scalp with headache. General sense of heaviness and exhaustion with pains. Headaches may be brought on by anticipatory anxiety.	Stress. Movement. Heat. Sunlight. Smoking. Humidity.	Passing large amounts of urine. Bending forwards. Perspiring. Lying with head propped-up on pillows.	**Gelsemium**
Headaches that are brought on by bright sunlight, before or after periods, or by severe coughing fits.	Severe bursting headaches. Pains lodge in top of the head or over eyes. Depressed and withdrawn with headaches.	After periods. Mental effort. Talking. Sympathy. Noise. Touch. Sunlight.	Cool, fresh air. Cool bathing. Resting with head elevated. Skipping meals. Being left in peace.	**Nat mur**
'Morning after' headache with nausea and irritability.	Suitable for headaches that follow over indulgence in food, coffee and alcohol. Heavy feeling in the back of the head with nausea and constipation. Feels worst first thing in the morning. Painfully sensitive to noise.	Waking. In the morning. Cold, draughty conditions. Stress. Being disturbed. Smoking.	As the day goes on. Being left in peace. Warmth. Sound sleep.	**Nux vomica**

Type of headache	General symptoms	Worse from	Better for	Remedy name
Headaches with exhaustion brought on by skipping meals.	Hypoglaecemic headaches that are improved by eating small amounts regularly. Shooting pains over one eye (usually the left) with nausea and dizziness. Feels worse being indoors and better for fresh air. Feels depressed, desperate and unable to cope.	Before a period. In pregnancy. Morning and evening. Falling asleep. Stooping. Sex.	Becoming warm in bed. Warm compresses. After a sound sleep. Vigourous exercise in the fresh air. Pressure.	**Sepia**
Severe, throbbing headache that is aggravated by the slightest movement.	Bursting headache that may be brought on by dehydrated state with accompanying dry mouth and skin, and constipation. Pains begin above left eye and move to base of skull. Terribly sensitive scalp with pains from light touch.	Warm, stuffy rooms. Movement. Stooping. Coughing. Eating. Touch. Exertion.	Firm pressure. Cool surroundings. Peace and quiet. Cold drinks. Keeping as still as possible.	**Bryonia**
Headaches brought on by atmospheric changes, e.g. before a thunderstorm, hunger pangs, fright or shock.	Aching over one eye brought on by hunger pangs. Throbbing pains follow fright or emotional shock. Dizziness which is especially severe on waking.	Lying on painful side. Shock. Cold air. Sudden atmospheric changes. Morning and evening. Mental effort.	Massage. Eating. After sound sleep. Bathing face in cold water. Cold drinks.	**Phosphorus**
Right-sided cluster headaches with dizziness and nausea.	Bursting, pulsating headaches with burning discharge from the eye of the affected side. Headaches set in at puberty, pregnancy or the menopause. Symptoms are severely aggravated by stuffy, overheated atmospheres.	Lack of fresh air. Keeping still. Evening and night. Eating rich, fatty foods. Lying down. Before a period.	Gentle exercise in fresh, cool, open air. Cold compresses. Pressure to painful part. Company. Sympathy. Having a good cry.	**Pulsatilla**

Type of headache	General symptoms	Worse from	Better for	Remedy name
Recurrent sick headaches from low blood sugar levels.	Dizzy headache in forehead which is aggravated by stooping. Throbbing, heavy sensation in crown of head, or a feeling of constriction around brain. Has to eat regularly in order to keep headaches and tiredness at bay.	Becoming over-heated. Too much physical effort. Mid-morning. Standing. Sweet foods.	Fresh air. Movement. Walking.	**Sulphur**

Seek Prompt Medical Help In Any Of The Following Situations:

■ Recurrent or daily headaches that occur on waking each morning.

■ Headaches that last for more than a day at a time.

■ Headaches that are accompanied by stiff neck, high temperature or light sensitivity.

■ Nausea or drowsiness following a head injury.

■ If there is severe pain, nausea or vomiting on bending the head forwards.

■ If painkillers are being taken on a regular basis for recurrent headaches.

■ Nausea, vomiting, blurred vision and severe pain from a headache affecting the area within and around one eye.

Indigestion

Indigestion can arise in varying degrees of severity for a number of different reasons. It is a common symptom of an overstressed lifestyle and the poor eating habits that usually go with it. Indigestion and heartburn also often occur in pregnancy, especially towards the later months as increasing pressure is put on digestive organs.

Since indigestion can be indicative of a deeper, underlying problem, it is best to seek professional advice if symptoms do not improve after sensible changes have been made in lifestyle and diet. It also must be stressed that the solution does not lie in short-term masking of symptoms by taking antacids on a constant basis, since this can only provide temporary relief and will do little to get to the root of the problem.

The appropriate homoeopathic remedy selected from the table below may do a great deal to resolve the discomfort of an occasional bout of indigestion. However, if indigestion symptoms have become persistent, it is best to seek help from a homoeopathic practitioner. This is advisable because homoeopathic remedies are intended for short-term use only: if they need to be taken on a regular basis to maintain improvement, this suggests that professional help is needed in order to deal more effectively with the problem. It is also important to stress that mild or infrequent bouts of indigestion often respond to simple, positive adjustments in diet and lifestyle that tackle the problem at its root cause.

Practical Self-Help

■ It is very easy to forget that the process of digestion begins before food reaches the stomach. Chewing allows it to be ground down into small pieces, while saliva provides lubrication and the opportunity for the secretion of digestive enzymes in the mouth. As a result, the importance of chewing food thoroughly cannot be overemphasized. If a meal is bolted down quickly, the stomach has to work much harder in order to do its job. The result is often discomfort, acidity and excess wind.

■ Certain foods have a reputation for being difficult to digest and should be avoided or eaten in moderation if indigestion is a problem. The foods most likely to cause indigestion include: cabbage, sprouts, raw onion or peppers, red meat with rich sauces, full fat hard cheeses, and pungent or highly-spiced dishes such as curries or chillies. Well-known irritants to the stomach lining include strong coffee, tea, alcohol (especially spirits) and cigarettes. Easily-digested foods include home-made vegetable soups or purées, crisp, lightly steamed vegetables, non-acid fruit, salads, pasta, fish and chicken. Always make sure to drink enough water: aim for six to eight large glasses daily.

■ Eat meals at regular intervals, avoiding large gaps in between. This becomes especially important at times of stress when the natural inclination is to wolf snacks down as quickly as possible, while going without proper food for lengthy intervals. This leads to a potentially disastrous situation for the indigestion sufferer, due to the combination of digestive problems associated with partially-chewed food, and the build-up of wind that arises from going without regular meals. The unfortunate result is often discomfort, leaden feelings in the stomach, queasiness and bloating.

■ Make time for meals rather than hurrying food down while watching television, reading the newspaper or scanning documents relating to work. Without becoming solemn about it, eating should be a time for relaxation and enjoyment. By relaxing when we eat, the meal we have is likely to be savoured fully and digested more easily.

■ Avoid eating when feeling tense or uptight. If an irritating or stressful situation has arisen, take a few minutes to relax and unwind before attempting to eat a meal. For information on simple relaxation techniques see the section on *Basic Self-Help Techniques For Stress Management* in **Chapter 8: The Stresses Of Modern Living: How To Cope**.

■ Be aware of the health problems that may be associated with the long-term or over-use of antacids. These include an increased risk of water retention and high blood-pressure in those who use products based on bicarbonate of soda, while those who use aluminium-based formulations may experience constipation. There is also a fundamental problem associated with habitual antacid use called *acid rebound*. This is a syndrome where excess acid is diluted temporarily by the use of antacids in order to ease discomfort in the stomach. However, the body responds by producing extra acid in order to compensate, with the result that stomach symptoms feel worse than ever. A vicious circle ensues, with long-term medication being needed in order to remain in a comfortable or stable condition.

Homoeopathic Help

Type of indigest-ion	General symptoms	Worse from	Better for	Remedy name
Indigestion that is linked to anticipatory anxiety.	Indigestion with abundant amounts of wind passing upwards and downwards. Severe rumbling and gurgling with distension that feels much worse for pressure of clothes. Acid or burning sensation travels from the stomach into the throat.	Anticipatory 'nerves'. Cold food or drinks. Tight waistband. Bread cabbage or beans. Stress. In the afternoon.	Being occupied or diverted from worrying. Warm food or drinks. Gentle exercise in the fresh air.	**Lycopodium**
Indigestion with severe wind that is relieved by belching.	Heavy, unpleasant sensations in stomach with violent burping. Severe bloating and swelling around the waist that follows eating anything. Feels faint and uncomfortable in overheated rooms.	Stuffy, airless surroundings. Tight clothes. Movement. Alcohol.	Being fanned. Fresh, open air. Passing wind. Sleep.	**Carbo veg**

Type of indigestion	General symptoms	Worse from	Better for	Remedy name
Acid indigestion with burning in the stomach.	Burning sensations and nausea are relieved by sips of warm drinks. Anxious, tense perfectionists who demand a great deal of themselves. Vomiting and diarrhoea are a frequent consequence of anxiety.	Cold surroundings. Cold food and drinks. At night. Worrying about health.	Warm rooms. Sips of warm drinks. In company.	**Arsenicum alb**
'Morning after' indigestion with constipation and headache.	Indigestion that follows an excess of alcohol, cigarettes or food. Nausea with headache that lodges in the back of the head. Feels very sick but has difficulties vomiting or passing a stool. Digestive problems follow from overuse of painkillers.	In the morning. Being stressed. Noise. After eating. Disturbed sleep. Cold, draughty conditions.	Sound sleep. As the day goes on. Warmth. Being left undisturbed.	**Nux vomica**
Indigestion and nausea after eating rich, fatty foods.	Digestive problems caused by eating too much pork, cheese or cream. Stomach pains are worse for jolting or jarring. Warm food and drinks disagree. Dry mouth without thirst. Heavy, leaden feeling in stomach with 'repeating' of food eaten hours before.	Overheated, stuffy rooms. Lying down. Resting. Dairy products.	Cool, fresh air. Gentle movement. Cool food and drinks.	**Pulsatilla**
Indigestion with terrific thirst for cold water.	Severe belching with heavy sensation in stomach that is much worse for eating. Nausea and discomfort are much worse for movement. Irritable, headachy and bad-tempered with sensitive stomach.	Warmth. Movement. Stooping. Eating. Vegetarian dishes.	Cool drinks. Cool surroundings. Peaceful conditions. Drawing knees up.	**Bryonia**

Type of indigest-ion	General symptoms	Worse from	Better for	Remedy name
Indigestion that is better for eating.	Stomach upsets accompany or are brought on by emotional stress. Hiccoughs after eating with cramping, spasmodic pains. Craves raw, sour or indigestible foods.	Emotional shock or upset. Strong smells. Coffee. Smoking. Stooping.	Breathing deeply. Eating. Sour foods. Pressure.	**Ignatia**
Pressure and burning in stomach that is aggravated by eating.	Craving for sour, acid foods or pickles. Acidity in stomach is made worse by smoking. Unpleasant-tasting belches with a sense of something rising into throat. Indifferent, apathetic or depressed when unwell.	Morning and evening. Standing. Stooping. Touch.	Vigorous exercise. Being warm in bed. Drawing limbs up. Fresh air.	**Sepia**

Seek Prompt Medical Help In Any Of The Following Situations:

■ If indigestion is persistent and does not respond to self-help measures.

■ Persistent loss of appetite for no apparent reason.

■ Weight loss for no obvious reason.

■ If nausea and discomfort begin to trigger bouts of vomiting, especially if there are any signs of blood in the vomit.

Influenza

Anyone who has experienced a bout of flu will know the difference in severity between influenza and a cold. Flu is an extremely debilitating illness which can embrace a variety of severe symptoms. These may include: general sensations of malaise or unwellness, high fever, aching limbs, shivering, sore throat, nasal discharge, severe cough, nausea and loss of appetite. Further complications may arise from a bout of flu, including bronchitis, sinus pain, depression and a lingering sense of weakness or exhaustion.

However, there are a number of practical steps we can take to boost our immunity in an effort to prevent flu developing in the first place, plus a variety of strategies that can be employed in order to minimize the complications of a bout of influenza, and speed up the rate of recovery.

Practical Self-Help

■ If you are in contact with flu sufferers and wish to boost your overall immunity, the following measures may be of help:

■ Take a Vitamin C supplement in order to help your body fight infection. Although this vitamin can be obtained from the diet, few of us eat raw fruit and vegetables in large enough quantities to be therapeutically useful within this context. Take one gram (1000mgs) a day while you are exposed to infection, ideally divided into four doses of 250 mgs over twenty-four hours. If you experience digestive problems such as acidity or diarrhoea, or if you have a history of kidney stones, reduce the dosage.

■ Increase foods in your diet that are high in vitamin C. Especially rich sources include raw peppers, tomatoes and citrus fruit. Remember that this vitamin is very easily destroyed by cooking, or oxidation if food is prepared and left to stand for a long period of time before eating. As a result, vitamin C content is best preserved by eating fruit and vegetables as quickly as possible after they have been washed, scrubbed or chopped. Also make a point of eating raw fruit or vegetables in order to maximize vitamin content. Steaming is the best method for cooking vegetables since it preserves their taste and texture, and does not have the drawback of essential nutrients leaching into the cooking liquid.

■ Avoid food and drinks that compromise the liver, since we are dependent upon the healthy function of this organ for efficient de-toxification of our bodies. Alcohol is especially damaging to the liver as well as depleting our bodies of vitamin C. Therefore, if we are trying to increase levels of this vitamin in order to boost immunity, it makes sense not to drink alcohol at the same time. Convenience instant foods also include colourings and preservatives which put extra strain on the liver. These are added in order to prolong shelf-life and make the appearance and texture of food more appealing. Foods that are high in fat should also be kept to a minimum, as well as red meat and refined (white) flour and sugar.

■ Foods that appear to improve levels of well-being and increase resistance to infection include frequent helpings of fresh fruit, vegetables, whole grains, garlic, fish, and complete proteins from pulses and grains. As much water as possible should be drunk in order to support the de-toxifying functions of the body, while coffee and strong tea should be avoided.

■ If early symptoms of flu have developed such as shivering, aching muscles, and a general feeling of unwellness, it is best to rest as much as possible at this stage in order to support the body in its fight against infection.

■ Avoid extreme changes of temperature when feverish. Adapting to sharp variations in external heat or cold increases the risk of chill, and puts extra strain on the body at a time when it needs all the support it can get.

■ Don't force yourself to eat in the early stages of illness if appetite is diminished. At this stage it is much more important to drink sufficient quantities of fluid in order to keep the temperature down. Although water is best, warm or chilled herbal teas may also be soothing or appealing.

■ Avoid dairy products and milky drinks as much as possible since they are thought to contribute considerably to mucus production. Sugary foods should also be kept to a minimum for the same reason.

■ If coughing or tightness in the chest is a particular problem at night, avoid sleeping completely flat and prop yourself up on two or three pillows. If sips of cool drinks are also soothing, keep a glass of water by the side of the bed.

■ Where there is a history of chest or sinus involvement as a complication of flu, ensure that garlic tablets are taken at the earliest opportunity. Two tablets should be taken three times a day until mucus production has ceased or slowed down dramatically.

■ By taking adequate time to recover fully from a bout of flu, complications are likely to be reduced and the overall recovery time should be shorter. Although it can be inconvenient or difficult to take time off work, the value of doing this when appropriate becomes obvious if we consider the long-term problems associated with post-viral syndrome.

Homoeopathic Help

Type of flu	General symptoms	Worse from	Better for	Remedy name
Rapid, violent onset with very high fever (most likely to be needed in the initial 48 hours of illness).	Sudden emergence of symptoms with very sore, red throat and dry, hot skin. Temperature is so high that skin radiates heat. Full, rapid pulse. Restless, irritable and sensitive to light, noise and movement.	Jarring movement. Noise. Bright light. Cold draughts of air. Being disturbed.	Resting propped-up in bed. Moderate warmth. Peace and quiet.	**Belladonna**
Rapid onset of symptoms after exposure to chill (most likely to be needed in the first 48 hours of illness).	Terrible anxiety and restlessness with onset of illness. High fever with hot head and chilled body. Flushes of heat alternate with bouts of shivering. Oversensitivity to pain leads to restlessness and desperation. Very thirsty for large quantities of cold water.	Extreme variations of temperature. Overheated rooms. At night. Alcohol.	Fresh air. After a sound sleep. Perspiration.	**Aconite**

Type of flu	General symptoms	Worse from	Better for	Remedy name
Slow, insidious development of symptoms over days.	Characteristic flu symptoms of heaviness, shivering and heavy, aching limbs. Droopy, heavy eyelids with glassy eyes. Dusky-red complexion with very dry, cracked lips. Constant need to lie down with aversion to making any kind of effort.	Becoming overheated. Direct sunlight. Cold draughts. Thinking of symptoms.	Fresh air. Stimulants. Perspiring. Passing water.	Gelsemium
Irritable and headachy with slow onset of illness.	Bad-tempered and discontented with general feeling of unwellness. General sense of dehydration with flushed, dry skin, thirst for cold water and constipation. Severe headache which is aggravated by movement of any kind.	Warmth. Stuffy rooms. Physical effort. On rising after lying or sitting. Initial movement after rest.	Keeping as still as possible. Cold drinks. Pressure to painful areas. Perspiring.	**Bryonia**
Flu symptoms with severe aching deep in the bones.	Weak, restless and chilly with bruised sensations in muscles of limbs, chest and back. Generally sluggish and nauseated. Sore, aching chest from persistent coughing.	Chill. In the morning. Lying on painful area. Movement. Sight or smell of food. Coughing.	Perspiring. Vomiting. Being spoken to.	**Eupatorium**
High temperature with extreme chilliness and restlessness.	Anxious, shivery, prostrated and terribly cold. Burning pains are better for warmth. Tight, wheezy chest and dry, irritating cough are worse at night: must sit up for relief. Nasal discharge is clear, scanty and acrid: burns the nostrils.	At night. Being alone. Cold food or drinks. Chilly surroundings. Exertion.	Resting propped-up in bed. Warmth. Hot water bottle. Company. Sips of warm drinks. Fresh air.	**Arsenicum alb**

Type of flu	General symptoms	Worse from	Better for	Remedy name
Severe sore throat and swollen glands which are worse at night.	Extremely restless, uncomfortable and anxious. All symptoms are exaggerated in bed at night. Sweaty, shivery and aching all over with marked discomfort in glands. Greenish-yellow nasal discharge and phlegm.	Extreme heat or cold. At night. Perspiring. Damp cold conditions. Becoming heated.	Resting. Moderate temperatures.	**Mercurius**
Weepy with well-established flu symptoms.	Thick, yellowy-green discharges from nose and chest. Loose, productive cough at night which is dry in the morning. Although chilly, feels much worse for stuffy surroundings and heat in general. Dry mouth with no thirst.	Warm, airless conditions. Resting. Warm food and drinks. Feeling neglected. At night.	Cool, fresh air. Gentle movement. Cool food and drinks. A good cry.	**Pulsatilla**
Extreme restlessness and depression with flu that gets much worse at night.	Tosses about in bed at night trying to get comfortable. Difficulty in sleeping from aching muscles with resulting agitation and depression. Feels generally worse for keeping still and better for gentle movement Hard, inflamed glands and thick, green mucus discharges.	Cold and damp. At night. Keeping still.	Warmth. Warm shower or bath. Gentle movement that does not exhaust.	**Rhus tox**

Seek Prompt Medical Help In Any Of The Following Situations:

■ If a sore throat occurs in anyone who has previously suffered rheumatic fever.

■ If sore, aching muscles and general malaise are accompanied by stiff neck and severe headache and light sensitivity.

■ High temperature in babies, very young children or the elderly.

■ Persistent high fever and exhaustion in an otherwise fit and healthy adult.

■ If symptoms are especially severe and do not respond to self-help measures.

■ If recovery is very slow and a bout of flu leaves extreme fatigue, depression and poor resistance to infection in its wake.

Psoriasis

See section on *Eczema* for an explanation of why it is best not to self-prescribe for chronic skin conditions such as psoriasis.

Sinusitis

Sinusitis is a painful and often distressing condition that may involve any combination of the following symptoms:

■ A constant sense of obstruction or blockage in the nose that makes breathing difficult.
■ Recurring headaches that affect the areas around the eye sockets, bridge of the nose or cheekbones.
■ A sense of pressure or fullness in the face and head on stooping or bending forwards.
■ A recurring, offensive taste in the mouth and/or unpleasant smell in the nostrils.
■ Mucus may be thick, yellowish-green and difficult to shift.

Chronic, or long-term problems with sinusitis are best treated by a homoeopathic practitioner for the most positive outcome to ensue. However, the occasional, mild bout of symptoms may respond to the following self-help measures in combination with an appropriately-selected homoeopathic remedy.

Practical Self-Help

■ Avoid foods that are thought to encourage mucus production. These include dairy foods such as milk, cheese, yoghourts and milk-based dishes such as puddings or rich sauces. Sugary foods and drinks may also contribute to the problem.
■ If a cold occurs, try to minimize possible sinus complications by using garlic supplements (two tablets three times a day) and vitamin C (one or two grams daily while cold symptoms are present). Drink frequent glasses of water, and keep the diet as light as possible by eating fresh, steamed vegetables, salads, soups, fresh fruit and fruit juices.
■ Open windows in order to give an adequate supply of fresh air in centrally-heated surroundings, and prevent rooms from becoming too dry by placing

bowls of water near each radiator. If nasal passages are particularly blocked up, sitting in a steam-filled bathroom may be very helpful.

■ Resist the temptation to blow the nose too vigorously, which can make discomfort and pain worse. Instead, clear nasal passages by blowing gently into a paper tissue which can be disposed of. This is preferable to using handkerchiefs which may serve to perpetuate a bacterial infection.

Homoeopathic Help

Type of sinusitis	General symptoms	Worse from	Better for	Remedy name
Yellow-green, thick, bland mucus with blocked nostrils that are aggravated by stuffy rooms.	Headaches with sinus inflammation that feel better for fresh, open air. They are also eased by gentle exercise out of doors. Generally weepy, depressed and out of sorts with illness. Stuffed-up nasal passages in the evening and at night. Mucus discharges flow freely in the morning.	Stuffy, heated rooms. Lying down. Warm compresses. In the evening and at night. Feeling neglected.	Fresh, cool, open air. Cool compresses. Gentle exercise out of doors. Having a good cry. Sympathy.	**Pulsatilla**
Inflamed sinuses with persistent pain at the root of the nose.	Stringy, greenish ropy nasal discharge that is very difficult to dislodge. Unpleasant smell in nostrils from impacted mucus. Pains and pressure at bridge of nose and above the eyes.	Cold damp conditions. Fresh air. Sleep. Bending forward. Alcohol.	Warmth. Pressure. Movement.	**Kali bich**
Thick yellow mucus with terrible sensitivity to cold air.	Foul-smelling nasal discharge with constant sneezing or nasal obstruction in cold conditions. Sore pains at bridge of the nose. Pains also affect the bones of the face. Irritable and bad-tempered when ill.	Cold, draughty conditions. Uncovering. Touch. Noise. Making an effort. At night.	Warmth. Wrapping up the head snuggly. Humidity.	**Hepar sulph**

Type of sinusitis	General symptoms	Worse from	Better for	Remedy name
Sinus pain with foul, yellow-green mucus and bad breath.	Constant sneezing with nasal discharge that is too thick to run. All discharges are increased and smell unpleasant. These include sweat, phlegm or saliva. Teeth and ears ache with inflamed sinuses.	Extreme changes of temperature. At night. Perspiring. Becoming chilled.	Moderate temperatures. Resting.	**Mercurius**
Dry, blocked nose with sinus pain.	Loss of sense of smell with persistently blocked nostrils. Sinus complications follow recurrent colds that are difficult to clear. Problems follow becoming chilled and damp.	Cold, damp air. Noise. Light. Touch. Jarring movements.	Wrapping the head up warmly. Warm, humid conditions.	**Silica**
One-sided sinus pain with yellow nasal discharge.	Severe pains around eye sockets that make eyes feel tired and heavy. Blood-streaked nasal discharge is alternately profuse or dry. Nasal passages feel swollen with oversensitive sense of smell.	Lying on painful side. Lying on back. Cold, fresh air. Morning. Evening.	Sleep. Bathing face in cool water. Being massaged.	**Phosphorus**

Seek Prompt Medical Help In Any Of The Following Situations:

■ Severe sinus pain that does not respond to self-help measures within a few hours.

■ High temperature and general feelings of unwellness accompanying sinus pain.

■ Nasal mucus that is offensive, yellow or green.

■ Sinus problems that occur on a recurrent basis which refuse to respond to self-help measures.

Sore Throats

These may vary from a mildly inflamed or painful throat that occurs as a precursor to a head cold, to full-blown tonsillitis. The latter can be a severely toxic illness, often resulting in feverishness, prostration, headaches and vomiting. With severe throat infections, the glands in the neck often become greatly enlarged and painful.

Pharyngitis occurs when the part of the throat between the tonsils and the vocal cords (pharynx) becomes inflamed as a result of viral or bacterial infection. Although symptoms resemble those of tonsillitis, they occur in a milder form. *Laryngitis*, on the other hand, is the result of bacterial or viral infections that attack the voice box (larynx), which is situated at the top of the wind pipe. Infection usually follows a sore throat or cold, leading to symptoms of hoarseness, loss of voice and feverishness.

Practical Self-Help

■ Lubricate the throat well by drinking frequently and sucking pastilles containing glycerine. However, remember that lozenges containing camphor, eucalyptus or menthol should be avoided when using homoeopathic medicines, since aromatic substances such as these may interfere with the chosen remedy's action. Instead, select pastilles that have a fruit-flavour base such as blackcurrant.

■ Avoid activities that are likely to irritate or inflame the throat, such as smoking or spending lengthy periods in a smoky atmosphere. Rest the voice as much as possible and avoid extreme changes of temperature.

■ If the throat is very painful, gargle at frequent intervals with a **diluted** solution of **Hypercal** (Hypericum and Calendula) tincture. In order to make a suitable gargle, dilute ten parts of water to one part of tincture. Other possible options include a solution of lemon juice and honey, or salt and water.

■ Use a vitamin C supplement in order to support the body in fighting infection. See the *Practical Self-Help* hints in the section on *Influenza* for general advice on dosage, as well as other tips which may be applicable for flu-like symptoms.

■ Humidify the atmosphere by using a custom-made humidifier, or place bowls of water at strategic points near each fire or radiator.

■ Ensure that fluid intake is high in order to keep the temperature down, and to support the body in flushing toxins out of the system. Avoid tea and coffee which have diuretic properties (they encourage fluid-elimination), and concentrate instead on water, fresh fruit juices, warm drinks of lemon and honey or herb teas. The latter may be drunk warm or as a long drink after being cooled in the fridge.

■ Rest as much as possible, ideally in bed. By taking time off when appropriate, recovery is likely to be speeded up in the long run.

Homoeopathic Help

Type of sore throat	General symptoms	Worse from	Better for	Remedy name
Early stage of sore throat that develops after exposure to cold air.	Throat symptoms develop rapidly and violently after chill or severe trauma. Terrible restlessness and feverishness with oversensitivity to pain. Wants to swallow but this increases pain and distress.	Warm rooms. After exposure to cold winds or draughts. At night. Extreme, or abrupt changes of temperature.	After sound sleep. Moderate temperatures.	**Aconite**
Initial stage of severe sore throat with bright red inflammation and very high fever.	Symptoms develop rapidly and violently. Irritable and very mentally and physically sensitive to sensory stimuli. Throat looks bright red, skin is dry, hot and red. Craves lemon drinks and must sit forward to swallow. 'Strawberry tongue' covered in small red spots.	Chill. Drinking. Talking. Empty swallowing. Bright light. Noise. Jarring movements.	Resting propped-up in bed. Moderate warmth.	**Belladonna**
Early stage of sore throat with puffy, water-logged appearance.	Severe stinging pains in throat with pink, glossy swelling. Throat puffs up rapidly in early stages. Terrific sensitivity to warmth in any form which makes symptoms much worse. Restless and fidgety when ill.	Warm drinks. Warm wraps or compresses. Resting. Touch.	Cool bathing. Cool drinks. Moving about.	**Apis**
Sore throat with loss of voice and hoarseness.	Thirsty for cold drinks with burning pains in throat. Constant impulse to clear the throat with marked sensitivity to cold air or change of temperature. Chest involvement may accompany sore throat with dry, tickly, wheezy cough.	Sudden change of temperature. Talking. Evenings. Being alone. Anxiety.	Cool drinks. Sleep. Reassurance.	**Phosphorus**

Type of sore throat	General symptoms	Worse from	Better for	Remedy name
Laryngitis from emotional trauma.	Constant hoarseness or sore throat dating from bereavement or other emotional shock. Persistent sensation of having to swallow over a lump or swelling in throat. Constricted feeling leads to choking. Ulcerated tonsils with stitching pains extending to the ear between swallowing.	Touch. Cold air. Smoking. Emotional stress or strain.	Keeping occupied. Eating. Swallowing.	**Ignatia**
Established sore throat with foul breath and increased saliva.	Feverish, restless and sweaty with sore throat and hard, swollen glands. All discharges are increased and smell offensive. Tongue may be swollen so that it takes imprint of teeth around the edges. Very easily chilled or overheated.	At night. Becoming chilled or overheated. Warmth of the bed. Sweating.	Moderate temperatures. Rest.	**Mercurius**
Established sore throat with extreme sensitivity to draughts of cold air.	Extremely sore, ulcerated throat with swollen glands. The slightest chill or draught of cold air causes great distress. Painful, sharp, sticking sensation in the throat as though a fish bone or splinter was lodged there.	Draughts of cold air. Uncovering. Touch. Exertion. At night.	Warmth. Warm wraps to head. Humidity.	**Hepar sulph**
Severe inflamed and swollen tonsils that are worse on the right side.	Dark or bluish-red inflammation of throat with whitish-grey spots on tonsils. Burning pains in throat are much worse for swallowing and warm drinks. Throbbing pains in right tonsil with hoarseness.	Movement. Damp, cold conditions. Hot drinks. Warmth.	Resting.	**Phytolacca**

Type of sore throat	General symptoms	Worse from	Better for	Remedy name
Left-sided sore throats that are much worse on waking.	Symptoms affect the left side, or may begin on the right and move to the left. Constricted feelings in the throat are made worse by touch or any pressure around the neck from clothing. Empty swallowing is more painful than swallowing food.	Waking from sleep. Mornings. Warmth. Empty swallowing. Hot drinks. Pressure on the throat.	Cool air. Cool drinks. Swallowing food.	**Lachesis**
Sore throats that move from right to left	Discomfort and pains in throat are made worse by cold drinks. Recurrent sore throats with inflamed tonsils. Constricted sensations as though a ball were sticking in the throat.	Cold food and drinks. Becoming overheated. On waking. Between 4–8 p.m. Eating.	Warm drinks. Movement. Being occupied or distracted.	**Lycopodium**

Seek Prompt Medical Help In Any Of The Following Situations:

■ Severe sore throat in anyone who has previously suffered from rheumatic fever.

■ If there are any signs of rash or high temperature.

■ Pus formation or ulceration of the tonsils.

■ Severe pain in the throat that makes swallowing difficult.

■ Sore throats in small children with persistent high temperature.

■ Any signs of breathing difficulties or drooling should be investigated as quickly as possible.

Vomiting

The causes of vomiting can be enormously varied. It may be one of the main symptoms associated with food poisoning (usually combined with diarrhoea), or it can occur as a result of a high temperature, irritation of the stomach from overindulgence in alcohol, or as a complication of a toxic condition such as appendicitis. Possible psychological triggers for vomiting include emotional shock or trauma, anticipatory anxiety before a stressful assessment, or induced vomiting associated with eating disorders such as bulimia.

In acute episodes of food poisoning, the vomiting reflex ensures that anything which needs to be expelled from the stomach is removed with speed and vigour. However, bouts of vomiting in these circumstances may go on for an extended period of time, leaving the patient exhausted, sore and generally prostrated. In this sort of situation, where no further complications are present, the self-help suggestions given below may be of great help.

Homoeopathic prescribing within this context can also be of immense support in aiding the body to do whatever is needed more efficiently. As a result, the possible reactions that may occur are as follows: initially increased episodes of vomiting that resolve the situation. These may be followed by a long sleep, from which the patient wakes feeling much better. Alternatively, the appropriate homoeopathic remedy may rapidly put an end to dry retching that goes on beyond the point where it is serving any positive function.

Because vomiting may be indicative of a serious disorder, *always* seek prompt medical advice if there is any cause for concern. This is especially important if vomiting and/or severe diarrhoea occur in the very young or the elderly.

Practical Self-Help

■ Ensure dehydration does not occur by drinking enough fluid. This is of paramount importance when diarrhoea and vomiting happen simultaneously, since a dangerously large volume of liquid may be lost from the body within a relatively short time. Age groups especially at risk include babies, very young children and the elderly. If dehydration is suspected, the following symptoms may confirm the diagnosis:

 ■ Depressed fontanelle (the soft spot at the crown of the head of young babies).
 ■ Reduced or concentrated urine output.
 ■ Dry or unelastic skin tone. Test an area of skin on the back of the hand by pinching it between thumb and forefinger. If it takes a long time to spring back into shape, this may be an indication of dehydration.
 ■ Sunken or dry eyes with lack of tears.

In order to prevent dehydration, drink plenty of water or a very weak water and saline solution. This may be made by dissolving a quarter of a level teaspoon of salt and four level teaspoons of sugar in a pint of water. If this tastes unpleasant to the patient, use plain water instead, or very diluted fruit juice (avoid citrus flavours such as orange or grapefruit which may irritate the stomach further).
■ Because the body is attempting to clear the digestive tract of something toxic during a bout of vomiting and diarrhoea, it is best to avoid taxing the system further by eating. The nausea that often occurs between espisodes of vomiting

will usually ensure that someone is not tempted to eat until the problem has been resolved by the body. When the sickness has subsided, and the appetite returns, it is important to introduce foods that are very light and digestible. Avoid oils, fats, spiced dishes and tea or coffee. Opt instead for home-made vegetable broths, fruit juices, yoghourt and steamed fruit.

■ Many people prefer to be alone during a bout of vomiting, while others may become frightened and panicky when they are about to be sick. This is often the case with those who have seldom vomited. In this situation, placing a hand on the sick person's forehead may feel comforting, while it also provides support to the head.

■ Rinsing the mouth and sponging the face in cool water are often soothing after vomiting.

Homoeopathic Help

Type of vomiting	General symptoms	Worse from	Better for	Remedy name
Vomiting with pallor, prostration and terrific thirst for cold water.	Constant craving for very cold water which is vomited soon after drinking. Violent retching with forcible vomiting which feels worse for the least movement. Clammy, pale and sweaty during and after vomiting bouts. Often needed when vomiting and diarrhoea occur together.	Drinking. Making any effort. Touch. Pressure.	Warmth. Being covered. Lying down. Drinking milk.	**Veratrum alb**
Episodes of vomiting with chilliness and restlessness relieved by warmth.	Burning thirst: craves ice cold water that is vomited immediately. Distress from sight, smell or thought of food. Severe anxiety with sickness that is worse for being alone. Diarrhoea and vomiting occur together.	At night. Becoming chilled or cold. Cold drinks. Making an effort. Being alone.	Warmth. Sips of warm drinks. Lying propped-up in bed. Company. Wrapping up snuggly.	**Arsenicum alb**
Severe nausea and vomiting intensified by the slightest movement.	Terrible, constant nausea not relieved at all after vomiting. No thirst with foamy vomit. Tender, distended stomach and abdomen with intermittent, colicky pains.	Movement. Extreme changes of temperature. Overheated rooms. Lying down.	Resting. Keeping as still as possible. Fresh air. Keeping the eyes closed.	**Ipecac**

Type of vomiting	General symptoms	Worse from	Better for	Remedy name
Vomiting after over-indulgence in alcohol and/ or food.	Nausea and vomiting with 'morning after' syndrome. Terrible retching with difficulty in bringing vomit up. Irritable, cold-sensitive and headachy. Once vomiting is over, nausea is greatly relieved.	On waking. Cold draughts. Uncovering. Exertion. Noise. Touch. Pressure of waistband.	Uninterrupted sleep. Peace and quiet. Warmth. As the day goes on.	**Nux vomica**
Vomiting which occurs as soon as cold drinks become warmed in stomach.	Terribly thirsty for cold drinks which initially agree, but are vomited up as soon as they become heated by the stomach. Often needed for post-operative vomiting that occurs as a result of reaction to anaesthetic.	Lying on back. Cold air. Warm drinks. Talking. Mental effort.	Cool drinks. Sleep. Massage. Bathing or sponging the face in cold water.	**Phosphorus**
Nausea and vomiting with marked aversion to warmth.	Although very chilly, symptoms feel much worse in warm surroundings. Dry mouth with no thirst, and burning in stomach that are relived temporarily by cold drinks. Weepy and in need of sympathy and attention when sick.	Becoming overheated. Lying down. Stuffy rooms. Warm drinks. Chill.	Cool, fresh air. Cool drinks. Uncovering. Sympathy. Having a good cry.	**Pulsatilla**

Seek Prompt Medical Help In Any Of The Following Situations:

■ If dehydration is suspected, especially in the very young or the elderly.

■ If abdominal pains occur with vomiting, especially if they begin around the navel and move to the right hand side.

■ High temperature, headache, stiff neck, and light sensitivity with vomiting.

■ Any sign of fresh or dark, dried, 'coffee ground' blood in vomit.

■ If nausea and vomiting occur on a long-term, regular basis, and are accompanied by weight loss, diminished appetite and general malaise.

■ Nausea and vomiting following a head injury.

■ If there is severe pain in or around one eye with blurred vision.

■ Effortless vomiting without nausea that is accompanied by recurrent headaches on waking.

■5■

Homoeopathy And Sports Injuries

Appropriate homoeopathic prescribing can play a vital role in speeding up recovery of sports and exercise injuries. In many ways, the homoeopathic approach comes into its own in this context because it accelerates the natural healing process so effectively. This is of particular value to those of us who enjoy regular exercise, since effective homoeopathic treatment enables us to return to our leisure activities far sooner than we would if we relied on rest and mechanical support alone.

There is an additional bonus for sports enthusiasts who opt for homoeopathic treatment, namely the holistic perspective on health and well-being which this approach has at its centre. From this perspective, positive health and vitality are seen as attributes that can be supported or undermined by our lifestyles. Homoeopathic practitioners, in common with other therapists who adopt a holistic approach, put great emphasis on the role that preventative measures can play in reducing our risk of incurring health problems. As a result, homoeopathic patients usually develop a strong sense of which elements in their lifestyles enhance their experience of well-being, and which do the reverse.

This has a particular relevance to sports enthusiasts who respond positively to the holistic approach by focusing on measures that can be used to prevent injuries occurring. By doing so, they are likely to find that their overall performance and sense of body awareness improve substantially.

In addition, punishing and painful exercise routines are losing their appeal as the 'no pain, no gain' approach appears less persuasive or healthy. Instead, sports and exercise activities that enhance balance and harmony of mind and body are becoming increasingly appropriate to a holistic approach to health e.g. yoga, Pilates, Medau and T'ai Chi. Because activities of this kind are generally aimed at increasing body awareness, the risk of injury is reduced when compared to the frenetic and competitive aerobics classes that were fashionable in the eighties. The homoeopathic approach fits well within this context, providing a system of healing that enables mind and body to regain their equilibrium, while also gently restoring a sense of well-being and vitality.

After first aid measures have been taken, and medical advice has been obtained, homoeopathic prescribing at home can do a great deal to ease the pain and speed up the healing process of a sports injury. For information on selecting and using homoeopathic medicines, see **Chapter 2:** *Homoeopathy In The Home: How To Use This Book*.

Achilles Tendonitis

This condition results in pain which is situated just above the heel in the lower back of the leg. Pain in this area usually indicates that the Achilles tendon may be damaged or partly torn. There is also the possibility that the sheath that covers the tendon may have become inflamed. This condition would be diagnosed as *tenosynovitis*.

If the Achilles tendon becomes overstretched or partly ruptured, the pain can be excruciating. Unfortunately, it is also an injury that can occur very easily as a result of a sudden movement that jars or stretches the heel. People who are especially at risk include those of us who go on exercising in our forties and fifties at the same pace we did in our teens. Because degeneration of the Achilles tendon may have occurred by this time, it is at far greater risk of being damaged through vigorous sports or exercise activities.

Basic First Aid

■ Apply an ice pack to the painful area for fifteen-minute intervals in order to ease the pain and reduce swelling. If you do not have an ice pack to hand, wrap a handful of ice cubes in a towel or cloth, or apply a bag of frozen vegetables to the site of the pain.

■ Elevate the leg by propping it up on a pillow or cushion.

■ Support the injured tendon by wrapping a bandage around the heel. Although this should be firm enough to support the painful area, make sure that circulation to the toes is not impeded. Check their colour regularly in order to establish that they are pink. If they look discoloured, loosen the bandage immediately.

■ If the tendon has been ruptured, the foot will remain still when the calf muscle is squeezed gently while the casualty is lying on their stomach. If a rupture is suspected, medical help should be sought immediately.

Rehabilitation And Prevention

■ If pain in the heel occurs, do not run for at least two weeks in order to avoid tendon spasm. Avoid stretching exercises until the pain has totally gone, and concentrate instead on non-weight-bearing activities such as swimming.

■ Daily massage may be helpful in reducing swelling and encouraging circulation to the injured area.

■ Minor damage to the Achilles tendon may take up to three months to heal. After the injury has fully healed, build up the time spent exercising *very* slowly, alternating running and walking activities. It is vital not to expect that an exercise programme can be resumed at the level of commitment and stamina that existed before injury occurred.

■ Ensure that muscles are always fully warmed up and stretched before running or jogging. Many tendon injuries are caused by overstretching cold muscles.

■ Avoid running on hard or uneven ground. Choose resilient, grassy surfaces where possible. Also make sure that running shoes give good support and adequate cushioning.

Type of injury	General symptoms	Worse from	Better for	Remedy name
Initial pain and trauma of injury.	Indicated for physical and mental shock of injury. Severe pain, swelling and bruising. May also be used as a local application in cream form (providing skin is not damaged).	Movement. Touch. Jarring.	Lying down.	**Arnica**
Later stage of injury with sore, bruised pain.	Often required if **Arnica** has initially helped with pain and swelling, but residual soreness remains. Lame, heavy sensations in injured heel.	Over-exertion. Cold, damp conditions. Going up or down stairs.	Warmth. Massage.	**Ruta**
Pain in heel that is relieved by elevating the foot.	Terrible soreness and aching in damaged tendon. Intermittent pains that result in restless weariness.	Cold. Damp. Movement. Feet resting on the floor. Stepping down from a high step.	Rest. Elevating foot.	**Phytolacca**
Persistent bruising and pain which is not resolved by **Arnica.**	Throbbing, squeezing, aching pains in injured area. Distracting pain that is relieved by cold compresses and applications.	Touch. Heat. Warm bathing. Becoming heated in bed.	Continued motion. Cool locally applied.	**Bellis perennis**

Type of injury	General symptoms	Worse from	Better for	Remedy name
Pain in tendon that is made more severe by immobility.	Established phase of tendon injury with aching that is relieved by gentle movement. Painful restlessness that is much worse in bed at night. Cramping pains in calf muscles.	Cold and damp. Initial movement. Resting. Overexertion. At night.	Warmth. Warm bathing. Massage. Gentle movement. Support to the injured area.	**Rhus tox**

Seek Prompt Medical Help In Any Of The Following Situations:

■ **If pain is very severe and rupture of the tendon is suspected.**
■ **If pain and swelling do not respond to first aid measures.**
■ **Heel pain in anyone who has suffered damage to their Achilles tendon in the past.**

Muscular Overexertion

It is exceptionally common to suffer from muscular aches and pains when first beginning an exercise programme. This is most often due to overdoing things as a result of enthusiasm, or unawareness of the measures that can be taken to minimize the risk of muscular strain. However, it is important to distinguish between the transient stiffness that follows exercising muscles that have not been used before, and persistent muscular aches and pains. The former should pass quickly as muscles become toned and flexible, the latter indicates that action is needed in order to prevent an injury occurring.

Practical Self-Help

■ Always make sure that muscles are thoroughly warmed up before beginning strenuous activities such as running. If cold muscles are stretched, there is a strong chance that tears or other injuries may occur. Before warming up muscles by stretching, doing any of the following activities for three to five minutes will serve to increase circulation to the heart and muscles:

■ Walking up and down stairs.
■ Jogging on the spot.
■ Using an exercise bike for fifteen minutes.

■ If you are exercising indoors, always make sure that surroundings are kept at a moderate, comfortable temperature. This is especially important when following a programme that includes a relaxation section which involves lying down for a sustained period of time. As body temperature falls in response to relaxation, it is essential that surroundings are comfortably warm in order to prevent chills or muscle cramps.

■ If you are a newcomer to physical exercise, never be tempted to launch abruptly into an ambitious programme of jogging, walking or aerobics classes. Instead, slowly build up stamina and flexibility by beginning with short blocks of exercise that gradually expand in length and intensity in proportion to your level of fitness.

■ Make sure that you are experiencing an all-round improvement in fitness by enjoying a range of exercise activities. These might include cycling, walking or running to condition the heart and lungs, weight training to increase muscle strength, and yoga to promote flexibility, stamina, relaxation and body awareness. By also including sports activities such as swimming and tennis, the range should be sufficient to improve fitness of mind and body while also preventing boredom setting in. A varied fitness programme should also ensure that a limited range of muscles do not get over-taxed, strained or injured.

■ If muscles are aching, soak in a soothing, warm bath. You may want to add a few drops of essential oils that encourage muscular relaxation. These include Bergamot, Chamomile, Lavender and Rosemary. Remember to use these very sparingly (no more than two to three drops), and also bear in mind that Rosemary may antidote the effective action of homoeopathic remedies. A few drops of the same oils may also be used diluted in a carrier oil to massage aching muscles. One or two drops of essential oil may be added to every 5mls of carrier oil. Suitable bases for dilution of essential oils include cold-pressed almond, sunflower, peach or apricot kernel oil.

Homoeopathic Help

Type of muscular over-exertion	General symptoms	Worse from	Better for	Remedy name
Generalized muscle aches from excessive physical effort.	Aches all over after vigorous exercise. Often needed by those who overdo physical effort after being totally unfit. Bruised aching pain in muscles. Tosses and turns at night because bed feels too hard.	Touch. Movement. After sleep. Jarring.	Lying with head low.	**Arnica**

Type of muscular over-exertion	General symptoms	Worse from	Better for	Remedy name
Muscle aches that feel better for continued movement.	Terribly restless with aching muscles: tosses and turns at night in an effort to get comfortable. Limping from cramping in calves and pains down back of thighs. Warm bathing is soothing.	Damp, cold air. Uncovering. Beginning movement. Resting. Overexertion.	Warmth. Hot bathing. Massage. Support to painful part. Stretching. Continued movement.	**Rhus tox**
Muscle pains that are much worse for movement.	Painful, sore muscles that feel much better for resting. Slight touch is painful, but firm pressure is soothing. Exhausted, apathetic and irritable with pain.	Movement. Initial motion. Heat. Touch. Stooping. Coughing.	Rest. Keeping as still as possible. Firm pressure. Cool air.	**Bryonia**

Seek Prompt Medical Help In Any Of The Following Situations:

■ **If burning muscle pain is severe or persists longer than expected after exertion.**

■ **If swelling and severe pain are present and there is any suspicion that the muscle may have been severely strained or ruptured.**

Strains And Sprains

Strains and sprains commonly occur as a result of vigorous or violent exercise or sports activity. Those who are most at risk include mature exercise enthusiasts whose muscles and joints are subject to degenerative changes. The problem may be further compounded when someone decides that they lead too sedentary a lifestyle and launches into a challenging exercise programme very abruptly.

A *strain* occurs as a consequence of a muscle becoming overstretched during the course of excessively challenging exercise in those who are unused to it. Other possible triggers include exercising muscles that have not been warmed up, or violent sports that put an undue strain on muscles. If muscle fibres are traumatized, the damaged tissue contracts and often becomes engorged with blood. As a result, pain and swelling set in rapidly, alerting the body that something is wrong. In rare cases, severe trauma may result in a torn or ruptured muscle. Thankfully, this is a fairly rare occurrence, with most people suffering less severe damage as a result of vigorous exercise.

Slight strains should heal completely without leaving complications in younger fitness enthusiasts, but the healing process may take longer as one becomes older. Although minor strains may be treated successfully at home with sensible self-help measures and homoeopathic prescribing, a ruptured muscle requires prompt medical treatment in order to avoid possible serious consequences.

Practical Self-Help

■ Rest must be taken for as long as the pain lasts. Remember that persistent or severe pain in any part of the body is a sign that something is amiss. Not using a strained muscle is essential because it gives it a chance to heal and repair itself.
■ Firm bandaging may be helpful in supporting the injured muscle, but it is essential that the binding is not too tight. Always check that the strapping is not obstructing the free flow of circulation.
■ As soon as the pain has eased, make sure that the affected area is gently exercised. This is important in preventing the stiffness and lack of flexibility that can set in when a limb is kept immobile for a substantial period of time.

A *sprain* usually affects the knee, ankle, wrist or finger joints. Unlike strains, which affect muscular tissue, sprains are a result of torn ligaments (these are fibrous tissues that stabilize a joint in position). Sprains often occur after falls, or when excessive demands are put on a joint during vigorous exercise. The distress and trauma that follow can span the full spectrum of intensity from mild to agonizing pain.

Minor sprains need not cause a major problem provided sensible self-help measures are observed and the joint is used with care in the future. However, it should always be borne in mind that once such an injury has occurred, it leaves the affected joint vulnerable to repeated sprains in the future. As a result, it is wise to take precautions in order to avoid putting extra stress or strain on the damaged joint.

Practical Self-Help

■ If a minor sprain occurs, apply an ice pack to the injured area as quickly as possible. If this is not available, use ice cubes wrapped in a cloth or towel, or a bag of frozen vegetables may serve as a good substitute. However, always avoid using ice-cold compresses on any injured area where the skin is broken.
■ Rest the injured joint as much as possible while pain is present. Also support the painful area with a crepe bandage that provides comfortable pressure, making sure that it is not too tight.

■ If the knee or ankle joint has been sprained, keep the affected leg raised on a cushion while resting. This encourages the swelling to drain away.

■ Once the pain has eased with rest and support, begin to gently exercise the injured joint, making sure that any weight-bearing exercises are avoided.

Homoeopathic Help

Type of strain or sprain	General symptoms	Worse from	Better for	Remedy name
Initial pain and swelling following injury.	The first remedy to consider for bruising, swelling and pain following strains or sprains. Reduces inflammation as well as easing emotional shock and trauma following an accident.	Touch. Movement. Making an effort.	Lying with head low.	**Arnica**
Sprains affecting the knee, ankle and wrist joints.	Often indicated for inflammation and pain that follow stress of repetitive movement. Inflammation, pain and stiffness in affected joint.	Damp conditions. Rest. Pressure to injured joint. Touch. Walking out of doors.	Moving about indoors. Warmth.	**Ruta**
Established pain of strains or sprains made worse by movement.	Often required to resolve the situation if **Arnica** has initially reduced pain and swelling. Tearing, severe pains eased by keeping as still as possible and made more intense by the slightest movement.	Touch. Making a physical effort. Getting up from a sitting position. Movement.	Keeping completely still. Firm pressure to painful part. Warmth to painful area.	**Bryonia**
Established strains and sprains that are relieved by continued motion.	Follows **Arnica** well once it has ceased to be of use in easing pain and swelling. Severe pain in damaged joint or muscle that is much more uncomfortable resting in bed and eased by being up and about.	Cold and damp. Lying, standing or sitting still. Initial movement. Excessive physical effort.	Continued movement that does not exhaust. Warm bathing. Warm compresses.	**Rhus tox**

Type of strain or sprain	General symptoms	Worse from	Better for	Remedy name
Sprains and strains that are made more flexible and comfortable by cool bathing.	Pain and swelling in affected muscle or joint. Injured area feels hot to the touch but does not look red or inflamed. Stabbing pains increase from warmth of bed. Injured area may feel numb and cold.	Warm bathing. Becoming heated. Motion.	Cool compresses. Cool bathing. Cool air. Resting.	**Ledum**

If Any Of The Following Occur, Prompt Medical Help Is Required:

- A joint that remains unusable after twelve to twenty-four hours.
- Injured joints that cannot be straightened.
- Severe pain that is accompanied by marked swelling or distorted appearance of the affected joint.
- An injured limb that feels numb or cold, and has a discoloured appearance (bluish-tinged).
- Suspected sprains in young children. Very often fractures of the wrist are mistaken for severe sprains, since it can be difficult to differentiate between the two conditions in a small child.
- Persistent and severe muscle pain.
- Swelling in a painful muscle.

Sun/Heatstroke And Heat Exhaustion

The symptoms of sun/heatstroke usually set in after exercising in excessively sunny, hot or humid conditions. If you suspect the onset of this problem, medical help should be sought immediately in order to avoid an emergency situation developing. Possible symptoms may include the following:

- High temperature.
- Dry skin.
- Irritability.
- Restlessness.
- Dizziness.
- Nausea.
- Confusion or drowsiness.

- Quickened pulse.
- Breathing problems such as irregular breathing.

If dehydration occurs in hot or humid conditions, heatstroke may be preceded by *heat exhaustion*. Sports enthusiasts are clearly at risk of developing a problem with heat exhaustion if they neglect their fluid intake while perspiring during exercise. If this happens, they may become dehydrated very rapidly. The symptoms that are likely to occur include the following:

- Dizziness.
- Headache.
- Cramps in muscles.
- Rapid pulse rate.
- Faintness.
- Weakness and exhaustion.

If heat exhaustion is neglected, it may develop into full-blown heatstroke. Although very mild cases can be alleviated by sensible self-help measures, it must be stressed that a medical opinion should be sought in order to prevent the risk of heatstroke developing.

Practical Self-Help

Heat Exhaustion

- At the first sign of symptoms, rest as much as possible in shady, cool surroundings, elevating the feet a little higher than the body.
- Ensure that there is a good supply of fresh, cool air and loosen any restrictive clothing around the neck and waist.
- Make a *very weak* saline solution by dissolving half a level teaspoon of salt in a litre of water (roughly two pints). This drink may be sipped at regular intervals in order to rehydrate the body and help prevent muscle cramps by replacing the salt that will have been lost while perspiring.

Sun/Heatstroke

- The first priority must be to cool the body down as rapidly and gently as possible. However, take care not to resort to measures that may be too drastic in order to avoid sending the body into a state of shock. Encourage the casualty to lie down and loosen or remove clothing. Sponge the body down with cool water, or soak a sheet in cool water, wring it out, and wrap it around the body. If you have access to a fan, direct the cool stream of air towards the casualty.
- Keep exposure to light and noise to a minimum, and create an environment that feels as cool, airy and spacious as possible.
- Take the temperature of the patient at regular intervals in order to check that it is not escalating to a dangerously high level (103°F or above).

■ While assistance is being given to the patient, send for medical help. This is an urgent matter if any of the symptoms listed on p. 99–100 occur.

■ Once he or she has recovered, make sure that the patient is not exposed to extreme temperature changes, since they are likely to be vulnerable to a recurrence of the problem.

Prevention

■ Where possible, avoid exercising when the sun is at its strongest and hottest. This happens roughly between 11 a.m. and 3 p.m. The best times of day for exercising are the early morning or evening.

■ On hot days, protect vulnerable areas such as the head and neck with a hat or cap. Also ensure that a good quality sun block is worn even on cooler, less sunny days.

■ Build up gradual tolerance to the heat of the sun by initially exercising during the times of day suggested above.

■ If you suspect the onset of any symptoms, seek the shade as quickly as possible and begin the self-help measures outlined above.

Homeopathic Help

Type of sun/heat-stroke or heat exhaustion	General symptoms	Worse from	Better for	Remedy name
Sudden onset of symptoms that are eased by bending head backwards.	Severe restlessness with red, hot, dry skin. Pulsating pains move down the body from the head. Pain in temples with throbbing headache. Severe irritability with outbursts of violent temper.	Jarring. Bright light or objects. Checked perspiration. Draughts of cold air.	Resting propped-up in bed. Bending the head backwards. Light covering.	**Belladonna**
Rapid, violent onset of symptoms that are made worse by bending the head back.	Flushed, itchy skin with explosive pains that radiate in an upward direction. Severe headache with throbbing pains that are eased by contact with cool air. Ice packs may increase discomfort in the head.	Warmth. Jarring. Motion. Bending the head backwards.	Elevating the head. Uncovering. Cool, fresh air.	**Glonoin**

101

Type of sun/heat stroke or heat exhaustion	General symptoms	Worse from	Better for	Remedy name
Heat exhaustion with 'air hunger'.	Sudden onset of collapse from dehydration. Bluish-tinged, pale, clammy skin with cold body and hot head. Strong craving for cool, fresh air: wants to be fanned.	Chill. Pressure of clothes. Lack of fluid. Warmth.	Elevating feet. Being fanned. Cold drinks. Fresh, cool air.	**Carbo veg**
Heat exhaustion with severe cramp in muscles.	Chilliness and faintness with clammy, pale skin. Heavy, cold sweats with weakness and prostration. Cramp and twitching in muscles of toes, fingers and calves. Convulsions may occur if situation is neglected.	Motion. Touch. Raising arms.	Cool drinks.	**Cuprum**
Chills and sudden faintness with heat exhaustion.	Icy cold with alternating burning sensations. Clammy, bluish-tinged skin with muscle spasms and cramps. Violent headache with pallor, increased amount of urine and nausea.	Pressure. Touch. Cold drinks.	Being covered. Lying down.	**Veratrum alb**

Seek Prompt Medical Help In Any Of The Following Situations:

■ If the patient's temperature is raised to a dangerously high level (approaching 103°F or above) send for medical help immediately while attempting to bring the temperature down.

■ If there are any indications that the casualty is drowsy, confused or lapsing in and out of consciousness, emergency medical help is required.

■ Badly sunburnt skin accompanying heat exhaustion or sunstroke requires medical attention, especially if there is any sign of blistering.

■ Severe headaches that develop in anyone suffering from heat exhaustion or heatstroke suggest that medical help is needed.

■ If there is any suggestion that the patient is entering a state of shock, lose no time in obtaining expert medical help. Symptoms of shock might include any of the following:

- Irregular or feeble pulse.
- Clammy, pale or blue-tinged skin.
- Drowsiness, confusion or unconsciousness.
- Irregular or difficult breathing.

■ If heat exhaustion or heatstroke have occurred, always seek a medical opinion, even though the temperature has returned to normal.

■ Because heatstroke is a potentially very serious problem, always seek medical help if there is any cause for alarm about the casualty's condition. This is especially important with regard to children and the elderly, who may experience serious symptoms rapidly.

Tennis Elbow (Tendonitis)

Although this is a problem that is by no means confined to tennis players (any more than golfer's elbow is confined to golfers), it is a condition that may be brought on or aggravated by exercise which involves repetitive or violent movement.

In theory, tendonitis can occur anywhere in the body where a tendon attaches muscle to bone, but the most common places include the shoulders, heels, outside of elbows (where it is called tennis elbow), or the inside of elbows (where it may be referred to as golfer's elbow).

The initial reason for the problem may be a small injury which leads to damage and/or inflammation of the tendon. This results in pain and tenderness around the area of the damaged tendon, which is unlikely to have a chance to heal while it is in use. Once healing has taken place, scar tissue may form which could result in residual pain for months or longer.

Practical Self-Help

■ Keep the painful limb as still as possible for a few days, using a firm bandage and a sling for support. Always check that the pressure of the bandage is firm but not so tight that it restricts the flow of circulation in the affected limb.

■ Apply cool compresses or an ice pack to the painful area in an effort to ease the pain. However, avoid using ice-cold applications on broken skin.

■ Once the initial pain has eased, start to gently move the affected joint, avoiding any movements that feel stressful or that cause pain. This will prevent it stiffening up.

■ Make sure that you do not return to your normal exercise commitments until you are confident that the inflammation has fully recovered.

Homoeopathic Help

Type of tendonitis	General symptoms	Worse from	Better for	Remedy name
Initial phase of pain and trauma.	Strongly indicated when an injury has occurred in order to ease pain and reduce inflammation. Helps with both physical and emotional trauma of injury. **Arnica** cream may also be massaged into the painful area provided the skin is unbroken.	Touch. Motion. Shock. Jarring. After sleep.	Lying with head low.	**Arnica**
Tendonitis that is relieved by movement.	Often needed if **Arnica** has initially helped, provided general symptoms agree. Much worse for resting, especially in bed at night. Affected joint feels stiff and immobile.	Keeping still. At night. Cold or damp. Becoming chilled. Initial movement. Too much physical effort.	Warmth. Hot bathing. Continued gentle exercise. Changing position. Massage.	**Rhus tox**
Tendonitis that is relieved by cool bathing.	Affected joint feels numb and cold, but pain and stiffness are worse from contact with warmth. Tearing pains with weakness of the affected joint.	Warm air. Warm bathing. Movement. At night.	Rest. Contact with cool air. Cool bathing.	**Ledum**
Established tendonitis with pain from scar tissue.	Restlessness, soreness and severe aching in inflamed joint. Tendon becomes rigid with severe pain and stiffness on movement. Affected joint is much more uncomfortable when lain on.	Overexertion. Cold. Lying down.	Warmth. Gentle movement. Massage.	**Ruta**
Long-standing tendon problems from an old injury.	Often required if **Arnica** has initially eased pain and improved mobility, but has ceased to help. Sore, bruised, aching pains in tendon that drive to distraction.	Touch. Cold bathing. Hot bathing. Becoming chilled. Becoming overheated.	Gentle movement. Cold compresses.	**Bellis Perennis**

Seek Prompt Medical Help In Any Of The Following Situations:

- If pain is very severe and rupture of the tendon is suspected.
- If pain worsens and does not respond to first aid measures.
- Pain in anyone who has suffered damage to their tendon in the past.

■6■

Homoeopathy For Babies And Children

As a rule, children respond very positively to homoeopathic treatment. This is because young children and babies have usually not been subject to the drug regimes that many of us have experienced by the time we reach adulthood. It is also easier to get a clear picture of a child's symptoms if they have not been modified by drug therapy, or become confused with the side effects of conventional drugs.

Positive reactions to homoeopathic treatment are also forthcoming in many young children because their overall energy levels and responses to stimuli are so much stronger than those of adults. This is why many children fall dramatically ill with an acute infection one minute, seem extremely unwell for a short time, and are up and about within a day or so. This decisive response to acute illness is indicative of the vigorous immune reaction in response to infection that many children possess. It is this self-healing mechanism that an appropriately prescribed homoeopathic remedy stimulates into action, so that infections can be resolved as quickly and with as little discomfort as possible.

However, there are also children who never develop a clear-cut, vigorous reaction to illness, but seem to be in a state of constant, vague unwellness. This may be the result of poor genetic inheritance, inadequate nutrition, overuse of conventional medication, adverse reaction to vaccination, or a combination of factors such as these. They may have constant colds, ear infections or chest problems with poor energy levels and stamina. Other complications may include eczema, psoriasis, hayfever, asthma or digestive disorders. In addition, behavioural problems may also occur, including poor concentration, lack of confidence, severe temper tantrums or antisocial behaviour. These are children who require help and advice from a homoeopathic practitioner for the reasons outlined in the section below.

The Role Of Home Prescribing

For children in the robust state of health outlined above, who fall ill dramatically but recover rapidly and decisively, homoeopathic home-prescribing can be immensely helpful. Provided the parent is able to select the most appropriate homoeopathic remedy for their child's symptoms, the results should be extremely exciting and gratifying.

On the other hand, the children who have poor or insufficient vitality to deal with infections fall into a category that requires a different approach. This does not suggest that they cannot be helped by homoeopathic treatment. On the contrary, seeing the progress that these children can make during a course of homoeopathic treatment is often one of the most gratifying aspects of working as a homoeopathic practitioner.

If your child has a straightforward 'acute' condition (of short duration) and you feel you would like to prescribe an appropriate homoeopathic remedy, you will need to familiarize yourself with the information contained in **Chapter 2: Homoeopathy In The Home: How To Use This Book**. This will give you the basic, practical advice that is needed in order to select an appropriate remedy for your child. Even if you feel that you are not ready to prescribe for your child, he or she will benefit from the *Practical Self-Help* advice in each section. This information will provide you with simple, non-invasive measures that you can utilize in order to make your child more comfortable and speed up the natural healing process.

If you are at all concerned about getting out of your depth, refer to the pointers at the end of each section which suggest when professional medical advice may be needed. In addition, consult the following section, and always follow your instinct if you are in any way concerned about the health of your child. It is essential to stress that you should never be hesitant about calling on professional help: where the health of your child is at stake, always err on the cautious side.

How To Recognize The Seriously Ill Child

It is important to be aware that young children and the elderly share a tendency to become severely ill with astonishing rapidity. As a result, it is very important to identify at an early stage any symptoms which suggest that a potentially serious problem may be developing. By taking appropriate action as quickly as possible, emergency situations can often be avoided.

Even if none of the following symptoms are present, but you feel that your child is unwell, always follow your instincts and seek a professional opinion if you are uneasy about the situation. If you know your child intimately, you may be alerted to a change in his or her health well before specific symptoms of illness have emerged. This might consist of no more than a noticeable change in feeding pattern, different behaviour or altered cry. Although none of these need be an automatic cause for concern, they may be valuable early warning signs if there are additional reasons for anxiety about your child's condition.

If any of the following occur, medical help should be obtained as quickly as possible:

- Yellow-tinged skin and dark-coloured urine.
- High temperature which is accompanied by muscle spasms or spasmodic twitching.
- Difficult, noisy, irregular or shallow breathing.
- Blue-tinged lips, fingertips or fingernails, especially when associated with breathing difficulties or collapse.
- Severe or persistent headache, high temperature, stiff neck and light sensitivity.
- Distressing abdominal pains lasting for more than an hour.
- Persistent vomiting.
- Drowsiness or confusion.
- Rashes that appear suddenly or for no reason.
- Rapid or severe swelling around the face, throat and neck.
- If a head injury has occurred.
- Blood in urine, stools or vomit.
- Persistent diarrhoea, especially if accompanied by vomiting in babies or small children.
- Signs of dehydration, including:

  - Dry mouth.
  - Loss of elasticity or poor skin tone.
  - Reduced or concentrated urine output.
  - Dry or sunken eyes.
  - Dry skin.
  - Sunken fontanelle (soft spot at the crown of the head) in newborn babies.

- Childhood infectious illnesses such as whooping cough or measles in babies under six months of age.
- Symptoms of illness that appear suddenly and with severity.

Childhood Infectious Diseases

Because homoeopathic medicines are understood to act by stimulating the self-healing mechanism of the body, they are equally able to provide this support when dealing with viral as well as bacterial infections.

Unlike conventional medication, which has a limited amount to offer when faced with viral illnesses such as measles or chickenpox, homoeopathic treatment can do a great deal to support the child through each phase of illness, easing feverishness, general aches and pains, sore throats, eye sensitivity and discomfort, coughing, and providing relief from itching and skin irritation. Most important of all, effective homoeopathic treatment can speed up the progress of the illness as it supports the body in its fight against infection.

The appropriate homoeopathic remedy may be taken internally, while a soothing herbal preparation may be applied to the skin. This may come in the form of a tincture, lotion, cream or ointment which can ease irritation and itching of the skin, discourage infection and promote speedy healing. Information regarding appropriate creams, tinctures and ointments, and recommendations for their use is given in the *Practical Self-Help* sections.

The Vaccination Issue

The growing vaccination debate is one of the most emotive and challenging issues currently aired in medical circles. The conventional medical approach states clearly that vaccination is an essential way of protecting children from the potential side effects of contagious childhood illnesses such as measles, whooping cough or mumps. As a result, great energy and financial resources are put into promoting campaigns in an effort to ensure that the bulk of the childhood population is vaccinated. Although some children are exempt from vaccination because of contraindications such as a history of allergic reactions, immunistaion is presented as being essentially benign for most children.

However, there is an alternative viewpoint which suggests that there may be problems associated with vaccination that go beyond the extreme neurological reactions that happen in a small proportion of cases. Conditions as diverse as allergies, ear infections, recurrent respiratory problems, rheumatoid arthritis, behavioural difficulties, and an increased risk of developing irritable bowel syndrome in later life, may be related to an adverse reaction to vaccination.

Problems may also arise from the different mechanisms involved in developing naturally-acquired immunity as opposed to immunity that is induced as a result of vaccination. This is why many homoeopaths regard childhood illnesses as giving the child's immune system the opportunity for a 'trial run' which serves to strengthen immune function. When naturally-acquired immunity occurs, infections usually enter the body through the mucus membranes of the nose and mouth, before circulating in the bloodstream. When a child comes into contact with the measles virus, it is usually inhaled through the nose. In time, it begins to multiply, in the tonsils, adenoids and lymph nodes before entering the bloodstream. As a result, the virus has made contact with the liver, spleen, thymus, and bone marrow before symptoms begin to appear, making it possible for effective stimulation of the immune system to occur.

However, vaccines are injected directly into the bloodstream, without bringing into play the body's first line of defence via the nose, mouth, or throat. Because of this, the impact on the immune system is likely to be stressful and traumatic. If we also take into account the fact that infants are vaccinated at regular intervals when their immune systems are in the process of developing, the potential negative effects demand consideration.

Because of the emotive nature of this debate, it is essential that parents have enough material at their disposal to enable them to make a decision with which they feel at ease. Information may be obtained from the suggested reading list given at the back of this book, which will provide you with material that can be discussed with your GP and health visitor. You may also find it helpful to contact an organization called The Informed Parent. This provides a support group and information service for parents who want to obtain as much material as possible about vaccination.

It is important to bear in mind that there are a variety of flexible options open to you and your child with regard to vaccination. It is possible to administer vaccinations one at a time, select specific vaccinations while opting out of others, delay vaccination until the immune system is stronger, decide against vaccination, using homoeopathic treatment to help your child through childhood infections, or use homoeopathic treatment to help your child deal with any after-effects of vaccinations.

Chickenpox

Chickenpox is a viral infection characterized by a severely itchy rash that may spread over the trunk, back, arms, legs and face. The rash begins as an outbreak of red spots which rapidly acquire a blistered, watery appearance. The skin eruption may be preceded by a feverish, unwell stage with vague, non-specific symptoms which may resemble flu in adults. Once the rash is fully out, it will stay extremely itchy until the spots become dry (when the patient ceases to be infectious). Chickenpox has a long incubation period which may last between one and three weeks. Generally speaking, chickenpox in children is a mild, infectious disease with very few complications. However, it is best acquired in childhood, since the symptoms are usually more severe in adults.

Practical Self-Help

■ A great deal can be done to ease the severe itching of the rash, thus making your child much more comfortable and less distressed. Instead of calamine lotion (which may be initially soothing but quickly dries on the skin), **Hypercal** or **Urtica urens** tincture should be used diluted, or added to the bathwater. If the spots are maddeningly itchy or stinging, choose **Urtica urens**. If they are painful and there is a risk of infection from the skin being broken as a result of scratching, select **Hypercal**. Dilute one part of tincture to ten parts of boiled, cooled water, soak a cotton wool pad with the lotion and bathe the spots as often as needed. This is immensely soothing and will do a great deal to make the spots less irritable. You may also add either tincture to the bathwater in order to soothe and calm the irritation. However, warm bathing is best avoided in the early stages of the illness when the spots are still emerging, because it can leave your child feeling feverish and enervated.

■ Additional relief may also be obtained from soaking in an oatmeal bath. Place a handful of oats in a pouch of fine muslin or gauze and suspend it under the hot water tap while it is running.

■ After the spots have been bathed with diluted tincture as recommended above, frequently apply **Hypercal** or **Urtica urens** cream to the irritated skin. **Calendula** cream may also be useful if there is any risk of the spots becoming infected. Always choose cream rather than ointment when dealing with a chickenpox rash, because ointment may discourage the rash from drying out.

■ Trim young children's fingernails very short so that they are less likely to remove the tops from spots when scratching. Also explain to older children that they should try to rub rather than scratch the spots in an effort to avoid breaking the surface of the skin. If these measures are combined with homoeopathic prescribing and the use of appropriate creams as suggested above, the risk of severe scarring should be reduced.

■ Once the watery blisters have dried and developed a crust, make sure that you gently pat the skin dry after bathing rather than rubbing. By doing so, you are less likely to remove the crusts covering the spots.

■ If your child's appetite has disappeared in the early stages of illness, make sure that you give them plenty of fluid to drink. This is more important than encouraging your child to eat, since it will help keep their temperature down as well as guarding against dehydration. If your child remains hungry, prepare light, easily digested foods, e.g. broths, steamed or fresh fruit, or purées. This is suggested in order to avoid the nausea that may occur if heavy, or indigestible foods are given when there is any suggestion of feverishness developing.

■ Many parents are now aware that aspirin should not be given to children who are feverish when ill in an effort to bring the temperature down because of the potential risk of a child developing *Reye's Syndrome*. This is a serious illness which gives rise to the following symptoms:

■ Vomiting.
■ Feverishness.
■ Drowsiness.
■ Convulsions.
■ Unconsciousness.

Homoeopathic Help

Type of chicken-pox	General symptoms	Worse from	Better for	Remedy name
Early stage with rapid onset of fever.	Marked anxiety and restlessness with high temperature. Thirsty with high temperature and dry skin. Intolerant and panic-stricken with discomfort. Most likely to be indicated before the rash has emerged.	At night. Extreme heat or chill.	Sleep. Fresh air. Once a sweat breaks.	**Aconite**
Early stage of illness with violent onset and dry, flushed skin that radiates heat.	Extremely rapid onset of symptoms with very high temperature. Child may be on the verge of delirium. Pupils become dilated and pulse is full and rapid. Severe headache with throbbing pains. More irritable and less panicky than children needing **Aconite**.	Becoming chilled. Noise. Jarring movement. Bright light. Being disturbed.	Sitting propped-up in bed. Darkened rooms. Peace and quiet.	**Belladonna**
Chilly, restless and anxious in feverish stage.	Extreme mental and physical unease with restlessness when ill. Although feverish, feels extremely cold and cannot warm up easily. Rash may also be soothed by warmth. Diarrhoea and nausea accompany illness.	When alone. With the approach of night. Becoming chilled. Physical effort.	Warmth. Sips of warm drinks. Company. Sitting propped-up in bed. Gentle movement.	**Arsenicum alb**
Chesty cough with rash that is slow to emerge.	Persistent, rattly cough with unpleasantly coated tongue. Once rash breaks, eruptions are large and bluish-coloured. Severe irritability and bouts of bad temper once illness sets in.	Warmth. Bathing. Becoming heated in bed. Evenings. Lying down.	Cool conditions. Coughing up phlegm.	**Ant tart**

Type of chicken-pox	General symptoms	Worse from	Better for	Remedy name
Irritable itchy rash that is especially severe in bed at night.	Restless and unable to keep still with physical discomfort from itching. Extremely sensitive to cold and damp which makes everything feel worse. Despondent and desperate when ill, especially at night.	Cold and damp. At night. Keeping still. Scratching spots.	Warmth. Warm bathing. Gentle movement.	**Rhus tox**
Established stage of chicken pox with swollen glands and drenching sweats.	Terribly restless and sensitive to the slightest change in temperature. Discharges are increased and may be offensive: sweat, saliva, etc. Unpleasant, metallic taste in mouth. Large spots that look infected or pussy.	At night. Extreme heat or cold.	Moderate temperatures.	**Mercurius**
Ongoing, low-grade fever with clinginess and tearfulness.	Slow-developing rash or lingering, slight fever. Unusual symptom of dry mouth without thirst. Although chilly, there is a marked intolerance of heat and craving for cool, fresh air. Child is weepy and pathetic with a marked need for attention and sympathy.	Evenings and at night. Warm air. Warm bathing. Resting. Stuffy surroundings. Lack of attention.	Cool, fresh air. Cool locally applied. Gentle movement. Sympathy. Having a good cry.	**Pulsatilla**

Seek Prompt Medical Help In Any Of The Following Situations:

■ **If there are any indications that the eruptions are becoming pussy or infected.**

■ **Bleeding beneath the surface of the skin.**

■ **Breathing difficulties including shallow or rapid breathing.**

■ **Vomiting.**

■ **Convulsions.**

■ **Severe headache with stiffness of the neck.**

■ **Extreme prostration or weakness.**

■ **Chickenpox in children who are under a year old.**

Colic

Although not a serious condition in itself, severe or frequent baby colic is a problem that can leave parents at their wits' end. Symptoms include sharp pains in the stomach or abdomen, with babies often drawing their knees up to their chest in an effort to ease the pain. This commonly occurs after birth, and intermittent bouts may continue until a baby has reached the age the age of three months or ten weeks.

Fortunately, there is a great deal that can be done to ease the situation by following simple self-help advice, and also by the appropriate use of the indicated homoeopathic medicine.

Because homoeopathy can be very effective in easing the symptoms of baby colic, do not give up if you cannot prescribe effectively yourself from lack of knowledge, experience or confidence. In such a situation, consult a trained homoeopath who will be able to give a professional assessment of your baby's case.

Practical Self-Help

■ When breast-feeding, it is important to check if there are ingredients in your diet which may be aggravating your baby's colic. Possible culprits include hot spices such as chilli or curry, raw onions, peppers, cabbage, cauliflower, brussels sprouts, citrus fruits, grapes, dairy foods, chocolate, strong tea, coffee or alcohol.

■ When bottle-feeding, check that the teat on your baby's bottle is the right size. If it is too big for a new-born, or too small for an older baby, there is a strong chance that air is being swallowed with each feed which cannot be brought up.

■ Always make sure when preparing your baby's feed that the formula is being made according to the correct proportions. If it is too concentrated, your baby may cry because of excessive thirst from taking in too much salt. Too dilute a formula may lead to distress because hunger pangs are not being satisfied.

■ If you suspect that excess wind is causing distress, gently rub your baby's back or stomach. This serves the dual function of being very soothing as well as encouraging your baby to burp.

■ Constipation may contribute to problems with colic. If your baby has a tendency to be constipated, follow the advice given in the relevant section in **Chapter 4**: *The A-Z Of Common Ailments*.

Homoeopathic Help

Type of colic	General symptoms	Worse from	Better for	Remedy name
Colicky pains with great distress and irritability.	Scarlet-faced and furious with pains. Screams frantically and cannot be pacified. Doubles up with pain. Distension of abdomen that is not relieved by passing wind. Colic often occurs with teething and/or diarrhoea.	Night.	Being carried. Rocking. Hot compresses.	**Chamomilla**
Dry, bright red skin with colicky pains.	Bad temper with spasmodic pains, but not as extreme as **Chamomilla**. Intermittent pains that rapidly come and go. Bends backwards in order to ease pains. Skin on abdomen radiates dry heat.	Noise. Bright light. Touch. Jarring. Pressure of bedclothes. Lying on painful part.	Warmth. Bending backwards.	**Belladonna**
Colicky pains that are eased by pressure to abdomen.	Baby lies on its stomach or pushes fists into abdomen in order to ease pain. Discomfort sets in abruptly with infant doubling up, or pulling knees up to chest.	Release of firm pressure to abdomen. Being still.	Pressure. Warmth applied to painful area. Movement. Release of wind.	**Colocynthis**
Colicky pains with persistent, fruitless attempts at passing stools.	Colic brought on, or aggravated by breast-feeding mother eating spicy foods or drinking a lot of coffee. Infant is chilly, irritable and extremely sensitive to pain and discomfort. Colic is most severe on waking from sleep.	Touch or pressure. Lack of sleep. Eating. Exposure to chill or cold draughts of air. On waking.	Warmth. Rest. Sound, unbroken sleep.	**Nux vomica**

115

Type of colic	General symptoms	Worse from	Better for	Remedy name
Colicky pains that are intensified by the slightest movement.	Cross, irritable, and intolerant of warm surroundings with persistent constipation. Marked thirst with preference for cool, rather than warm liquids. Firm pressure and warm compresses applied to abdomen ease pain.	Hot, stuffy rooms. Movement. Light pressure or touch. Jarring movements.	Fresh, cool air. Lying still. Firm pressure to painful area.	**Bryonia**
Severe colicky pains that are relieved by arching back or stretching.	Colic with bouts of diarrhoea that do not ease the pain. Discomfort is centred around the navel. Often needed by breast-feeding babies whose mothers are drinking excessive amounts of strong tea.	Lying. Bringing knees up to chest. Feeding. At night.	Arching backwards. Stretching. Firm pressure.	**Dioscorea**
Colicky pains with severe abdominal rumbling, gurgling, and bloating after feeds.	Symptoms occur or become more intense in the afternoon, or after each feed. Pressure around the waist or abdomen causes great distress and discomfort. Colic may be aggravated by breast-feeding mother eating a diet that is too high in fibre, e.g. cabbage, beans and wholewheat items.	Afternoons. Cold drinks. After feeds. Touch or pressure. Becoming overheated. Waking from sleep.	Release of pressure around waist. Release of wind upwards or downwards. Warm drinks. Fresh air.	**Lycopodium**
Colicky pains that are eased by pressure and massage.	Symptoms may occur when teething. Infant produces an excessive amount of wind which frequently escapes downwards. Passing wind sometimes relieves discomfort of colic.	Chill. Cold liquids. Night. Tight clothing.	Bringing knees up to chest. Firm pressure. Warmth. Massage.	**Mag phos**

Type of colic	General symptoms	Worse from	Better for	Remedy name
Weepiness and clinginess with colic.	Infant is pathetic and very demanding of attention when in pain. Changeable bowel movements: no two stools look alike. Stuffy rooms intensify distress and discomfort, while cool, fresh air helps. Symptoms aggravated by mother eating too rich or fatty a diet.	Overheated rooms. Lack of fresh air. Evenings. Heavy clothing or bed covers. Keeping still.	Movement. Fresh, cool air. Removing covers. Attention and fuss.	**Pulsatilla**

Seek Prompt Medical Help In Any Of The Following Situations:

■ **If your baby seems unduly distressed.**
■ **If discomfort is accompanied by stubborn constipation, vomiting, diarrhoea or reduced flow of urine.**
■ **If you suspect that your baby is becoming dehydrated.**
Symptoms may include any combination of the following:

   ■ **Dry mouth.**
   ■ **Dry or sunken eyes.**
   ■ **Depressed fontanelle (this is the soft spot at the crown of a new-born baby).**
   ■ **Diminished amount of very strong-smelling, discoloured urine.**
   ■ **Reduced elasticity of the skin.**

Croup

An attack of croup can be an extremely frightening experience for both child and parent due to the tendency for acute symptoms to develop with rapidity and severity, usually at night.

One of the most alarming symptoms associated with an attack of croup is the sound that a child makes when breathing in. This hoarse, rasping sound is called *stridor* and is caused by the air passages becoming inflamed or swollen. Additional symptoms that usually accompany an attack of croup include hoarseness, sensitivity of the throat, discomfort in the chest, and a characteristic-sounding, hollow cough.

If your child is not suffering a cough or cold and suddenly develops *stridor*, seek medical advice straight away. This is important in order to check whether your child has inhaled a foreign object such as a peanut.

117

Practical Self-Help

■ At the first signs of an attack of croup, take your child into a steam-filled room which will enable him to breathe more easily. A steamy atmosphere can be easily and quickly created by filling the bath with hot water and running the shower, while the door and windows are shut. If you sit calmly with your child, encouraging them to take slow, even breaths, the inhaled steam should do a great deal to ease a mild attack of croup. However, a young child should never be left alone in a bathroom where the bath is filled with very hot water, since burns and scalds happen very easily. In order to prevent such an accident occurring, always make sure that someone is present with your child.

■ If a child panics during an attack of croup, this can make the symptoms more severe and distressing. Reassurance can be given in any way that you feel your child will best respond to: this could include cuddling, stroking, or speaking softly and calmly.

Homoeopathic Help

Type of croup	General symptoms	Worse from	Better for	Remedy name
Croup with extreme anxiety, panic, and restlessness.	Symptoms develop rapidly and violently: especially after exposure to dry, cold winds. Goes to bed fit and well and wakes abruptly from sleep with hoarse, dry coughing spasm. Breathing difficulties rapidly lead to terror and panic. Attacks tend to occur after midnight.	Cold, dry winds. After midnight. Cold drinks. Inhaling tobacco smoke.	Sweating. Fresh air.	**Aconite**
Loud coughing spasms prevent sleep or wake child before midnight.	Suffocative, harsh, dry cough with sense of breathing through a dry sponge. Breathing may be laboured or noisy on falling asleep. Characteristic sound of rasping cough resembles that of a saw being drawn through dry wood.	Touch. Cold drinks. Breathing in. Excitement. Speaking. Sugary foods or drinks.	Warm drinks.	**Spongia**

Type of croup	General symptoms	Worse from	Better for	Remedy name
Coughing spasms begin as soon as child's head hits the pillow.	Bouts of deep, barking, choking cough get worse after midnight. Croup may develop after measles. Holds sides in order to minimize pain in chest from repeated episodes of violent coughing.	Lying down. Warmth. After midnight. Talking. Cold food or drinks. Stooping.	Fresh air. Pressures.	**Drosera**
Terrible anxiety with croup that responds very well to reassurance.	Harsh, croupy cough with burning in throat and chest. Bouts of croup that have gone beyond initial, severe onset, but keep relapsing. Coughing brought on by change of temperature or by lying down.	Talking. In the evening. Strong smells. Change of temperature.	Touch. Reassurance. Warmth. Sitting up.	**Phosphorus**
Barking croupy cough which is intensified by exposure to cold air.	Croup develops or becomes more severe in the morning or evening. Exposure to cold makes everything worse. Suffers from the slightest uncovering: even of a hand or foot. Becomes irritable and bad-tempered with croup.	Chill. Cold draughts. Breathing out. Touch. Uncovering.	Warmth. Humidity. Being well-covered.	**Hepar sulph**
Croup with severe choking, suffocative spasms on entering deep sleep.	Reacts badly to any sense of pressure or constriction around throat and neck. Croupy coughing spasm may be set off by touching throat. Difficulty swallowing because throat feels constricted. Fear of going to sleep.	Warmth. Waking from sleep. Swallowing saliva. Tight clothes around neck.	Fresh cool air. Cool drinks or food. Motion.	**Lachesis**
Bouts of croupy cough with stringy, sticky, yellow mucus that is brought up with difficulty.	Gagging and breathless from the effort of coughing and loosening phlegm. Sense of heaviness and constriction in chest on waking. Raw pains radiate from under breast bone to back and shoulders.	Morning. Waking from sleep. Stooping. Sitting. Cold and damp. Undressing.	Movement. Warmth.	**Kali bich**

Seek Prompt Medical Help In Any Of The Following Situations:

■ Any child under five years of age who develops noisy, harsh or difficult breathing should be seen by your GP as quickly as possible.
■ Severe attacks of croup with breathing difficulties.
■ Signs of drooling or blueness around the lips.
■ If your child is extremely distressed and inhaling steam has not helped.
■ If self-help measures have not improved the condition within twenty minutes.

Earache

The misery of earache can affect adults as well as children, with one adult in thirty suffering from it every year. However, it is an even more common problem in childhood, with ear infections often occurring as a complication of the common cold. Children are more likely to suffer ear infections because the *eustachian tube* which joins the back of the nose and the ear cavity is shorter than in adults. As a result, infections can travel rapidly from the nasal passages to the ears. If we also consider that children's *adenoids* are more subject to inflammation, it is not surprising that ear, nose and throat problems are very common in childhood.

The common symptoms of acute ear infections include stabbing pains and a sense of obstruction or fullness in the affected ear, plus feverishness and partial loss of hearing. If a bacterial infection is left to run its course, there is a strong probability of a build-up of pus developing which can perforate the ear drum. If this occurs, a discharge will appear as the severe pain in the ear diminishes.

If you suspect that your child is suffering from ear problems, it is best to begin self-help measures as quickly as possible in an effort to ease pain and deal with inflammation. However, if you suspect that your child may be suffering from a bacterial infection, e.g. if earache accompanies tonsillitis, it is best to seek a professional medical opinion as well as proceeding with self-help measures.

Practical Self-Help

■ Avoid exposure to sharp, cold winds if you know that your child has a tendency to earache. On a cold, windy day always make sure that your child's ears are well-covered by a bonnet, hat or scarf if they are spending time out of doors.
■ If your child is diagnosed as having an ear infection, avoid contact with water until the ear is fully recovered.
■ Watch out for tell-tale signs which suggest that your baby may have ear problems. Common symptoms include rubbing or pulling the ear, especially if your baby is uncharacteristically distressed and weepy.
■ Make sure that your baby or infant has plenty to drink, especially if they are feverish. However, if an ear infection is combined with a generally congested

state of the nose and chest, avoid giving too much milk which can contribute to increased mucus production.

■ Many children find contact with warmth eases the pain of earache. Soothing compresses may be made from a warm hot water bottle wrapped in a towel or a flannel which has been well wrung out after being immersed in warm water. Always make sure that you use warm rather than boiling water in an effort to prevent accidental burns and scalds occurring if your children are very young. If your child prefers cool compresses, use a cool flannel, or a custom-made cool pack which can be kept in the fridge and wrapped in soft cloth before applying to the skin.

■ If a discharge begins to weep from the ear, always seek a professional opinion and examination rather than attempting to deal with the problem yourself. This is especially important if the discharge looks or smells unpleasant.

■ If ear infections and persistent colds are becoming a frequent occurrence, a great deal can be gained by seeking professional homoeopathic advice. Successful homoeopathic treatment appears to deal with the underlying weakness that is leading to repeated bouts of illness, stimulating your child's immune system to overcome infection more effectively.

Homoeopathic Help

Type of earache	General symptoms	Worse from	Better for	Remedy name
Right-sided earache that comes on violently and abruptly (early stage of illness).	High temperature with earache, with extremely bright red, hot, dry skin. Throbbing pains in ears and throat with swollen glands. Affected ear looks bright red and feels hot to the touch. Extreme irritability and bad temper in a usually placid child.	Noise. Movement. Bright light. Jarring. Chill. Excitement or stimulation.	Lying propped-up in a warm, darkened room. Warm compresses.	**Belladonna**
Earache that comes on rapidly after exposure to dry, cold winds (early stage).	Goes to bed as usual, but wakes from sleep with terrible earache and distress. Child is frantic and beside himself with pains. Extreme restlessness and anxiety when unwell. Thirsty when feverish with hot head and cool body.	At night. Exposure to chill or cold winds. Overheated rooms. Lying on the painful part.	Fresh air. Sweating. Moderate temperatures.	**Aconite**

Type of earache	General symptoms	Worse from	Better for	Remedy name
Rapid onset of earache with less violent symptoms than those requiring **Belladonna** or **Aconite**.	Often needed in the early stage of ear infections before discharge has been produced. Pulling, drawing, itchy sensations in the ear. Pains may be left-sided or worse in the left ear than the the right. Flushed or pale with earache.	At night. Effort. Noise. Jarring. Movement. Touch. Cool air.	Lying down. Cool compresses.	**Ferrum phos**
Terrible distress and screaming with earache.	Frantic weeping and temper tantrums with pain. Cannot be pacified or distracted: toys are thrown to the floor in frustration. One pale and one flushed cheek with feverishness. Earache may occur with teething problems.	Warmth. Overheated rooms. Touch. Noise. Bright light. Chill.	Being rocked or carried. Being taken for a drive in a car.	**Chamomilla**
Established stage of earache with thick, yellow-coloured discharge.	Extreme chilliness with marked dislike of cold draughts. Slight uncovering causes great distress and discomfort. Sticking, splinter-like pains in ears and throat with offensive discharge. Very irritable and bad-tempered when ill with aversion to being touched.	Chill. Cold draughts of air. Cold winds. Lying on sensitive side. At night.	Warm rooms. Wrapping the head up warmly. Resting in a warm bed.	**Hepar sulph**
Established ear infection with offensive green discharge and heavy perspiration.	Swollen glands and sore, ulcerated throat with ear infection. Drooling on the pillow at night from excess saliva. Complains of unpleasant taste in mouth: breath also smells offensive. Becomes extremely anxious and restless at night.	Extreme warmth or chill. At night. Becoming overheated in bed. Stooping. Touch.	Resting in moderate temperatures.	**Mercurius**

Type of earache	General symptoms	Worse from	Better for	Remedy name
Lingering symptoms of ear infection with clinginess and weeping.	Marked dislike of overheated, stuffy rooms despite chilliness. Ear troubles set in after chill or getting wet. Thick, creamy, yellowish-green discharge with swollen glands. Calm child becomes uncharacteristically demanding and attention-seeking.	Overheated rooms. Lack of fresh, cool air. Resting. Evenings. Humid conditions. Lack of attention.	Cool, fresh air. Gentle movement. Cool drinks. Cool compresses. Sympathy and attention.	**Pulsatilla**
Left-sided ear pain that comes on during sleep.	Severe sore throat with earache that wakes child from sleep. Constricted, swollen feeling in throat that is aggravated by pressure of clothes around the neck. Affected ear feels stuffed up or obstructed.	Warm rooms. Lack of fresh air. Warm drinks. Pressure of clothes around neck. Swallowing saliva. After sleep.	Cool surroundings. Fresh air. Loosening clothes around neck. Swallowing food or liquid. Cool drinks. Movement.	**Lachesis**

Seek Prompt Medical Help In Any Of The Following Situations:

■ If your child is extremely distressed and in severe pain.

■ Ear problems in babies that are accompanied by dehydration and/ or sunken or swollen fontanelle (the soft spot at the crown of the head).

■ If you observe seepage from the ear which is clear, pussy, blood-streaked or unpleasant-smelling.

■ Marked redness, inflammation, sensitivity or pain behind the ear.

■ If problems occur after your child has pushed a foreign object into his or her ear, do not attempt to remove it yourself but seek professional medical help. This is necessary because of the risk of a layperson inadvertently pushing the object further into the ear in an effort to help.

■ If your child has not responded to self-help measures within twenty-four hours, or if you suspect your child's overall condition is deteriorating.

German Measles

German measles is a relatively mild illness which usually causes little more distress than a rash and feeling under the weather. However, it is a contagious virus that can cause birth defects in the unborn child of a pregnant woman.

Common symptoms in the early stage of infection include: mild feverishness and slightly swollen glands behind the ears and at the back of the neck. The rash will emerge fairly rapidly once symptoms are under way (usually on the first or second day). It consists of reddish-pink, small, flat spots which usually appear initially on the face, spreading quickly to the rest of the body. The rash is not long-lasting and generally clears up by the fourth or fifth day of illness.

If your child has been diagnosed as suffering from German measles, it is essential that any friends who are pregnant should be informed. Once they have been told, they can avoid visiting until your child has fully recovered. Because German measles has an incubation period of three weeks before the rash appears, it may also be necessary to notify anyone who has been in contact with your child during this period.

Practical Self-Help

See the self-help suggestions given in the *Measles* section. You will find that the same principles apply, although German measles is generally an illness with milder symptoms. If your child is coping very well on their own, there is no need to prescribe a homoeopathic remedy. However, if they are distressed by their symptoms, the appropriate homoeopathic prescription will do a great deal to boost their energy levels so that they are supported through the course of their illness. As a result, they are likely to experience the minimum amount of distress and complications.

Homoeopathic Help

Type of German measles	General symptoms	Worse from	Better for	Remedy name
Rapid onset of illness with extreme restlessness and distress.	Required in the early stages before the rash emerges. Sore, sensitive eyes with runny nose. Thirsty with upset stomach and diarrhoea. Dry, irritating, croupy cough. Restless sleep with intensification of symptoms at night.	At night. Extreme heat or chill. Bright light.	Sound sleep. Rest.	**Aconite**
Violent, rapid onset of illness with extreme feverishness.	Temperature goes up rapidly with resulting bright red, hot, dry skin. Throbbing headache with rapid pulse. Muscles twitch and jerk in light, fitful sleep. Although drowsy, child is irritable from lack of sound sleep.	Bright light. Noise. Jarring movement. Chill.	Resting in a darkened room. Sitting propped-up in bed.	**Belladonna**
Flushed and feverish with red areas on cheeks.	Needed in the early phase of illness when symptoms are less intense than those requiring **Aconite** or **Belladonna**. Child tires easily with intermittent bouts of feverishness.	At night. Movement. Lack of sweat. Noise. Chill.	Resting. Cool compresses.	**Ferrum phos**
General state of congestion with thick, yellow mucus.	Well-established stage of illness with inflamed sinuses and swollen glands. Nasal discharge is stringy and thickened. Headaches occur from congestion of nasal passages and sinuses. Loose, rattly cough. Child becomes listless and apathetic.	Cold, damp conditions. Fresh air. After sleep. Hot weather. Stooping.	Warmth. Pressure to painful part. Movement.	**Kali bich**

Type of German measles	General symptoms	Worse from	Better for	Remedy name
Lingering symptoms with low-grade fever after rash has appeared.	Swollen glands and persistent cough that is alternately dry and loose. Thick, yellowish-green nasal discharge, with greenish phlegm from chest. Child is demanding, clingy and weepy.	Stuffy, overheated rooms. Resting. Warm food and drinks. Rich foods. In the evening and at night.	Fresh, open air. Cool compresses. Cool drinks. Sympathy and attention. Gentle movement.	**Pulsatilla**
Lingering symptoms after the rash has appeared with severe flushes of heat.	Great distress in warm conditions with a constant need to uncover, or to push feet out of bed covers. Feverishness with dry skin. Persistent greenish mucus from nose and phlegm from chest.	Warmth. Heat of the bed. Chill. Washing or bathing. Eating. After sleep.	Moderate temperatures.	**Sulphur**

Seek Prompt Medical Help In Any Of The Following Situations:

■ **Severe lethargy or distress**.
■ **Persistent headache, especially if accompanied by a stiff neck and/ or vomiting**.
■ **Severe symptoms in a baby of under six months of age**.
■ **Persistent or severe cough that does not respond to self-help measures**.
■ **Bleeding under the skin**.
■ **Breathing difficulties**.
■ **Marked discomfort or distress with eye symptoms**.
■ **If you are pregnant**.
■ **If your child develops German measles your GP should be notified**.

Measles

Measles is a viral infection that usually begins with a general period of feeling feverish and unwell, with a dry cough that may last for a couple of days. Once the temperature falls, characteristic small white spots are to be seen inside the mouth which resemble grains of salt. The fever may set in again as further slightly-raised, dull-red spots emerge on the forehead and behind the ears. These generally spread to the rest of the head and trunk, but do not usually affect the arms or legs. As the eruption comes out, the spots get larger and eventually join together. Other symptoms experienced during the early phase of measles may include a runny nose, earache, swollen glands, diarrhoea, light sensitivity and/or inflamed watery eyes.

Measles is a contagious viral disease which has an incubation period of approximately ten to fourteen days.

Practical Self-Help

■ Children who suffer from measles often complain of sore, light-sensitive eyes. If this happens, make sure that the stress is taken off your child's eyes by closing curtains and keeping the room as dimly-lit as possible.

■ If your child is not eager to eat, follow the recommendations given in the *Chickenpox* section. This may be especially relevant in the feverish stage of illness.

■ If the rash is irritable, it may be soothed by one of the preparations mentioned in the *Chickenpox* section.

Homoeopathic Help

Type of measles	General symptoms	Worse from	Better for	Remedy name
Early stage of illness with extreme feverishness.	Fever develops violently and rapidly. Skin is bright red, dry and very hot. Pupils become dilated and pulse is rapid. Painful throat makes drinking difficult. Throbbing headache with light sensitivity and tremendous irritability.	Noise. Bright light. Being disturbed. Jarring. Chill.	Sitting quietly propped-up in bed. Darkened rooms. Warmth.	**Belladonna**
Sudden onset of symptoms with extreme restlessness and distress.	Fever develops rapidly, violently and without warning. Terrible restlessness and fear with high temperature. Marked sensitivity to pain drives child frantic. Very tender, sensitive eyes with runny nose and hard, croupy cough.	At night. Extreme warmth or chill.	Open air. Sound sleep.	**Aconite**

127

Type of measles	General symptoms	Worse from	Better for	Remedy name
Rosy-red, waterlogged rash with extreme sensitivity to heat.	Stinging, burning rash that is soothed by contact with anything cool. General swelling of face, eyes and eyelids which have a 'water bag' appearance. Itchy and fidgety with illness.	Warm bathing. Warm air. After sleep. Resting. Touch.	Cool bathing. Cool air. Gentle movement.	**Apis**
Marked eye sensitivity and discomfort with measles.	Distressing sensitivity to light with painful, burning watering eyes. Bland discharge from the nostrils. Dry, hoarse cough. Nose and eye symptoms feel more comfortable in the open air.	Warmth. Bright light. Approach of evening.	Fresh open air. Wiping eyes.	**Euphrasia**
Gradual, insidious development of illness with severe cough.	Slow-developing temperature with flushed, dry skin. Severe headache which is much worse for the slightest movement. Persistent dry, tickly cough with marked thirst for cold drinks. Child is bad-tempered and withdrawn.	Movement. Warmth. Being disturbed. Eating.	Cool surroundings. Keeping still. Fresh air. Cool drinks. Pressure to head or chest if painful.	**Bryonia**
Lethargic and exhausted with general shivering and aching.	Illness takes days to emerge with increasing weariness. Chills alternate with high fever. Flushed puffy face with heavy, drooping eyelids. Lack of interest and apathy towards everything: just wants to be left in peace and quiet.	Making an effort.	Warmth. Passing large quantities of urine. Fresh air.	**Gelsemium**
Established stage of measles once the rash has emerged fully.	Alternating dry and loose cough which is productive in the morning and irritating at night. Dry mouth without thirst. Thick, bland, yellowish-green discharges. Pathetic, clingy and very weepy with illness.	Heat. Stuffy rooms. Resting. Eating.	Cool, fresh air. Cool food and drinks. Gentle movement. Having a good cry.	**Pulsatilla**

Type of measles	General symptoms	Worse from	Better for	Remedy name
Measles with extreme chilliness and diarrhoea.	Terrible restlessness that gets worse as night comes on. Irritable, burning rash eased by warm bathing. Nausea and severe diarrhoea intensified by cold drinks. Dry, wheezy, troublesome cough relieved by being propped-up on pillows. Child is fretful, fussy and very anxious.	Night Cold food or drinks. Being chilled. Being alone.	Sips of warm drinks. Warm surroundings. Warm compresses. Gentle movement. Sitting propped-up in bed. Company.	**Arsenicum alb**
Measles with terribly irritating rash that is much worse for warmth.	May be indicated when the rash is fully out: especially if it reacts very badly to heat and bathing. However, it should not be repeated frequently because of its very deep-acting nature in skin conditions.	Warmth. Becoming heated in bed. Chill. At night. Waking from sleep. Eating.	Fresh, cool conditions. Lying down.	**Sulphur**

Seek Prompt Medical Help In Any Of The Following Situations:

■ Measles in children of less than six months old.

■ If fever doesn't subside as the rash fully emerges.

■ Extreme lethargy or weakness with feverishness that does not resolve itself.

■ Any sign of breathing difficulties or severe cough.

■ Extreme light sensitivity with signs of potential eye infection.

■ Persistent or severe headache, especially if combined with vomiting and/or stiff neck.

■ Bleeding under the skin or from any orifices of the body.

■ Ear infection.

■ If your child develops measles your GP should be notified. He, in turn, will register all cases with the local health authority.

Mumps

Mumps is an unpleasant viral childhood illness which is characterized by painful, swollen glands in the face. It usually begins with a child feeling generally unwell with a raised temperature. The *parotid glands* located under the ears become tender and swollen as well as the *salivary glands* under the tongue and the jaw. If the latter happens, swallowing and opening the mouth become very painful. The glandular swelling may often affect one side of the face, spreading to the other as the course of the illness develops.

Mumps has an incubation period of two to four weeks and is generally not as contagious as measles.

Practical Self-Help

■ Make sure your child has plenty of fluid to drink, avoiding any citrus flavours that may may make the salivary glands feel more tender. If your child is not keen to drink, make lollipops from non-acidic bases such as apple juice, or encourage your child to eat as much fluid-filled fruit as possible, e.g. melon.

■ Some children with mumps feel more comfortable if warm pads are applied to the tender areas of the face. Commercially-produced heat pads may be used, or you can make your own by wrapping a hot-water bottle in a towel. Alternatively, soak a flannel in warm water and wring it out well before applying it to the painful areas.

■ If your child is having difficulty opening his or her mouth, drinks should be given through a straw, and foods should be blended. Soups and broths are also easier to eat than solid food if the mouth and jaw are tender. Liquid foods of this kind have an added bonus of being easier to digest.

■ If your child has mumps, it is important that they should avoid contact with adults who have not suffered from the illness. Although not extremely contagious, if mumps is contracted by an adult the symptoms can be much more severe and distressing than they are in childhood. Women may suffer a complication of inflammation of the ovaries (called *oophoritis*), while men may develop painful swelling of the testicles (*orchitis*). There is also a small chance of men being made infertile if they develop mumps as adults.

Homoeopathic Help

Type of mumps	General symptoms	Worse from	Better for	Remedy name
Extreme restlessness and anxiety with onset of illness.	Rapid onset of illness with great physical and emotional distress. Feverish and thirsty with burning head and chilled body. Burning, stabbing pains are intensified by chill. Child is fearful and panicked by symptoms. Indicated for initial symptoms of *orchitis* in adults.	Extreme heat or chill. Warm rooms. At night.	Fresh air. After sleep. Sweating.	**Aconite**
Rapid, violent onset of symptoms with very high temperature, headache and irritability.	Abrupt descent into illness with extreme feverishness and very bright red, dry, hot skin. Painful and sensitive throat and glands with great difficulty in swallowing: has to bend forward to swallow liquids. Right side may be more affected than the left.	Noise. Touch. Movement. Bright light. Chill. Stooping.	Resting propped-up in bed. Warmth.	**Belladonna**
Slow, insidious development of illness with extreme sensitivity to movement.	Although drowsy and lethargic by day, child cannot sleep at night. Marked thirst for large drinks of cold water with dry skin, mouth and lips. Irritable, constipated and headachy: can't be bothered to do anything.	Movement. Sitting up. Warmth. Physical effort.	Keeping as still as possible. Cool surroundings. Cool drinks. Perspiring.	**Bryonia**
Left-sided glandular pain and swelling that moves to the right.	Severe sense of constriction in throat that is made much worse for tight clothes around the neck. Child finds it easier to swallow food than saliva on its own. All symptoms are much worse when waking from sleep.	Warm drinks. After sleep. Tight collars. Warm surroundings. Empty swallowing.	Cool food and drinks. Cool, airy surroundings. Loose clothing around neck. Swallowing food.	**Lachesis**

Type of mumps	General symptoms	Worse from	Better for	Remedy name
Extremely puffy, swollen glands with marked aversion to heat in any form.	Rosy-red, puffy swellings in glands with stinging pains. 'Water bag' swelling of eyelids: lips and face may also look taut and swollen. Child is irritable, fussy and fidgety.	Warm bathing. Warm compresses. Overheated rooms. Resting. After sleep.	Cool bathing. Cool compresses. Contact with fresh, cool air. Gentle movement.	**Apis**
Mumps with severe swelling of glands making movement of the jaw very difficult.	Speaking, eating and drinking are very difficult due to stiff, enlarged glands. Tonsils are painful and swollen with irritating dryness at the back of the throat. Thirsty, flushed and feverish. Weak and sweaty with illness.	Sweating. Left side. Cold.		**Jaborandi**
Extreme restlessness with mumps that is intensified at night.	Terrific sensitivity to cold and damp with aching in limbs: tosses and turns constantly. Painful swollen glands which may be worse on the left side. Cold sores on the lips may emerge with illness. Child is morose and depressed, especially at night.	Keeping still. At night. In bed. Cold, damp air.	Warm bathing. Warm wraps. Gentle movement provided it does not lead to overexertion.	**Rhus tox**
Mumps with shooting pains in the ears when swallowing.	Tense, hard glands adjacent to the ear and below the jaw. Difficult swallowing from pain in glands and dryness in throat. Tonsils and uvula look swollen, puffy and dark red. The right side may be more severely affected than the left.	Warmth of bed. Cold. At night. Hot drinks.	Moderate warmth that does not overheat.	**Phytolacca**

Type of mumps	General symptoms	Worse from	Better for	Remedy name
Established stage of mumps once fever has subsided.	Bad breath with unpleasant metallic taste. Increased saliva with swollen tongue. Profuse, unpleasant-smelling perspiration. Child becomes extremely anxious and restless with the approach of night.	Extreme heat or chill. Cold draughts. Perspiring. At night.	Moderate temperatures. Resting.	**Mercurius**
Established stage of mumps with weepiness and clinginess.	Indicated for low-grade symptoms that persist once fever has subsided if general symptoms agree. Dry mouth without thirst. Discomfort is much worse in warm, stuffy surroundings or from warmth of bed.	At night. Stuffy rooms. Heavy covers. Resting. Warm food and drinks.	Fresh, cool surroundings. Gentle movement. Cool food and drinks. Firm pressure. Sympathy and affection.	**Pulsatilla**

Seek Prompt Medical Help In Any Of The Following Situations:

- **If vomiting is accompanied by abdominal pains.**
- **Marked weakness or lethargy.**
- **Problems with vision or hearing.**
- **Distressing, severe headache with very stiff neck.**
- **Convulsions.**
- **If your child develops mumps your GP should be notified.**

Nappy Rash

Nappy rash can vary in severity from a mild skin eruption which causes little distress to an inflamed or spotty rash which covers an extensive area of the genitals, buttocks or thighs. It is often irritated by chemicals that are present in urine and/or faeces, and by traces of detergent that may be left in poorly-rinsed towelling nappies.

It is best to treat the rash when it first appears, in order to avoid the possible complication of your baby developing a fungal infection. Although homoeopathic treatment can be very effective in dealing with nappy rash, it is important to stress that the remedies listed below should only be used for the occasional, mild outbreak. If your baby is suffering from severe or recurrent episodes of this problem, it is best to seek help from a homoeopathic practitioner.

Also take care when using deep-acting remedies such as **Calc carb** and **Sulphur**. These can promote a long-term, deep-seated, positive action when they match the characteristic symptoms of the patient. As a result, they should not be repeated frequently or over an extended period of time. If you are in doubt, always stop giving the remedy and wait for a few days in order to observe the reaction that is taking place. Alternatively, if you are feeling confused or unsure about how to proceed, consult a professional practitioner.

Practical Self-Help

■ Leave your baby without nappies for regular periods of time. Exposing the affected skin to the air can promote healing. However, always ensure that the room temperature is kept comfortably warm in order to prevent your baby getting a chill.

■ Change nappies frequently.

■ Avoid using plastic pants which can aggravate the problem by sealing in moisture. Experimenting with different types of nappy liners and throw-away nappies can be helpful in enabling you to find the best combination for your baby.

■ Use soap powder instead of biological formulations when washing towelling nappies. Also, make sure that they are thoroughly rinsed so that traces of detergent are not being left in the fibres.

■ Avoid giving your baby acidic or sugary fruit juices which can irritate an already sensitive skin.

■ Apply **Calendula** ointment to the affected area after each nappy change.This will help soothe the skin, as well as easing redness and inflammation. If your baby is sensitive to the lanolin base of the ointment, opt instead for **Calendula** cream which is lighter, and more easily-absorbed. **Hypercal** cream or ointment, a combination of **Hypericum** and **Calendula**, may be used if your baby is in great discomfort or distress from nappy rash.

■ Always make sure that you dry the affected area thoroughly after each nappy change, before applying the appropriate cream or ointment.

Homoeopathic Help

Type of nappy rash	General symptoms	Worse from	Better for	Remedy name
Nappy rash that is soothed by contact with cool air.	Rash looks rosy-red, shiny and very sore. Touch causes great distress as does contact with heat in any form. Baby is fidgety and restless.	Warm rooms. Hot weather. Resting. Warm clothing. Touch. Becoming damp.	Contact with cool air. Cool compresses. Removing nappy. Movement.	**Apis**
Burning hot nappy rash that is irritated by urinating.	Skin quickly becomes hot and severely inflamed. Baby cannot sleep at night because of irritation of skin: drowsy during the day. Is generally hypersensitive, restless and irritable.	Passing water. Chill. Touch. Movement.	Warmth.	**Cantharis**
Irritated skin that is relieved by warm compresses.	Although rash is burning, itchy and inflamed, baby is soothed by contact with warmth in any form. Digestive problems may accompany rash. Baby is very restless, distressed and fretful with itching.	Chill. Cool compresses. Exertion. At night.	Warmth. Warm bathing. Warm compresses. Movement.	**Arsenicum alb**
Extremely itchy nappy rash that causes great distress and restlessness at night.	Flaky, burning, maddeningly itchy spots that make baby toss and turn in a desperate effort to get comfortable. Exposure to cold and damp causes great distress while being rocked or carried is soothing.	Chill. Damp. Keeping still. At night. Overheating. Warmth of bed.	Being carried. Moderate temperatures.	**Rhus tox**

Type of nappy rash	General symptoms	Worse from	Better for	Remedy name
Bright red, hot, angry-looking rash with dry skin (early stage of rash).	Skin is so hot and inflamed that it radiates heat. Rash appears with suddenness and severity: disappears as rapidly. Placid baby becomes extremely irritable, fractious and bad-tempered.	Jolting or jarring. Lying on irritated skin. Touch. Disturbance or loud noise.	Rest. Peaceful surroundings.	**Belladonna**
Nappy rash in large babies with a tendency to clammy, sour sweats.	Pale, sweaty skin with cracks and chaps. Slow or late experience of developmental milestones, e.g. closure of fontanelles, teething, etc. Generally sluggish system leads to constipation.	Overheating. Chill. Exertion. Contact with cold air. Change of weather. At night.	Moderate warmth. Dry conditions. When constipated.	**Calc carb**
Terribly red, itchy rash that is very sensitive to bathing.	Rash is especially distressing on getting warm in bed: baby is very restless and tries to get limbs out of covers. Raw-looking rash that may bleed from repeated scratching. In common with **Calc carb**, this remedy should not be repeated frequently.	Warmth. Contact with water. Stuffy, overheated rooms. Becoming chilled. Sugary foods.	Cool surroundings. Contact with fresh, cool air.	**Sulphur**
Moist nappy rash with poor healing skin that cracks and weeps.	Itching and discomfort is especially severe in folds of skin around genital area. Skin reacts very badly to becoming overheated. Baby has poor-quality, misshapen or brittle nails.	Becoming cold. Dampness. Overheating. At night.	Exposure to air.	**Graphites**

If nappy rash does not respond to self-help measures, or if your baby is subject to regular or severe bouts of the problem, professional advice should be consulted.

Teething

Problems with teething vary a great deal from baby to baby, with some experiencing great distress while others take it in their stride. Although the first teeth (called milk teeth or incisors) appear during the first year, they are likely to cause little disturbance apart from minor swelling and inflammation of the gums. Possible additional symptoms may include dribbling or drooling from the mouth, as well as a tendency to chew on firm objects such as a teething ring or fingers.

However, the first and second molars, which are the next to appear, are far more likely to cause distress. These should emerge any time between the ages of one and three. Common symptoms include swelling, heat and inflammation of the gums and cheek on the affected side of the mouth, as well as a general state of irritability and weepiness from pain.

Practical Self-Help

■ Firm pressure is usually soothing to inflamed, painful gums. Either rub the sensitive gums gently, or let your baby gnaw on biscuits which are especially manufactured for this purpose. However, if your baby is chewing on anything, always watch what is happening in order to ensure that there is no risk of choking.

■ Contact with cool items is often soothing to babies with inflamed, sensitive gums. Teething rings are available with a cavity which can be filled with cool water and kept in the fridge when not in use. Alternatively, give your baby a cool, clean flannel to suck on.

■ Where possible, avoid using sedative formulations. Once an appropriate homoeopathic remedy has been selected and administered, relief from pain and distress should follow very swiftly. However, if you are finding it very difficult to differentiate between homoeopathic remedies, or if you have given what appears to be a well-indicated remedy and it fails to act, seek professional advice. Caring for and comforting a very distressed, teething baby can be a fraught affair, sometimes making it very difficult to select an appropriate homoeopathic remedy with confidence and clarity of thought. A homoeopathic practitioner has the necessary emotional objectivity, as well as professional experience, to choose a suitable prescription for your baby.

Homoeopathic Help

Type of distress with teething	General symptoms	Worse from	Better for	Remedy name
Desperate frustration, anger and howling with teething pains.	Cannot be pacified: throws toys around in frustration. Colic and loose, greenish, watery stools with teething: infant draws knees up to chest. Generally flushed with one pale and one red cheek.	Becoming overheated. Chill. At night.	Being rocked, carried or driven in a car. Moderate warmth. Cool locally applied.	**Chamomilla**
Teething with inflamed, spongy gums that bleed easily.	Offensive-smelling breath with inflamed-looking gums. When teeth emerge, they are of poor quality enamel. Dental cavities develop rapidly. Irritability and restleness with difficulties sleeping at night.	Touch. Lying down. In the fresh air.	Firm pressure. Warmth. Warm food. Movement.	**Kreosotum**
Teething with terrible anxiety and restlessness.	Symptoms are especially severe at night, with infant waking from sleep in a state of great distress. Generally feverish state with hot head and cool limbs and body. Startled expression with oversensitivity to pain.	Chill. Contact with cold air. Touch. At night.	Sound sleep. Moderate, even temperatures.	**Aconite**
Teething with extreme feverishness and flushed, hot, dry skin.	Symptoms develop suddenly and violently. Bright red, hot, inflamed gums which cause great distress. Right-sided ear pain with teething. Light sleep with muscle spasms and jerking. Normally placid, easy-going infant becomes irritable and cross.	Noise. Bright light. Jarring movement. Touch. Chill.	Darkened, quiet rooms. Warmth.	**Belladonna**

Type of distress with teething	General symptoms	Worse from	Better for	Remedy name
Digestive problems with teething, including excessive production of wind and diarrhoea.	Teething occurs later than expected: other milestones may also be delayed, e.g. crawling, walking or talking. Difficulty in assimilating calcium and other nutrients from food, with attendant weight or stamina problems.	Effort. Physical demands. Movement.	Warm bathing. Moderate warmth. Rest.	**Calc phos**
Persistent ear or catarrhal problems with teething.	Difficult to rest at night because of stuffed-up nose: breathes through mouth instead. Mucus is thick, yellowish-green and bland. Weepy, clingy and demanding with pains. Unlike babies requiring **Chamomilla**, infants in **Pulsatilla** state respond well to attention and distraction.	Stuffy, overheated rooms. Lack of fresh air. Lying still. Evening and night. Warmth.	Cool, fresh air. Cool surroundings. Cool drinks. Cool compresses. Gentle movement. Attention and sympathy.	**Pulsatilla**
Delayed, difficult teething in large, sweaty, pale infants.	Teething problems in infants who are generally slow, sluggish and chilly. Cold, sour-smelling sweats are common: scalp and feet are especially clammy. Slow digestion with easy weight gain and constipation. Mild-tempered, placid infants become obstinate, wilful and stubborn when teething.	Overheating. Physical effort. Chill. Dairy products.	Moderate warmth. Resting. When constipated.	**Calc carb**

Seek Professional Advice In The Following Situations:

■ **Persistent digestive or catarrhal problems when your infant is teething**.

■ **If your baby is pulling or rubbing one or both ears**.

■ **If distress and pain do not respond to self-help measures**.

■ **Always resist the temptation to put ill-defined or vague symptoms down to teething problems. If you suspect your teething baby is unwell, always seek professional medical advice**.

Whooping Cough

Whooping cough can be an extremely distressing and frightening experience for both children and parents. It is a contagious illness that affects the lungs, resulting in clogging of the airways with thick mucus that can only be dislodged with great effort.

The initial symptoms of whooping cough resemble those of a cold and may include raised temperature, cough and nasal discharge. However, unlike a cold which should clear up within four or five days, a child with early symptoms of whooping cough will get worse. During the next stage, the nasal discharge thickens and the cough becomes more severe and distressing.

Once this phase is well under way, a child develops the characteristic 'whoop' when coughing. This normally happens at the end of a coughing bout when the child may be gasping for breath, and may be accompanied by vomiting. It is not uncommon during a severe episode of this kind for a child to become extremely flushed, or for the face to become tinged with blue. The latter may happen if the body is short of oxygen. This phase may continue for two to three months with symptoms gradually diminishing in intensity as the disease progresses. However, a child may be left with a residual, low-grade cough for several months.

Whooping cough has an incubation period of one to two weeks.

Practical Self-Help

■ Although the coughing bouts may be very alarming, it is essential to refrain from giving cough-suppressants in an effort to prevent the cough occurring. It is vital that the coughing reflex is allowed to happen because it is attempting to expel mucus from the lungs. If this mechanism is compromised, the lungs are likely to become clogged with mucus, making breathing much more difficult.

■ If your child vomits with whooping cough, it is best to give small, easily-digested meals after a coughing spasm. Also make sure that your child has plenty to drink, especially if they are not keen to eat.

■ Babies are normally most comfortable lying on their stomachs over your knees during a coughing bout. Make sure that their faces are unobstructed so that they can cough freely, and pat their backs gently in order to assist them. Children are generally most comfortable sitting upright with their backs supported.

■ Although it may be very difficult, try to be as calm and reassuring as possible when your child has a coughing bout. Fear and panic during a severe episode of coughing can make the sense of suffocation worse, which can aggravate the situation. On the other hand, if your child can relax as much as possible, the bout of coughing should be over faster and with less distress.

Homoeopathic Help

Type of whooping cough	General symptoms	Worse from	Better for	Remedy name
Whooping cough with terrible nausea and bouts of coughing ending in vomiting.	Child becomes tense, stiff and breathless during a bout of coughing. Rattly, wheezy chest when coughing. Severe bouts lead to pale, bluish skin colour and nosebleeds. Child is terribly sensitive to movement which makes everything worse.	Damp conditions. Lying flat. Motion. Overheating. Eating.	Fresh air. Cool drinks. Resting.	**Ipecac**
Severe coughing bouts with cold, clammy, bluish-tinged skin.	Child is exhausted and prostrated by whooping cough. Craves fresh air during and after bouts of coughing: relieved by being fanned. Burning, raw sensation in throat and chest. Hard, dry cough rapidly becomes loose and productive.	At night. Stuffy rooms. Heat. Talking.	Fresh, open air. Being fanned. Loosening clothes. After sleep.	**Carbo veg**
Vomiting of clear, stringy, tenacious mucus at end of coughing bout.	Coughing fits may be brought on by overheated, stuffy rooms. Child swallows constantly in an effort to clear the throat of mucus. Face becomes reddish-purple from the effort of coughing. Very sensitive to any sense of irritation in throat.	Heat. Lying down. Touch. Pressure of clothes. Irritation in throat. Brushing teeth. Rinsing mouth.	Cool drinks. Walking. Bathing with cool water.	**Coccus cacti**

Type of whooping cough	General symptoms	Worse from	Better for	Remedy name
Coughing bouts begin after a distressing smothering sensation.	Episodes of coughing follow each other in quick succession. Vomiting stringy mucus after coughing spasms. Cough is brought on by eating. Body temperature fluctuates: too hot when covered, chilled when uncovered.	Inhaled air. Eating. Change of air.	Warmth.	**Corallium rubrum**
Coughing bouts begin as soon as child lies down.	Severe coughing spasms with vomiting, cold sweats and nosebleeds. Tickling and irritation in throat. Choking coughing fits continue for a long time.	After midnight. Lying down. Heat. Cold food. Talking. Laughing. Stooping.	Fresh air.	**Drosera**
Child bend backwards during coughing spasms in an effort to bring up mucus.	Breathlessness before coughing spasms. Rattling, congested chest with very little mucus raised. Vomits or sleeps after coughing bouts. Child has to sit up in order to breathe.	Warmth. Tantrums. Lying down. Becoming too hot or chilled. Movement. Drinking milk.	Bringing up mucus. Sitting up. Vomiting.	**Anti tart**
Aching, brushed sensations in chest from coughing.	Child becomes distressed before coughing bouts anticipating the discomfort it will bring. Presses hands against chest in an effort to hold it still in order to minimize pain.	During sleep. After exertion. At night. Cold, damp conditions.	Resting with head low.	**Arnica**
Coughing spasms with easily-raised mucus.	Cough dries up in cold air, becoming looser in warm surroundings. Sits forward in order to feel more comfortable during coughing bouts. Suffocative, choking feelings before vomiting.	Cold air. Becoming overheated. Exertion. Between 2–3 a.m. Dehydration. Touch. Movement.	Warmth. Sitting leaning forwards with elbows on knees. During the day. Fresh air.	**Kali carb**

Seek Prompt Medical Help In any Of The Following Situations:

■ If whooping cough occurs in a baby under six months of age.

■ Severe breathing difficulties, wheezing, or laboured, accelerated breathing alternating with bouts of coughing.

■ Distressing chest pain.

■ Confusion or drowsiness.

■ Severe headache.

■ If self-help measures are not relieving the situation and you feel that the health of your child is deteriorating rather than improving.

■ It is wise to be aware that whooping cough is a potentially serious illness in very young babies and children. If you suspect that your child is showing the early symptoms of whooping cough, notify your GP. He or she may want to arrange for an examination in order to confirm the diagnosis.

■ Refer to the *Cough* section for further indications that might suggest the need for professional help.

■7■
Homoeopathy For Women

Many women are drawn to the holistic approach of homoeopathic medicine because of its emphasis on treating the whole patient on emotional, mental and physical levels. If we consider the wide range of physical and emotional symptoms covered by the diagnostic label of premenstrual syndrome, the homoeopathic approach to treatment makes a great deal of sense in dealing with women's problems.

When treating a patient with PMS, her homoeopath will strive to select the most appropriate remedy that covers the symptoms as a whole, rather than giving one remedy for fluid retention, another for breast tenderness, an extra remedy for headaches, and something else for irritability and mood swings. Because homoeopathic medicines work by stimulating energy levels, enabling the body to regain a sense of balance and harmony, problems involving hormone imbalances often respond well to the homoeopathic approach.

However, homoeopathic treatment for women is not limited to dealing with conditions such as hot flushes, painful periods, PMS or heavy menstrual bleeding. The potential range of conditions that may be treated with homoeopathy is extremely wide and varied, including migraines, fatigue, recurrent colds, eczema, hayfever, irritable bowel syndrome, insomnia, cystitis, arthritis, anxiety and depression.

In addition, homoeopathic treatment has a great deal to offer in easing problems that may arise during pregnancy, including morning sickness, heartburn, constipation and haemorrhoids. Increasing numbers of women are making use of homoeopathy and other complementary therapies such as acupuncture or aromatherapy during labour and childbirth, while homoeopathic treatment can be of tremendous help in treating both mother and baby in the initial phase after delivery.

Deciding When To Prescribe

Generally speaking, the newcomer to homoeopathic prescribing should only attempt to treat conditions that fall into an 'acute' category. These are illnesses that have a limited life span and tend to clear up of their own accord, provided appropriate conditions are available to support recovery. Good examples of this kind of problem include stomach upsets, the common cold, and cuts and bruises.

However, many of the conditions discussed in this chapter fall into a category which is categorized as 'chronic'. This does not refer to the severity of the problem but is used to describe a long-term condition that is liable to repeated flare-ups over time. Unfortunately, these acute episodes, which often occur within the framework of a chronic condition, are unable to resolve the situation. The result is a long-term battle with a condition such as pre-menstrual syndrome, stress incontinence or painful periods.

Generally speaking, homoeopathic treatment for chronic problems is best obtained from a homoeopathic practitioner in order for the best outcome to be obtained. However, the advice given in the *Practical Self-Help* sections may be of great help in alleviating the condition while homoeopathic advice is sought.

It is also worth bearing in mind that it is sometimes appropriate to self-prescribe a well-indicated homoeopathic remedy for an acute bout of a chronic condition such as cystitis. If you suffer from mild or infrequent bouts of cystitis, and you can select an appropriate homoeopathic remedy with confidence, you may be able to do a great deal to ease the situation by self-prescribing. However, if you suffer from regular bouts of severe cystitis, this is an indication that the situation is a full-blown, chronic condition and you should seek professional advice.

See **Chapter 2:** *Homoeopathy In The Home: How To Use This Book* for more detailed information about assessing the condition to be treated, selecting and taking the indicated remedy.

Urogenital Problems

Cystitis

Cystitis is a very common complaint in women, especially during pregnancy. Although some women find that they have a single attack that is successfully treated and never appears again, many others are subject to recurrent episodes of the condition.

Cystitis occurs because the bladder has become inflamed, usually as a result of bacterial infection travelling up the urethra. Symptoms include: a frequent, urgent desire to pass water, passage of very concentrated, dark-coloured, strong-smelling urine, stinging or burning on passing urine, feverishness, abdominal discomfort, and a general feeling of being unwell.

The odd bout of cystitis may be effectively treated by selecting an appropriate homoeopathic remedy from the table below, and following the self-help advice for an acute episode of infection. However, if you are subject to very severe or recurrent problems with cystitis, it is best to seek advice from a homoeopathic practitioner who will want to address your underlying predisposition to the condition, rather than limiting treatment to the short-term easing of immediate symptoms.

Practical Self-Help

■ At the first twinge of discomfort, drink a large glass of water, repeating the process every hour until symptoms have eased.

■ Drinking cranberry juice can do a great deal to ease the discomfort of cystitis by making urine more alkaline. If you feel early symptoms of cystitis developing, drink a glass of cranberry juice at hourly intervals until discomfort has eased. Once the acute phase of infection has passed, drink a glass of cranberry juice twice daily until you are sure the problem has gone.

■ If cranberry juice is not available, home-made barley water is also an excellent, soothing, alkaline drink to take during a bout of crystitis. Two tablespoonfuls of a pearl barley should be added to a litre of water, then boil and strain the liquid, which should be cooled in the fridge until needed. Unfortunately, commercially-produced barley waters are not a suitable substitute. These contain a large proportion of sugar with added citrus flavouring, which can lead to increased irritation of the bladder.

■ If possible, take it easy during the acute phase of cystitis. This is particularly important if you feel generally feverish and unwell at the beginning of an attack. By resting during this phase it is often possible to overcome the problem more effectively and rapidly.

■ Avoid the following items during a bout of cystitis, since they are likely to aggravate the problem: citrus fruits, sugary foods and drinks, caffeinated soft drinks, coffee, tea and alcohol. If you suffer from recurrent bouts of cystitis these foods and drinks are best avoided altogether, or taken in very infrequent or moderate amounts.

■ If you have a tendency to develop cystitis, never put off the urge to pass water. If urine is allowed to build up, it can encourage infection of the bladder and kidneys. Also make a conscious effort to empty your bladder completely each time you pass water.

■ Guard against constipation by drinking a large glass of water at regular intervals through the day. Also make sure that you include lots of high fibre foods in your diet.

■ Eat regular portions of fresh fruit and vegetables daily, avoiding those that have a reputation for aggravating cystitis. These include grapes, citrus fruits, strawberries, spinach, tomatoes, asparagus, potatoes and raw carrots.

■ If sugary foods and drinks are a regular feature of your diet, make a special effort to cut down. This is especially important if you suffer from thrush as well as cystitis, since sugar intake can aggravate both conditions. Explore alternative soft drinks which are naturally sweetened with fruit juices rather than artificial sweeteners or white sugar. Also watch out for 'hidden' sugar content which may be labelled as corn syrup, glucose or dextrose.

■ If you suffer from recurrent bouts of cystitis, emptying the bladder before and after intercourse can be a positive way of discouraging repeated infection. Washing the genital area gently with warm water (without the addition of strongly-perfumed bubble bath or soap) can also be very helpful.

■ Always wipe from front to back after passing a stool. This is an important way of avoiding transferring bacteria from the anus to the urinary tract.

■ Avoid wearing tight trousers, tights, leggings, or nylon underwear that favour the growth of bacterial or fungal infections. Instead opt for loose-fitting clothes made from natural fibres such as cotton or linen.

■ If recurrent bouts of cystitis are a problem, taking a vitamin C supplement can be a helpful way of discouraging infection. However, it is best not to take vitamin C routinely in high doses (over a gram a day) for an extended period of time if you suffer from kidney stones.

■ Garlic supplements are thought to possess valuable anti-bacterial properties, aiding the body in fighting the effects of a broad range of micro-organisms, including those that may lead to urinary tract infections.

■ If you suffer from frequent bouts of cystitis and use a diaphragm, it may be helpful to consider an alternative form of contraception. Diaphragms that fit very snuggly have a tendency to interfere with the free flow of urine from the bladder. The balance of micro-organisms in the vagina can also be adversely affected by the presence of a diaphragm or cap. This imbalance can encourage the growth of E coli, which is one of the most common causes of bladder infections.

Homoepathic Help

Type of cystitis	General symptoms	Worse from	Better for	Remedy name
Cystitis with chilliness, shivering and anxiety.	Terrible physical and mental restlessness when ill. Severe burning sensations on passing water that are relieved by contact with warmth, e.g. hot water bottle. Nausea and/or diarrhoea may accompany cystitis.	Chill. Cool surroundings. At night. Cold drinks. Alcohol. Physical exertion.	Warmth. Sitting propped-up in bed. Sipping warm drinks. Gentle movement. Company. Fresh air to the head and face.	**Arsenicum alb**

Type of cystitis	General symptoms	Worse from	Better for	Remedy name
Cystitis with stinging pains and general state of fluid retention.	Minimal or absent thirst with fluid retention. Stinging, scalding urine that has to be passed straight away. Terrific sensitivity to heat when unwell. Fussy, fidgety and irritable with cystitis.	Warmth. Warm compresses. Contact with warm air. Resting. Touch. Pressure of clothes. At night.	Cool compresses. Contact with cool air. Uncovering. Continued movement.	**Apis**
Violent attacks of cystitis that set in abruptly with severe burning pains.	Scalding sensations before, during and after passing urine. Distressing, constant urge to pass water: a few drops are passed each time. Discomfort in kidneys as well as bladder. Exhausted, chilly and shivery with feverishness.	Coffee. Passing water. Drinking. Movement.	At night. Warmth. Massage.	**Cantharis**
Initial stage of severe cystitis with abrupt onset.	Feverish with rapid rise of temperature: skin is dry, hot and flushed. Pains and discomfort are intensified by jolting or jarring. Drowsy by day and restless at night. Traces of blood may be present in urine. Irritable, restless and easily disturbed when ill.	Being disturbed. Noise. Bright lights. Jarring. Chill. Pregnancy.	Warmth. Peaceful surroundings. Sitting propped-up in bed. Darkened rooms.	**Belladonna**
'Honeymoon' cystitis or symptoms that follow catheterization during surgery.	Distressing sensation of being unable to fully empty the bladder: a few drops seem to remain. Stinging, burning pains that continue after urine has been passed. Dark, concentrated urine is passed with great effort. Easily angered and irritable with cystitis.	Early morning. Touch or pressure. Intercourse. Surgery or 'high-tech' birth.	Resting. Warmth. Eating.	**Staphy sagria**

Type of cystitis	General symptoms	Worse from	Better for	Remedy name
Cystitis that is brought on by exposure to damp and cold.	Chilly, but craves fresh air and cool conditions. Urgent need to pass water: if it is delayed, urine is passed involuntarily. Thrush may be present with cystitis. Discomfort and urgency are much worse when lying down or resting. Tearful and in need of sympathy when ill.	Warmth. Stuffy surroundings. Warm food or drinks. Resting. Being alone.	Cool, fresh air. Cool drinks. Gentle exercise. Company. Having a good cry. Sympathy.	**Pulsatilla**
Cystitis with extreme cold sensitivity and irritability.	Indicated in situations of 'burn out' where there is overconsumption of alcohol, coffee and junk foods. Spasmodic pains in bladder and bowel. Burning and itching accompanies passage of urine.	Cold surroundings. Draughty conditions. Coffee. Alcohol. After eating. Touch. Lack of sleep.	Sound sleep. Peace and quiet. Warmth.	**Nux vomica**

Seek Prompt Medical Help In Any Of The Following Situations:

■ If there is any suggestion of pain in the hollow of the back or sides, accompanied by vomiting and/or high temperature.

■ If urine is tinged with blood.

■ If symptoms are severe or persistent and do not respond to self-help measures.

Thrush

Although it is considered a minor problem, the symptoms of genital thrush can cause a great deal of distress, irritation and frustration. Problems arise when the micro-organism *candida albicans* spreads, and an overgrowth occurs. Although it is normally kept in check by the friendly bacteria that live in the gut, if a factor is introduced that upsets this balance in microflora, candida begins to colonize areas where it shouldn't be found.

Antibiotic treatment is a major culprit in undermining the balance in the gut between friendly and not-so-friendly bacteria. Because antibiotics often wipe out the microbes that have a positive role to play, as well as the bacteria that are being targeted by the drug, the result is often an overgrowth of candida. Antibiotics can also have a deleterious effect on the acid-producing bacteria in the vagina that keep candida in check, leading to symptoms of genital thrush. Additional factors that can cause similar problems include the use of vaginal deodorants, douches or strongly-perfumed bubble baths that can interfere with the action of acid-forming bacteria. Hormonal fluctuations in pregnancy, or in users of the contraceptive pill, can lead to changes in vaginal conditions which permit symptoms of thrush to arise. Those who suffer from diabetes are also susceptible to bouts of vaginal thrush.

The following are common symptoms of vaginal thrush:

- Irritation and itching of the vagina and vulva.
- Increased need to pass water.
- Soreness and/or burning when passing urine.
- Painful sensitivity during intercourse.
- A thick, white, creamy or yellowish, yeasty-smelling discharge that resembles the appearance and texture of cottage cheese.

If candida overgrowth is widespread, the following symptoms may also occur:

- Pre-menstrual syndrome including mood swings, breast enlargement and tenderness, fluid-retention and fatigue.
- Problems with digestion, including alternating diarrhoea and constipation, heartburn, indigestion, bloating of the abdomen and a tendency to hypoglycaemia (low blood sugar levels).
- Urinary tract infections.
- Food sensitivities or allergic reactions.
- Joint pains.
- Chronic exhaustion.
- Unexplained skin rashes and disorders.

If you suffer from mild and infrequent episodes of vaginal thrush, an appropriately-selected homoeopathic remedy combined with basic self-help measures should do a great deal to alleviate the immediate irritation and distress. However, if you suffer from the more general symptoms of *candidiasis* (overgrowth of candida), treatment should be sought from a trained homoeopathic practitioner, who will have the necessary expertise to deal with the problem at a more fundamental level.

Practical Self-Help

- If thrush is a recurrent problem, it is best to avoid the foods and drinks that can aggravate the condition. These include alcohol, tea, cheese, sugar, sweetened drinks, malted foods, white bread, red meat that has been treated with growth hormones and antibiotics, mushrooms, vinegar, pickles, and any foods or drinks that have been fermented. Foods to concentrate on instead include whole foods (as close to their unrefined state as possible), fruit, fresh vegetables, pulses, brown rice, natural live yoghourt, fish, herb teas or tisanes, and four or five large glasses of mineral water daily.

■ In order to relieve itching and irritation, take a salt bath (add a tablespoonful of common salt to your bathwater) or douche with a solution of half a teaspoon of vinegar and a cup of water. Natural yoghurt, used straight from the fridge, is also very soothing when applied to the irritated area.

■ Steer clear of scented or highly-perfumed foam baths, bath oils, soaps and vaginal deodorants, which can make irritation worse.

■ Wear loose-fitting underwear made from natural fibres such as cotton. Avoid tight-fitting synthetic underwear, tight jeans, tights, or leggings which create a moist, warm environment that favours the growth of *candida albicans*, the micro-organism that causes thrush.

■ If you use a barrier method of contraception, you may have a sensitivity to the condoms, creams or gels that you are using if you suffer recurrent problems with thrush.

■ Garlic supplements may be very helpful in acting as an antifungal agent. Because it is often anti-social to eat enough fresh garlic in the diet to be therapeutically helpful (many people are very sensitive to the smell of garlic), odourless supplements can be immensely useful. Two tablets of concentrated, powdered garlic should be taken three times daily while an acute attack of thrush is present. This may be cut down to a maintenance dose of one concentrated tablet a day once the immediate problem has receded.

■ Well-established or recurrent symptoms may respond well to supplementing with acidophilus, caprylic acid, or oil of evening primrose.

■ If you suspect your immune system is functioning below par as a result of stress, supplementing with vitamin C and B complex is likely to be helpful. One to three grams of vitamin C may be taken daily during an acute episode of thrush, reducing the dose to a level of bowel tolerance if loose stools occur. Also ensure that you obtain a non-yeast-based formulation of B complex.

■ It is important to avoid the temptation of using over-the-counter creams which have a localized anaesthetic effect. These will only mask the symptoms for a short while, without having any effect on the source of the problem. It is also possible to develop a sensitivity to the cream, which can irritate the problem further.

Homoeopathic Help

Type of thrush	General symptoms	Worse from	Better for	Remedy name
Thrush that occurs mid-way through menstrual cycle.	Bouts of thrush with sensitivity, itching, burning, and swollen sensation in vagina. Discharge may be hot, irritating, bland, thin, or like egg white. Sensation as though warm water is flowing down thighs.	Uncovering. Warmth. After a period. Touch.	Cool conditions.	**Borax**
Thrush with burning sensation that is soothed by warmth.	Irritation and discomfort are eased by general contact with warmth and warmth locally-applied. Discharge is burning, thin, watery, and clear. Vulva feels very inflamed and sensitive. Anxious, restless and exhausted when ill.	Cold conditions. Cold drinks. At night. Alcohol.	Warmth. Sips of warm drinks. Warmth locally applied. Gentle movement.	**Arsenicum alb**
Thrush with thick, offensive, irritating, yellowish discharge.	Disinclination for intercourse because of sensitivity and dryness of vagina. Extreme itching which is aggravated when walking. Exhausted, depressed, irritable and stressed with symptoms.	Mornings. Before periods. Sitting still. Emotional strain.	Vigorous exercise in the fresh air. In bed. Eating. Sound sleep. In the afternoon.	**Sepia**
Thrush with painful dryness of vagina.	Thick discharge like uncooked egg white, or thin, clear, watery discharge. Aversion to intercourse because of painful, burning dryness of vagina. Depressed, withdrawn, and despondent with symptoms.	Warmth. Lack of cool, fresh air. Touch. Sympathy. After sleep. During or after a period.	Cool, fresh conditions. Cool compresses and cool bathing. Skipping meals. Gentle movement.	**Nat mur**

Type of thrush	General symptoms	Worse from	Better for	Remedy name
Thrush with chilliness and low back pain.	Urgent desire to pass water with general sensitivity of vagina. Thrush is aggravated before a period and becoming chilled. Itchy, burning discharge with cramping pains in muscles.	Cold or chill. Overheating. Physical effort. After pregnancy. After intercourse. Touch. Movement.	Fresh air. Warmth. During the day.	**Kali carb**
Thrush with thick, sour-smelling, smarting discharge.	Thrush with sluggish metabolism, weight gain, and persistent constipation. Aggravation of symptoms leading up to and after a period, with cravings for sugar or dairy foods. Poor stamina with constant exhaustion and flushing after slightest physical effort.	Chilly, cold conditions. Bathing. Physical effort. At night.	Moderate warmth. When constipated.	**Calc carb**
Thrush with very itchy discharge that causes awful restlessness at night.	Difficulty sleeping from itching when warm in bed. Cool bathing eases itching. Vaginal discharge is very apparent when passing water. Alternating hot and cold sensations with perspiration and a marked dislike of cold draughts.	Extreme changes of temperature. Becoming overheated in bed. Humidity. Touch.	Resting. Moderate temperatures.	**Mercurius**
Recurrent thrush with symptoms of pre-menstrual syndrome.	Thrush occurs before a period, at puberty, or during pregnancy. Thick, yellowish, bland discharge with marked discomfort and irritation from becoming warm. Severe mood swings, weepiness, and craving for sympathy and affection when unwell.	At night. Warmth. Stuffy conditions. Dairy foods. Resting. Becoming heated in bed.	Cool, fresh air. Cool locally applied. Gentle movement. Uncovering. Having a good cry. Sympathy.	**Pulsatilla**

Type of thrush	General symptoms	Worse from	Better for	Remedy name
Extreme itching that is worse for contact with heat in any form.	Severe or recurrent thrush with itching that affects perineum (area from vulva to anus). Heavy, offensive, yellow or white discharge which is very marked before a period. Irritability with tendency to recurrent headaches.	Washing or contact with water. Becoming warm overheated in bed. Sugary foods. Chill. Standing. During the menopause.	Moderate, steady temperatures. Res	**Sulphur**
Thrush with terrible burning and smarting that is felt deep in the vagina.	Great discomfort with irritating, offensive, yellow vaginal discharge that stains underwear. Pulling, or dragging sensations in back or genital area. Very irritable and restless with discomfort.	Walking. Standing. Chill. Cool bathing. Lying down. Touch.	Sitting. Warmth.	**Kreosotum**

Seek Medical Advice In Any Of The Following Situations:

■ If self-help measures failed to improve the situation.

■ If you are subject to severe or recurrent bouts of thrush.

■ If vaginal irritation or discharge appears for the first time, it is wise to seek a medical opinion in order to establish that it is thrush. By doing so, other possible reasons for infection can be ruled out.

Gynaecological Problems

Pre-Menstrual Syndrome

The range of symptoms covered by the definition of pre-menstrual syndrome (PMS) is extremely wide, with a variety of problems affecting emotional and physical health falling within this diagnosis. The severity of emotional symptoms connected with PMS can be astonishing, with many women finding that they are relaxed and well-balanced for one half of the month, but they become emotional time-bombs during the second half of their monthly cycle. Rapid mood swings from depression to euphoria, irritability, violent outbursts of anger, tearfulness, and self-destructive feelings of lack of self-esteem can emerge at this time. Additional problems often include poor concentration, apathy, lack of drive, difficulties with co-ordination, low libido, and general mental and physical exhaustion.

If we add to this list the range of physical problems that can emerge at this time, the problem of PMS is one that clearly needs to be taken seriously. Physical symptoms may include breast tenderness and enlargement, a general state of fluid-retention with fingers, feet and waist being especially affected, food cravings and irregular appetite, pains at ovulation (mid-cycle), severe period pains, migraines and/or headaches, acne, insomnia, cystitis and thrush. Bouts of PMS can vary from mild to severe episodes of physical and emotional imbalance. Although intermittent, the latter can seriously affect the quality of our lives, diminishing our pleasure and zest for living.

However, there are positive steps to be taken which can do a great deal to ease the problems of PMS. Unlike conventional medicine, which tends to limit itself to advice about hormone therapy, diuretics, use of tranquillizers and/or anti-depressants for extreme emotional symptoms, the alternative perspective takes a much broader view of the situation.

Alternative practitioners such as homoeopaths, herbalists or acupuncturists regard each case of PMS as being unique to the patient who is suffering the symptoms. In other words, although there are common symptoms of PMS that many women suffer from, such as irritability, mood swings, fluid-retention or poor concentration, there will be individualizing aspects to these symptoms that make them unique to the patient. For example, one PMS sufferer may experience extreme irritability that is eased by being in sympathetic and attentive company, while another may find that they are made much more on edge by supportive company, and considerably relieved by being left alone.

Practitioners who approach the problems of PMS from a holistic perspective are also likely to give general advice on positive steps that can be taken to improve overall levels of health and vitality. This might include information on helpful dietary changes, exercise, relaxation, and general advice on stress reduction. Some of this advice is included in the *Practical Self-Help* section below, since it may alleviate mild or infrequent symptoms of PMS.

In addition, occasional doses of a well-selected homoeopathic remedy may do a great deal to relieve the distress of immediate symptoms. However, if your symptoms are well established, severe, or do not respond to self-help measures, it is better to consult professional advice rather than attempting to deal with the problem by yourself.

Practical Self-Help

■ Certain foods can contribute to mood swings, fluid-retention and fatigue. These include caffeinated drinks (coffee, tea and cola-type, fizzy sodas), carbonated, sweetened drinks, foods with a high sugar content such as biscuits, cakes, or puddings, alcohol, salt, processed 'instant' meals, and foods which contain large amounts of artificial flavourings and preservatives. Try to drastically cut down, or ideally eliminate these foods from your daily intake, introducing the following dietary items instead.

■ Make sure that foods are as nutritious as possible by choosing to eat items that are as close to their natural state. Of course, this is not a suggestion that foods should be eaten raw when they need to be cooked to be palatable, such as raw lentils or uncooked, wholemeal bread dough! It applies instead to the importance of obtaining foods that have not been freeze-dried, tinned, irradiated, or processed by the addition of chemicals in order to artificially preserve their shelflife well beyond their natural life-span. By choosing whole grains, pulses, fresh fruit and vegetables (ideally eaten steamed or raw), seeds and nuts (unsalted), live natural yoghurt, fresh fruit juices, and small portions of cheese, fish or poultry if we are not vegetarians, we are far less likely to suffer from the symptoms that result from a diet that is mainly comprised of junk foods. These symptoms correspond to many of those suffered by pre-menstrual women and include persistent headaches, low or erratic energy levels, fluid retention, abdominal bloating, constipation, jitteriness, poor concentration and irritability.

■ Cutting down caffeine intake is much easier than it used to be, due to the increasing range of alternatives to tea and coffee now available on the market. Thankfully, the days are gone when the only beverages on offer to those who wanted to avoid caffeine were peppermint tea or dandelion coffee. These days, the choice of herbal teas available has widened enormously, with combinations of herbal flavours appearing that are delicious and refreshing. These can be infused and taken as a hot beverage, or served in tall glasses with added pieces of diced fruit as a cooling summer drink.

■ An excellent range of soft, carbonated drinks is also available for those who want to avoid alcohol, added sugar or caffeine. Although they can be expensive, they provide an excellent alternative to wine when drunk with a meal, and do not have the unpleasant after-taste of low-calorie drinks that rely on artificial additives as sweeteners.

■ Drink four or five large glasses of filtered or mineral water daily, in order to guard against dehydration which can make symptoms of PMS worse. This is especially important if you work in a modern office block with central heating and air conditioning. When combined with double glazing, the result is a hermetically-sealed environment with poor ventilation and a very dry atmosphere. Keep a bottle of mineral water on your desk if it is not convenient to take regular short breaks.

■ Avoid salted foods such as crisps, nuts, and 'instant' meals that include a high proportion of sodium. Explore alternative seasonings to add to your meals, for example ground sesame seeds, toasted herbs such as basil, or seasoned pastes such as tahini. This is especially important if you suffer from fluid retention or high blood-pressure.

■ If you suffer from fuzzy-headedness, fatigue, erratic energy patterns, mood swings and difficulty in concentrating, you may have low blood sugar levels (hypoglycaemia). This is a condition commonly experienced by PMS suffers, and measures that can be taken to stabilize blood sugar levels can be of great benefit in also alleviating symptoms of PMS. To combat this problem, eat small amounts at regular intervals (every two hours if necessary) whenever symptoms appear. Avoid sugary foods that initially give a rush of energy, but quickly leave the body depleted again, leading to a craving for more sugar. Instead, choose a piece of fruit (fruit sugar has a less erratic effect on blood sugar levels than refined, white sugar), a slice of wholemeal bread, rice cakes or raw vegetables. Also avoid other items that have an adverse effect on blood sugar levels, encouraging them to rapidly peak and trough. These include strong, sweetened tea and coffee, chocolate, fizzy sweetened drinks, biscuits and cakes.

■ If you experience mood swings, anxiety or depression, take up a form of exercise that you find enjoyable, challenging and absorbing. This should ideally be an activity that involves regular, rhythmic working of the muscles, e.g. running, walking or low-impact aerobics classes. Regularity is as important as the length of time spent enjoying the activity. Aim to do one half-hour session a minimum of three and a maximum of five times a week. If you are a beginner, build up slowly from ten minute to fifteen, twenty, and finally thirty minute sessions. Exercise of this kind has a beneficial effect on the heart and lungs, but also has an important bearing on emotional health and well-being. This is because it produces pleasure-giving chemicals in the brain called *endorphins* which have a natural, anti-depressant effect. As a result, regular exercise can have a vital role to play in alleviating emotional imbalances and mood swings, as well as improving self-esteem and general well-being as new physical challenges are being met.

■ If stress levels are high, and you feel that they are contributing to your problem, explore relaxation techniques or meditation. If you want to combine learning how to relax with an exercise programme that will encourage overall suppleness and muscular strength, attend a yoga class. A good yoga teacher will teach you how to breathe from your abdomen in order to induce a state of relaxation, as well as general techniques that can be employed for relaxing specific muscle groups.

■ Take care when using a vitamin B supplement. Although B6 is recommended as being helpful in alleviating symptoms of PMS, there is a possibility of toxic side effects arising if this vitamin is taken in high dosage on a regular basis. If supplementing with vitamin B, it is preferable to choose a complex formulation which provides the full range of B vitamins which work best together.

■ Oil of evening primrose, a good quality multivitamin and multimineral formulation, and extra vitamin C, may also help alleviate symptoms of PMS. It is often helpful to supplement your diet with extra nutrients if you feel it has been of a poor quality in the past. However, once the quality of your daily food intake has improved, it should not be necessary to rely on supplements on a long-term basis.

Homoeopathic Help

Type of pre-menstrual syndrome	General symptoms	Worse from	Better for	Remedy name
Deep depression with low sex drive and indifference.	PMS develops after pregnancy, especially if gap between pregnancies has been short, allowing too little time for recovery. Dragging down sensations: pelvic contents feel as though they are about to fall out. Severe mood swings: screaming and shouting alternates with weepiness and apathy.	Any time in menstrual cycle. Touch. Skipping meals. Mornings. Sitting still. Emotional demands.	Vigorous, rhythmical exercise in the fresh air. Walking. Elevating legs. Eating small amounts often.	**Sepia**
Pre-menstrual syndrome with reliance on stimulants, sedatives or alcohol to cope.	General state of physical and emotional 'burn out' from excessively high stress levels. Reliance on coffee to keep going and alcohol to relax. High convenience food intake with resulting constipation, headaches and indigestion. Irritable and snappy before painful periods.	Lack of sleep. On waking. Coffee. Alcohol. Cigarettes. Chilly surroundings. Stress.	Peace and quiet. Warmth. Sound, uninterrupted sleep. Later in the day.	**Nux vomica**

Type of pre-menstrual syndrome	General symptoms	Worse from	Better for	Remedy name
Pre-menstrual syndrome with severe fluid retention.	Sluggish metabolism with chilliness, constipation, breast tenderness and enlargement. Severe backache with general state of tension. Bag-like swelling around eyes, especially around upper eyelids. General state of catarrhal congestion with recurrent sinusitis. Anxiety, panic attacks and inability to sleep before periods.	Chill or cold, draughty conditions. Touch or pressure. Coffee. Early morning.	Fresh air. Daytime. Warmth. Sitting bending forwards with hands supported on knees.	**Kali carb**
Pre-menstrual syndrome with severe headaches and fluid retention.	Recurrent headaches or migraines occur before or after periods. Fluid imbalance leads to dry skin and lack of lubrication in vagina. Craving for salty foods before periods. Dry, cracked lips and cold sores when run down. Weepy, depressed and withdrawn with marked dislike of sympathy and displays of affection.	Touch. Sympathy. Being seen to cry. Heat. Exposure to sunlight.	Being left alone. Peace and quiet. Cool, shady surroundings. Rest. Skipping meals.	**Nat mur**
Pre-menstrual syndrome that is relieved as soon as bleeding begins.	Severe pains at ovulation. Symptoms build in intensity as period approaches with violent mood swings and severe disruption of sleep pattern. Left-sided migraines or headaches improve as soon as period begins. Flow is dark, heavy and clotted.	Becoming heated. Stuffy, airless rooms. Warm bathing. Becoming chilled. Tight clothes around neck or waist. After sleep. Before a period. The left side.	Cool, fresh air. As soon as bleeding begins. Movement.	**Lachesis**

Type of pre-menstrual syndrome	General symptoms	Worse from	Better for	Remedy name
Pre-menstrual syndrome with abdominal bloating and strong craving for sugar.	Constipation alternates with diarrhoea. Rumbling and gurgling in gut with need to pass excess wind. Sensation of gas passing through vagina. Periods are painful and heavy with clotted, dark-coloured flow. Depressed, irritable, insecure, and anxious before periods.	In the afternoons. Becoming chilled or overheated. Restrictive clothes around waist. High-fibre diet. Overexertion. Anticipating speaking in public.	Moderate warmth. Fresh air. Gentle exercise out of doors. Loosening a tight waistband. Being occupied.	**Lycopodium**
Pre-menstrual syndrome with enlarged, painful breasts.	Sluggish metabolism, chronic constipation, weight gain and poor physical stamina intensified before a period. Although chilly, easily overheated with clammy sweat on head and feet. Craves sweets, eggs, milk or indigestible foods. Easily frightened and upset before periods.	Becoming chilled or damp. Cool bathing. Physical or emotional strain. Fresh air.	Moderate warmth. When constipated. Resting.	**Calc carb**
Pre-menstrual syndrome with weepiness and craving for sympathy.	Although chilly with cold hands and feet, warm surroundings are not tolerated well. Nausea, indigestion, diarrhoea, backaches or headaches may occur before or during irregular periods. Recurrent problems with vaginal irritation and discharge. Changeable moods with a tendency to be very weepy in sympathetic company.	Overheated rooms. Lack of fresh air. Rest. At night. Being too warmly clothed. When alone. Rich, creamy foods.	Fresh, cool air. Cool surroundings. Gentle exercise in the fresh air. Having a good cry. Sympathetic company.	**Pulsatilla**

Type of pre-menstrual syndrome	General symptoms	Worse from	Better for	Remedy name
Severe depression with pre-menstrual syndrome that is very intense before a period.	Tension headaches that start at the nape of the neck and extend to the top of the head. Painful periods with shooting, intermittent pains that increase as the flow gets heavier. Severe mood swings with black depression and jitteriness. Unable to control emotions.	Chill. Exposure to cold or damp air. Before or during a period. At night.	While eating. Warmth. After diarrhoea. Walking.	**Cimic**

Seek Medical Help In Any Of The Following Situations:

■ **Severe or well-established symptoms.**

■ **If emotional imbalance is causing great distress, or if there is any suggestion of suicidal feelings being apparent.**

■ **Persistent vaginal discharge, especially if intercourse has become painful.**

■ **Irregular bleeding or 'spotting' between periods.**

■ **If self-help measures have not improved the situation.**

Painful Periods

Although painful periods can occur at any time during the years of fertility, there are certain stages when this is problem is most likely to emerge. Many young women find that the initial phase of menstruation can be difficult, with periods being both irregular and painful. However, the situation can change after pregnancy and childbirth, with periods becoming increasingly less traumatic. Alternatively, many women who experience painful periods in their teens', discover that they become far less distressing once they reach their mid-twenties.

The symptoms of painful periods can vary enormously, with some women experiencing the odd, nagging cramp, while others are totally incapacitated by severe pain. When it is severe, the intensity of pain is hard to imagine if we have not experienced this form of distress.

Additional symptoms that often accompany painful periods include the following:

- Vomiting.
- Diarrhoea.
- Fainting.
- Dizziness.
- Drenching perspiration.
- Headaches or migraines.
- Fatigue and exhaustion.
- Severe mood swings including tearfulness and/or irritability.

Conventional medicine either offers prescription of the contraceptive pill as a way of suppressing the natural monthly cycle of ovulation and bleeding, or drugs which interfere with the synthesis of *prostaglandin*, which has been implicated in causing spasms of the womb.

However, it is important to bear in mind that if we are unhappy with the conventional medical approach to this problem, there are a number of positive self-help measures we can explore in order to improve the situation. This is generally a more attractive option to those of us who prefer to a take a pro-active stance with regard to management of health problems.

If you suffer from mild or infrequent period pains, a well-indicated homoeopathic remedy selected from the table below can do a great deal to ease the immediate situation. However, if you suffer from extremely severe or well-established period pains that have not responded favourably to self-help measures, it is best to consult a homoeopathic practitioner.

Practical Self-Help

- Relaxation techniques can be a valuable tool in combating the distress of painful periods. By learning to breathe from the abdomen rather than the upper chest, it is possible to induce a general state of muscular relaxation. Because most of us respond to pain by tensing or guarding our muscles, thereby making the pain worse, focusing on regular, rhythmic abdominal breathing can be an important way of breaking the vicious circle of general tension. Because anxiety is often an attendant problem to severe pain, breathing from the abdomen is immensely helpful in acting as a natural tranquillizer and calming influence.
- Investigate alternative methods of pain relief such as using a TENS (transcutaneous electrical nerve stimulation) machine. This is an immensely effective, simple way of providing pain relief, often used in pain clinics to ease the distress of those who suffer pain on a chronic (long-term) basis. The TENS

machine consists of a small, battery-operated unit (about the size of a personal cassette player), to which two or four pads are attached. Once they are placed over the site of the pain and the machine is switched on, a small electrical current passes between the pads. The amount of electrical stimulation can be adjusted by the user until a gentle tingling is felt. Once this point is reached, the pain should rapidly subside. Treatment with TENS provides a very attractive alternative to the use of conventional painkillers, since it offers the possibility of pain relief without the potential side effects of liver damage or stomach bleeding. TENS machines are understood to work by providing low-level electrical stimulation that slows down or stops pain messages reaching the brain and nervous system. TENS machines are not limited to treating menstrual cramps, since they can also provide effective relief for back pain, joint pains, post-surgical discomfort and labour pains.

■ Increasing the amount of vigorous exercise taken on a regular basis can also help a great deal with painful periods. Brisk walking, cycling, jogging and swimming stimulate the circulation as well as improving all-over fitness. If stress is contributing to period problems, regular, rhythmic exercise will also help channel the excess adrenalin that is produced when feeling stressed and anxious. As a result, it is possible to unwind more easily and sleep more soundly.

■ If constipation or fluid-retention are recurrent problems, they may contribute to painful periods. Guard against constipation by eating a high-fibre diet that includes a large proportion of fresh fruit, vegetables and whole grains, and drink plentiful quantities of water. If fluid-retention is problematic, avoid foods that have a high salt content, and avoid adding extra salt to your meals. Take regular exercise to stimulate the circulation, and include fresh parsley in your diet as a natural diuretic.

■ If painful periods occur with general symptoms of PMS (see the **Pre-Menstrual Syndrome** section in order to establish whether this could be the case), consider using the following supplements: oil of evening primrose, vitamin B complex, vitamins E and C.

■ If warmth eases the pain, try soaking in a warm (not hot) bath, or applying a heat pad or hot water bottle to the area where the pains are located. A lower back massage can also feel very soothing and comforting when pains are severe.

Homoeopathic Help

Type of painful periods	General symptoms	Worse from	Better for	Remedy name
Period pains that are relieved as soon as bleeding begins.	Severe cramps and symptoms of PMS that occur in the days leading up to a period. Left-sided ovarian pains at mid-cycle. Period pains extend to back and radiate down thighs. Flow is dark in colour and contains clots. Emotionally volatile before periods.	Warmth. Stuffy rooms. After sleep. Tight clothes. During puberty or menopause.	Cool, fresh air. Gentle movement. Once flow begins. Loosening clothes.	**Lachesis**
Chilly, anxious, and restless with period pains.	Vomiting and/or diarrhoea occur with severe pains. Contact with cold makes distress worse, while warmth eases pains. Constantly restless when in pain: exhausted from constant tossing about, but can't stop. Anxious, fussy and fidgety with pains.	At night. Chill. Physical demands. Being alone.	Warmth. Hot water bottle locally applied. Sips of warm drinks. Gentle movement. Company.	**Arsenicum alb**
Period pains with severe constipation from over use of painkillers.	General state of muscular tension from excessive stress levels. High caffeine intake makes pains worse. Severe abdominal cramps and muscle spasms feel better for firm pressure. Extreme irritability and outbursts of anger.	Stress. Cold draughts. Coffee. After eating. Touch. Lack of sleep.	Warmth. Rest. Sound sleep. Firm pressure. Bending double.	**Nux vomica**
Irregular periods with gushing, bright-red bleeding.	Periods come too frequently with violent, labour-like pains. Bearing down sensation with cramps as though contents of pelvis are about to fall out. Profuse, bright-red, clotted flow that feels hot and gushing.	Jarring movements. Lying on painful area. Bright light Noise.	Warmth. Resting propped-up in bed. Peace and quiet.	**Belladonna**

Type of painful periods	General symptoms	Worse from	Better for	Remedy name
Period pains with awful nausea that is aggravated by slightest movement.	Steady, oozing flow of bright-red blood with intermittent gushes. Faint feeling with pain leads to prostration and collapse. Squeezing, pinching cramps around navel, or pains flit from left to right side.	Extreme heat or chill. Eating. Touch. Humidity.	Fresh air. Resting with eyes shut. Firm pressure. Keeping as still as possible.	**Ipecac**
Period pains with frustration and intolerance of pain.	Period arrive early with heavy, dark, clotted flow. Hot and thirsty with pain. Vomits with severe cramps before and during period. Pains radiate to the back and extend down the thighs. Frantic, inconsolable, and abusive with pains.	Heat. Cold draughts. Coffee. Before and during periods.	Moderate temperatures.	**Chamomilla**
Period pains which increase with the flow.	Irregular periods: often too early. Shooting, flitting pains which extend across the lower abdomen and radiate down the thighs. Heavy, dark bleeding with severe clotting. Terribly restless with constant need to change position. Terribly depressed with PMS.	Becoming chilled or damp. Initial movement after rest. During a period. At night.	Warmth. Fresh air. Eating. Diarrhoea. Walking.	**Cimic**
Waves of pain that begin and end abruptly with periods.	Weakness and faintness with pains that build rapidly in severity. Although movement does not give much relief, keeping still feels worse. Doubling-up with pains. Marked agitation and anger with those who try to help.	Damp cold. Anger. Keeping still. Drinking iced water when heated.	Firm pressure. Bending double. Warm compresses or applications.	**Colocynthis**

Type of painful periods	General symptoms	Worse from	Better for	Remedy name
Delayed periods with severe PMS.	Period arrives late, with cutting pains that are aggravated by resting. Scanty flow with flitting pains that are changeable in nature. Craves cool, fresh air although chilly. Headaches and digestive problems occur premenstrually. Weepy and in need of sympathy, affection and support when distressed.	Resting. Warm, stuffy rooms. At night. Warm clothes.	Gentle exercise. Fresh, cool air. Having a good cry. Sympathetic company. Firm pressure.	**Pulsatilla**
Bearing-down pains during period with sensation of or actual prolapse	Scanty flow with a sensation as though pelvic contents are about to fall out. Standing or walking intensify discomfort. Delayed periods with severe depression, exhaustion and apathy.	Before a period. Emotional demands. Sitting still.	Fresh air. Vigorous exercise. Having a sleep. Pressure. Becoming warm in bed.	**Sepia**

Seek Medical Help In Any Of The Following Situations:

■ **Extremely severe period pains.**

■ **Long-term problems with painful periods.**

■ **If previously trouble-free periods have become painful and/or irregular for no obvious reason.**

Homoeopathy For Pregnancy And Childbirth

Morning Sickness

Anyone who has experienced the problems of morning sickness will know that this can be a distressing and trying aspect of early pregnancy. Although the symptoms generally occur within the first twelve weeks of being pregnant and disappear around the end of the third month, some of us are unlucky and suffer symptoms right through the entire pregnancy.

The term 'morning sickness' is rather misleading, since it suggests this is a problem that is restricted to the morning. While many women find that this is the case, there are some who experience sickness in the evening, and others who are unfortunate enough to feel sick and nauseated all day.

However, morning sickness is not an inevitable occurrence, since some women discover that they either experience no sickness at all in the first three months, or suffer from no more than the odd pang of nausea from time to time. As we can see, there are wide variations in the possible severity and frequency of symptoms that may arise in early pregnancy.

Many women find that making use of the simple, self-help measures suggested below is enough to ease the problem of morning sickness. If symptoms are mild or intermittent in nature, it can also be helpful to use an occasional dose of an appropriate homoeopathic remedy. However, if they are persistent or severe in nature, it is far better to consult a trained practitioner who will have the necessary experience to deal with your morning sickness within the broader context of your overall health.

It is also essential to stop self-prescribing if you discover that you need to take a homoeopathic remedy on more than an infrequent or short-term basis to obtain relief. Always remember that homoeopathic remedies should *never* be taken on a routine basis over an extended period of time, but should only be needed for a brief period in order to promote the desired relief of symptoms.

Practical Self-Help

■ If morning sickness is especially severe on getting out of bed, get into the habit of keeping some biscuits and water readily to hand in the bedroom. Make sure that you eat one or two biscuits and have a drink as soon as you sit up. It is important to do this on a regular basis while nausea is present, since sickness is more likely to occur if the stomach is empty. It is also important to get out of bed slowly, gradually getting used to being in an upright position. By taking things slowly in this way, dizziness and disorientation are less likely to be a problem.

■ Even if you feel nauseated, it is important to avoid going for long periods of time without eating. As suggested above, having an empty stomach makes morning sickness worse. This is due to the volatile nature of blood sugar levels in pregnancy, which can rapidly plummet to a very low level if meals are missed. This leads to unpleasant symptoms of dizziness, difficulty in concentrating, disorientation and severe nausea. In order to guard against this situation developing, it is important to have a small snack every couple of hours, and to make a conscious effort to eat at mealtimes. It is best to avoid snacking on foods and drinks that may make blood sugar levels more unstable in the long run, and to choose items that are nutritious and sustaining without piling on the calories. Snacks that should be avoided include sugary biscuits, cakes, fizzy sweetened drinks, chocolate, coffee and crisps. Ideal snacks include sticks of raw vegetables, pieces of fresh fruit, fruit juices that do not include added sugar, and rice cakes with toppings of low-fat cheese or vegetable-based pâtés and spreads. It is also very important to avoid becoming dehydrated by drinking four of five large glasses of mineral or filtered water daily.

■ Try to keep your daily intake of food as light and easily-digestible as possible. It can be very difficult to find the time or enthusiasm to prepare meals that involve a great deal of effort and planning when pregnant, especially if this is your second or third pregnancy. However, it is possible to benefit from choosing cooking methods that produce foods that are nutritious and easily-digestible such as stir-frying, steaming, baking or poaching. Methods to be avoided include deep or shallow frying, roasting and boiling. Avoid foods that are high in saturated fat such as red meat, cream cheeses, bacon and cream. Opt instead for whole grains, fish, poultry, fresh vegetables, unroasted nuts, seeds and live yoghourts. Home-made soups and broths can also be extremely palatable if nausea is a problem with heavier dishes.

■ Bolting or eating food 'on the run' can contribute to digestive problems, making nausea worse, Although boring, it is important to make a conscious effort to chew each mouthful thoroughly before swallowing it.

■ If dairy foods make your nausea worse and you have to avoid them, it is important to check that your calcium intake is high enough. Good alternative sources of calcium include green, leafy vegetables, e.g. broccoli or spinach, wholegrains and almonds. If you are vegetarian, also make sure that you are having enough iron from pulses, nuts and seeds.

■ Morning sickness can sometimes be linked to an unspoken anxiety or uneasiness about being pregnant. However much a baby is wanted, unexpected emotions can come to the surface during pregnancy which may be surprising or distressing. If this is the case, it is important to appreciate that it is not uncommon and many mothers have been taken unawares by such feelings before or after the birth. Talking about these emotions is enormously helpful, since it can lead to positive insights being gained about the source of distress, fear or anxiety. The appropriate person to talk to might be a close friend or family member, or a professional counsellor, alternative practitioner or GP.

■ It is best to avoid tea, coffee, smoking and alcohol when pregnant. Because these irritate the lining of the stomach, they can make digestive problems more acute. Smoking and drinking alcohol or coffee may also have more serious effects on the unborn child, such as increasing the risk of low birth-weight or the incidence of miscarriage. Even if they have previously been ardent tea or coffee drinkers, many women find that they are instinctively repelled by the smell and taste of tea or coffee during their pregnancy. Thankfully, a wide variety of tea and coffee substitutes are now available which are palatable and caffeine-free. If you enjoy herbal teas, choose blends that give you a variety of flavours rather than sticking to one preparation, and experiment with grain-based coffee substitutes if you want to find a palatable alternative to coffee. Also experiment with the new range of carbonated, soft drinks that are marketed as a substitute for wine. They do not have the overly-sweet taste of apple of grape juice, which makes them much more suitable for drinking with a meal.

Homoeopathic Help

Type of morning sickness	General symptoms	Worse from	Better for	Remedy name
Morning sickness with craving for savoury foods.	Headaches with morning sickness that are improved by lying still. Vomits white, slimy liquid. Craves, or has absolute dislike of fatty, slimy, or starchy foods. Can't stand being fussed over when feeling ill: wants to be left alone. Repressed anxiety, sadness or depression about pregnancy.	Warm or hot surroundings. Hot sunlight. Noise. Displays of affection. Sympathy and attention.	Fresh, cool air. Cool compresses. Resting. Being left in peace and quiet.	**Nat mur**
Persistent, terrible nausea that is not relieved after vomiting.	Hot or cold, clammy perspiration with nausea. Difficult vomiting with empty retching and watery saliva. Nausea is not relieved by eating, but is made very much worse by the slightest movement. Pale and prostrated with morning sickness.	Movement. Stooping. Vomiting. Strong smells. Eating.	Fresh, cool air. Rest. Keeping still.	**Ipecac**
Morning sickness that is eased by eating small amounts frequently.	Symptoms are at their worst in the mornings. Distressing headache and dizziness accompany empty sensation in stomach. Sour or tart flavours appeal when hungry. Awful sensitivity to smell of cooking. Nausea is relieved by eating, but rapidly comes back when stomach is empty. Exhausted, depressed and irritable when pregnant.	Long gaps without eating. Cooking smells. On waking. Becoming chilled. Thought of food. Emotional demands of family.	Being warm in bed. Fresh air. Eating small amounts often.	**Sepia**

Type of morning sickness	General symptoms	Worse from	Better for	Remedy name
Nausea and morning sickness with severe chilliness.	Although terribly chilly when feeling ill, warm, stuffy rooms make things worse. Sickness occurs in the morning and/or at night. Nausea follows eating rich, fatty or creamy foods. Weepy and in need of cheering up.	Lack of fresh, cool air. Warmth. Warm food or drinks. Resting. Mornings and evenings.	Cool, fresh air. Cool compresses. Gentle movement in fresh air. Sympathy and encourage-ment. After a good cry with someone sympathetic.	**Pulsatilla**
Morning sickness with terrible chilliness and need for warmth.	Prostrated, faint and restless with nausea and vomiting. Sips of warm drinks help, while cold food or drinks make things worse. Terribly anxious and fearful about state of health of herself and the baby.	Chilly surroundings. Eating or drinking even a little. Cold food or drinks. Being alone. Untidy surroundings.	Warmth. Sitting propped-up in bed. Warm body with cool, fresh air to head and face. Small sips of warm drinks. Company.	**Arsenicum alb**
Severe bouts of vomiting with morning sickness.	Unpleasant, copious amounts of saliva with nausea and vomiting. Forcible, profuse vomiting with paleness and profuse clammy sweat. Tremendous thirst for cold drinks after vomiting. Exhausted and faint with a need to lie down.	Movement. Pressure of clothes or covers. After drinking. Sweating.	Resting. Lying down. Cool surroundings.	**Veratrum alb**

Type of morning sickness	General symptoms	Worse from	Better for	Remedy name
Morning sickness with vomit that is very difficult to bring up.	Although nausea is relieved once vomiting has occurred, being sick is very difficult with lots of gagging and empty resting. Indicated for morning sickness in tense, irritable, overstressed women who 'burn the candle at both ends' in order to cope with work and domestic demands.	Cold, draughty, conditions. Mornings. Spicy foods. Coffee, alcohol, and cigarettes. Lack of good quality sleep. Mental and emotional strain.	Lying down. As the day goes on. Warmth. Sound, uninterrupted sleep. Peace and quiet.	Nux vomica

Seek Medical Help In Any Of The Following Situations:

■ If symptoms of morning sickness do not respond to self-help measures.

■ Severe, persistent or long-lasting morning sickness.

Heartburn

Heartburn is a commonly-occuring problem experienced by pregnant women, especially during the last few months. During pregnancy, the muscle that normally closes off the upper part of the stomach from the gullet becomes relaxed and there is every likelihood of digestive juices rising into the gullet from time to time. This is further aggravated by the growing foetus pressing on the stomach as the pregnancy gets well under way. As a result, the common symptoms of an unpleasant taste in the mouth, 'repeating' and burping of food eaten hours before, burning in the centre of the chest, and acidity in the stomach and gullet, are likely to arise.

It should be possible to minimize the symptoms of heartburn by sensible changes in diet and lifestyle alone. However, if heartburn follows an overly-rich meal or period of over-indulgence, one or two doses of an appropriately-selected homoeopathic remedy should resolve the problem speedily, and with the minimum amount of distress.

If digestive problems pre-date your pregnancy, or if severe or persistent heartburn does not improve by using self-help measures, it is important to seek a professional opinion.

Practical Self-help

■ Avoid foods that tend to be difficult to digest. These include foods that are high in fat such as full-fat hard cheeses, fried foods, greasy snacks such as crisps and nuts, and meals that are prepared with rich, creamy sauces as accompaniments. Other foods that may cause problems include raw onions, peppers, tomatoes, citrus fruits such as oranges or grapefruit, or beans and pulses.

■ Eat small portions of easily-digested foods often through the day, rather than having large gaps in between mealtimes. Also avoid eating heavy or large meals late at night which can result in bouts of severe heartburn overnight. This occurs because the digestive system is unable to work as efficiently at night as it does during the day, due to the slowing down of all bodily functions while we sleep. As a result, a large meal eaten late at night can take a very long time to digest, causing great discomfort in the process.

■ Opt for foods that are appetizing, light, and easy on the digestive system. These include home-made soups and broths, steamed vegetables, grilled fish or poultry (avoiding the skin which is high in fat), and plenty of filtered or bottled water. If raw fruit aggravates your symptoms of heartburn, try lightly steaming pieces of fruit with a little added honey.

■ If you enjoy muesli but find it difficult to digest, try soaking it overnight in a little milk or fruit juice. This allows the starch in the cereals to be partly broken down into sugar, making it easier to digest. Alternatively, try switching to a cooked breakfast cereal like porridge.

■ Avoid tea, coffee, alcohol, spicy foods and cigarettes, all of which irritate the stomach lining. Experiment with soothing herb teas such as fennel, chamomile or peppermint, bearing in mind that peppermint may interfere with the action of homoeopathic remedies. As a result, it is best to drink an alternative herb tea if you are having homoeopathic treatment.

■ Avoid eating snacks 'on the run', and always try to relax and enjoy your food when eating. This is an important way of avoiding heartburn, since it encourages the process of digestion to happen more smoothly. Because digestion begins in the mouth when digestive juices and saliva are mixed with the food, it is also very important to chew each piece of food thoroughly.

■ If heartburn is especially problematic at night, try propping yourself up on two or three pillows. However, this should be avoided if you have any problems with swollen or puffy ankles.

Homeopathic Help

Type of heartburn	General symptoms	Worse from	Better for	Remedy name
Burning pains that are soothed by warm drinks.	Severe discomfort and burning in the stomach with nausea, chilliness, and mental and physical restlessness. Small sips of warm drinks help: gets up at night to make a cup of tea. Anxious, fussy and fidgety with symptoms.	Cold or chilly surroundings. Cold food or drinks. Making an effort. At night. When alone.	Warmth. Frequent sips of warm drinks. Being propped-up on pillows in bed. Company.	**Arsenicum alb**
Heartburn with acidity that rises into the throat.	Discomfort and burning extend from the stomach to the throat. Frequent burping that raises a little acid each time. Very conscious of gurgling and rumbling in stomach and abdomen. Quickly full when eating, with great difficulty in finishing a meal.	Cold food and drinks. Large meals. High-fibre diet. Becoming overheated. Restrictive clothing. Afternoons. Anticipating an important event.	Warm food or drinks. Loosening clothes. Distraction from symptoms. Moderate warmth. Fresh air.	**Lycopodium**
Heartburn that follows a period of eating badly or extreme stress.	Heartburn may be accompanied by headache, nausea, constipation and a generally 'toxic' feeling after eating junk foods or drinking too much coffee. Unpleasant, sour taste in mouth with persistent burping. Irritable and anti-social with digestive problems.	Becoming chilled. On waking. Noise or loud music. Lack of sleep. Drinking coffee or alcohol. Mental or physical stress.	Warmth. Sound, undisturbed sleep. Having a nap. Passing a stool. By evening.	**Nux vomica**

Type of heartburn	General symptoms	Worse from	Better for	Remedy name
Heartburn after eating fatty meat or very rich foods.	Severe nausea and heartburn follow an overly-rich meal. Red meat with high fat content, e.g. pork, creamy sauces, ice cream, fried foods, or cream cakes make heartburn worse. Although mouth is dry, thirst is absent. 'Repeating' of foods eaten hours before when burping. Tearful and weepy when unwell.	Becoming overheated. Warm foods or drinks. Lack of fresh air. Lying down. Evening and night. Heavy clothes or bed covers.	Cool, fresh air. Cool drinks or food. Walking in fresh air. Uncovering. Sympathy. After a good cry.	**Pulsatilla**
Heartburn which is made more intense by eating.	Sensitivity to water in pregnancy: the sight or thought of water induces nausea and sickness. Uneasiness in stomach aggravated by putting hands in warm water. Unpleasant, empty, sinking sensation is made worse from feeling anxious.	Lying flat. Becoming anxious or upset. Warm food or drinks. Dehydration. Salty foods.	Sleep. Cool drinks until they become warmed by stomach. Massage. Reassurance.	**Phosphorus**

Seek Medical Help In Any Of The Following Situations:

■ **Severed or persistent heartburn or indigestion.**
■ **Symptoms that do not respond to self-help measures.**

Labour and Childbirth

Homoeopathy, in common with other holistic therapies such as acupuncture, has an extremely positive role to play in childbirth. When used appropriately, it can do a great deal to calm panic and anxiety, stimulate flagging energy levels and ease pain during labour. It also has a vital role to play in the days following delivery, when pain from episiotomy, bruising, and volatile emotions can distract from the excitement and exhilaration of getting to know your baby. When homoeopathic remedies are used within this context, they can do a tremendous amount to speed up physical and emotional recovery.

Although some midwifery diploma courses now include introductory sessions in alternative therapies, it is still difficult to find a midwife who is also qualified to use homoeopathy. If you want to use homoeopathic remedies during your labour, it is best to consult a homoeopathic practitioner. You can then decide whether you want your homoeopath to attend your labour, or if you prefer to rely on homoeopathic remedies selected by your partner.

If you choose the latter course of action, your homoeopath may want to have a joint session with you and your partner. Within this framework you can discuss the problems you anticipate may arise, and your homoeopath can supply you with clear, concise information about the remedies that are likely to be most useful.

Although the second course of action is a popular one, it must be stressed that it is not usually as helpful as having your homoeopath at the birth. Attending a birth is one of the most powerful emotional experiences we are likely to witness, with the result that it is often very difficult for a partner to be objective enough to choose the appropriate homoeopathic remedy. A homoeopath, on the other hand, will have the necessary experience to differentiate between suitable remedies, as well as the necessary degree of professional objectivity.

Once you have made your decision, you will need to inform your consultant that you intend to use homoeopathic remedies during your labour. If you want your homoeopath to be present during the birth, this must also be discussed with your consultant, who may want to meet with your practitioner. If you are planning to have your baby at home, you will need to raise these issues with your GP and midwife.

In the following table you will find a description of the homoeopathic remedies that are often indicated in labour. This is done in order to give an impression of the potential usefulness of homoeopathic remedies within this context, rather than to encourage self-prescribing.

Type or stage of labour pains	General symptoms	Worse from	Better for	Remedy name
Fearful anxiety at onset, or second stage of labour.	Terrible anxiety and physical and mental restlessness. Pain seems unbearably strong. Often indicated in fast, violent labour. Either feels she wants to die, or feels terrified she is about to die.	Touch Examination. Extreme warmth or chill.	Uncovering. Fresh air.	**Aconite**

Type or stage of labour pains	General symptoms	Worse from	Better for	Remedy name
Labour slow to start, or feeble pains that keep stopping and starting.	Pains are changeable and intermittent once labour is underway. Baby may be in difficult or breech position. Distress is intensified by warm, stuffy, airless rooms. Weepy, hopeless and despondent in labour.	Lack of sympathy. Warmth. Lack of fresh air. Keeping still.	Fresh, cool air. Cool compresses to forehead or face. Moving. Sympathy and encourage-ment.	**Pulsatilla**
Weak labour pains with slow or insufficient dilation of cervix.	Long, slow, arduous labour. Severe, unproductive labour pains that fly about in all directions. Weak, feeble labour pains with shivering and trembling. Although chilly, craves fresh air. Irritable and exhausted during labour.	Cold air. Becoming chilled. Becoming exhausted.	Fresh air.	**Caul**
Backache labour that is relieved by massage to the back.	Labour pains relieved by firm pressure to back, or squatting with elbows supported on knees. Pains radiate from hollow of the back to the buttocks. Severe wind and burping with contractions. Bad-tempered, bossy and irritable during labour.	Chill. Uncovering.	Warm surroundings. Firm pressure. Massage.	**Kali carb**
Vomiting in labour with violent retching as contractions occur.	Bruised, aching, exhausting pains during labour. Straining sensation during contractions as though about to pass a stool. Violent, persistent retching with great difficulty in raising vomit. Irritable, angry and abusive in labour.	Cool surroundings. Touch. Draughts of cold air. Uncovering.	Warmth. Peaceful surroundings.	**Nux vomica**

Type or stage of labour pains	General symptoms	Worse from	Better for	Remedy name
Frantic and impatient with with unproductive pains.	Unbearably painful labour pains that drive to distraction: feels she cannot go through with it. Slow dilation of cervix with severe pains in the back. Frustration with pain and slow progress lead to extreme outbursts of anger and abusive language.	Fresh air. Becoming overheated.	Sweating. Uncovering when too hot. Moderate warmth and warm applications.	**Chamomilla**
Rapid prostration and exhaustion in first stage.	Tires rapidly in the early stages of labour: fears that she doesn't have the energy to see it through. Heavy, exhausting labour pains affecting the back. Legs feel heavy, weak and wobbly. Contractions arrested when examined. Worn out expression with droopy eyelids and drowsiness.	Thinking ahead. Effort of contractions. Hot surroundings. Cold draughts.	Fresh air. Moving about. Sweating.	**Gelsemium**

After The Birth

Homoeopathic medicines can be astonishingly helpful in the days following delivery, aiding mother and baby to deal with the shock and trauma of the birth process on emotional as well as physical levels. This can be especially valuable in situations where the experience of giving birth has been quite different to what was envisaged.

Unfortunately, this unhappy situation often occurs when mothers prepare detailed birth plans in advance, outlining the medical assistance they will accept, and those techniques they want to avoid. If events take a difficult turn, and medical intervention is needed that was positively not desired, this can lead to overwhelming negative feelings. These may include anger, resentment, disappointment, guilt, and a sense of failure, which can cloud the excitement of the initial phase following birth for the new mother.

Homoeopathic prescribing in the days following delivery can also be of vital assistance in relieving the pain and discomfort of episiotomy and vaginal bruising. If further complications arise, such as mastitis, the appropriately-selected homoeopathic remedy, used in conjunction with practical self-help measures, can do a great deal to ease the condition.

Homoeopathic Help

Type of problem	General symptoms	Worse from	Better for	Remedy name
General aching, bruising, and soreness following delivery.	Immensely well-indicated for the physical and emotional shock that can follow childbirth. Promotes effective re-absorption of blood and healing of bruised tissue. Required in the first few days after childbirth.	Touch. Examination. Movement. Jarring.	Resting.	**Arnica**
Bruising to deep tissue that has not been resolved by **Arnica**.	Extremely sore, sensitive bruising that is eased in the first few days but not completely healed by **Arnica**. Tired and exhausted with throbbing, squeezing, aching pains.	Touch. Cold bathing. Warm bathing. Warmth of bed.	Continued movement. Cool compresses.	**Bellis perennis**
Slow-healing, extremely sensitive episiotomy or tear.	Use as an external application in cream or diluted tincture in order to ease pain and speed up healing. Add ten drops of tincture to bathwater or bidet and bathe the sensitive area. Alternatively, soak a sanitary towel in diluted tincture and apply to the perineum. Apply cream after bathing.	Cold or chill.	Resting. Gentle movement.	**Calendula**
Residual pains after forceps delivery or epidural.	Shooting, tearing pains in episiotomy or tear. Persistent back pain following epidural. Shooting pains radiate from damaged area. Extra-sensitive wounds or residual pain once wound has superficially healed.	Touch. Jarring. Exertion. Movement. After forceps delivery.	Massage. Lying on stomach.	**Hypericum**

Type of problem	General symptoms	Worse from	Better for	Remedy name
Sharp, stinging pains after episiotomy or Caesarian.	Strongly indicated after 'high tech' births where mother is physically and mentally stressed. Stitching pains in and around the wound which is exceptionally sensitive to touch. Emotionally traumatized with feelings of guilt, resentment and unexpressed anger at having been cheated out of the fulfillment of a natural birth.	Touch. Pressure of clothes or bed covers. Emotional stress. Passing water. At night.	Resting. Warmth.	**Staphysagria**

Mastitis

Mastitis is a painful condition that arises when a blocked duct in the breast develops into an abscess. The majority of women who experience this problem have recently given birth, and have been unable or chosen not to breast-feed. Infection is thought to enter the breast tissue through cracks in the nipples, infecting the milk ducts and glands. Symptoms may include the following:

■ Lumpiness or soreness in the affected breast.
■ Redness or inflammation of the skin above the lumpy tissue.
■ Glands adjacent to the affected breast may also become tender, e.g. in the armpit.

If feverishness develops in addition to the symptoms mentioned above, this may be an indication that the blockage has developed into mastitis. If this is the case, prompt professional help must be sought. Successful homoeopathic prescribing is immensely helpful within this context, since it may make treatment with antibiotics unnecessary. As a result, a mother may continue breast-feeding because homoeopathic remedies do not have any reported adverse effects on babies.

However, if the symptoms of a blocked duct are treated at an early stage with the aid of self-help measures and appropriate homoeopathic prescribing, it may be possible to prevent mastitis developing.

Practical Self-Help

■ Breast-feed frequently in order to encourage the expression of milk from the ducts. It may take a little while before you discover the position in which your baby feeds most happily and easily. If your baby does not want to feed as often as your breasts feel full, make occasional use of a breast pump in order to express excess milk.

■ Place your baby on the affected side first, making sure that this breast is thoroughly emptied at each feed.

■ Massage your breasts between feeds, and also gently stroke your breasts towards your nipple while your baby is feeding.

■ Make maximum use of the force of gravity in order to drain the affected duct. If you can hold your baby to your breast with the painful area in the uppermost position, this will encourage draining of the blocked duct.

■ Regularly swing your arms to encourage the flow of circulation, and make sure you do not become dehydrated. The best way of guarding against the latter is to make a point of drinking four or five large glasses of filtered water daily, in addition to hot drinks.

■ Check that your bra fits well, and that the cup size is adequate. If you are in doubt, most department stores have sales assistants who are happy to give advice about bra sizes.

■ At the first sign of trouble, use a simple hydrotherapy technique to ease discomfort and inflammation. Soak a flannel or small, soft towel in hot water and wring it out thoroughly. Apply this cloth to the affected breast, leaving it in place until it begins to feel cool. Replace it with another flannel that has been soaked in cool water for ten minutes. When this begins to warm, remove it and replace the hot flannel. Continue doing this for an hour or two.

■ If you are beginning to feel run down, ask for help from friends, neighbours or close relatives so that you can rest for a day or two. By taking bed rest in the early stages of illness, it is often possible to halt the problem without suffering complications.

Homoeopathic Help

Type of mastitis	General symptoms	Worse from	Better for	Remedy name
Rapid, violent onset of pain and inflammation.	Skin around the affected duct radiates heat and looks bright red: streaks of redness may run from the nipple along the surface of the breast. Terrific sensitivity to touch or jarring. Pains are severe lying flat in bed. Irritable and short-tempered with pain.	Least touch. Sudden, jolting movements. Lying on the painful side. Noise. Disturbance.	Sitting propped-up in bed. Warmth. Peace and quiet.	Belladonna

Type of mastitis	General symptoms	Worse from	Better for	Remedy name
Mastitis with sore, sensitive glands.	Generalized aching and shooting pains over the body. Breasts feel extremely tender and swollen and look deep or purple-red. Cracked, sore nipples with shooting pains that radiate from breasts to armpits. Exhausted, low and shivery with pains.	Becoming overheated. Becoming chilled. Touch. At night. Pressure to the right breast.	Lying on the left side or the stomach. Comfortable heat.	**Phytolacca**
Mastitis with marked sensitivity to movement.	Hard, sensitive breasts that are agonizingly painful when touched or moved. Although light touch is intolerable, there may be a desire to apply firm pressure to the painful area. Feels generally dry and dehydrated. Thirsty for long, cool drinks. Irritable and antisocial when unwell.	Warmth. Physical effort. Light touch. Jolting. Becoming overheated. Movement.	Cool surroundings. Keeping as still as possible. Firm pressure. Lying on the painful area. Long, cool drinks. Being left in peace and quiet.	**Bryonia**
Mastitis with pains and discomfort that are much worse at night.	Terribly restless and uncomfortable with mastitis: tosses about in bed trying to get comfortable. Glands may be generally inflamed and swollen. Sweaty and sensitive to the slightest variation in temperature. Anxious and trembly with pains.	At night. Chill. Becoming too hot. In bed. Sweating. Touch.	Resting. Moderate, stable temperatures.	**Mercurius**

Type of mastitis	General symptoms	Worse from	Better for	Remedy name
General glandular swelling with heat sensitivity and congestion of breasts.	Chilliness with intensification of symptoms from overheated, stuffy rooms. Firm pressure may ease the pain, but heavy clothes or bed covers make discomfort worse. Severe mood swings and weepiness as a result of the pain.	Overheated rooms. Lack of fresh air. In the evening. At night. Lying down. Warmth in any form.	Cool, fresh air. Opening a window. Gentle movement. Cool compresses or cool bathing. Firm pressure. Having a good cry in sympathetic company.	**Pulsatilla**
Inflamed breasts with very cracked sore nipples.	Breasts feel hard and very swollen. Cracks in nipples are very painful and distressing. Symptoms may be left-sided or worse on the left than the right. Unable to sleep at night from pain: drowsy during the day. Feverish with hot, flushed head and chilly hands and feet.	Chill. Becoming too hot. Damp. Lying on the left side. At night.	Wrapping up well. Rest. Fresh air.	**Graphites**

If Any Of The Following Occurs, Seek Prompt Medical Advice:

■ **Feverishness or general sense of unwellness.**
■ **If self-help measures have not stimulated a definite improvement within twenty-four hours.**

Post-Natal Depression

Although it is usual for the weeks or months following childbirth to be extremely emotionally charged, there are certain emotional reactions to the experience of pregnancy and motherhood that suggest that post-natal depression may be a problem.

If any of the following are especially intense, if they persist for an extended period of time, or if they appear to be gaining in severity, it is important to consider getting extra support from an alternative or conventional medical source:

■ Severe, persistent anxiety about your own health, or the health of your baby.
■ Diminished confidence or self-esteem.
■ A sense of being unable to cope with day-to-day tasks at home or at work.
■ An inability to be refreshed by sleep when you have the chance to relax.
■ Persistent involuntary tearfulness, or feelings of depression which descend without warning.
■ Physical, mental and emotional exhaustion that is not temporarily relieved by periods of rest or relaxation.
■ Persistent apathy, indifference or emotional numbness.

Most mothers will recognize many of the symptoms described above as being familiar emotional reactions to the responsibilities and demands of motherhood. However, if these sensations become persistent, or seem to be intensifying rather than diminishing over a reasonable period of time, extra help may be needed to deal positively with the problem.

If mood swings or depression occur soon after childbirth, occasional doses of an appropriately-selected homoeopathic remedy, plus the self-help advice given below, may help enormously. On the other hand, if depression is becoming a long-term problem it is more appropriate to seek professional help. This may come from a conventional or alternative medical source. If you are uneasy about the drawbacks associated with the use of tranquillizers, or do not feel at ease about taking anti-depressants, the latter course of action is well worth exploring. Whichever you choose to take, always make sure that you are frank about how you are feeling, so that the maximum help and support can be given to you.

Practical Self-Help

■ Acknowledge your feelings, rather than following advice that suggests a 'stiff upper lip' approach is best. The latter is likely to cause more long-term complications rather than encourage the resolution of emotional problems in a constructive way.
■ Talk as much as you need to with someone you can trust. This could be a close family member, a good friend, your GP or your alternative therapist. If you feel that you need a more formal framework in which to explore your feelings, you may find counselling immensely helpful. This can be especially the case if you have unresolved emotions about your experience of childbirth, which you feel may be inhibiting the bonding process between you and your baby.

■ Try to keep in contact with some of the mothers you met at ante-natal or relaxation classes. It can be immensely therapeutic to compare notes with someone who is likely to be going through similar problems, especially if this is your first baby.

■ If you live in an area which is fairly remote from friends or family, make a point of using the telephone in order to keep in touch.

■ Depression can often spring from a feeling of loss of identity: a sensation many new mothers experience. It is essential to recognize these emotions when they arise and ask for help. By getting the necessary support, you can make sure that you spend some time away from your baby. The amount of time may be relatively short, but it will give you the opportunity to do something for yourself. Choose to do whatever you find most pleasurable: this could be as simple as having a long bath, going to the hairdresser's or having lunch with a friend.

■ If you frequently feel irritable, tense and on edge, have a regular back or full body aromatherapy massage. Apart from feeling wonderfully relaxed by the massage, a trained aromatherapist will be able to select a blend of oils for you which will encourage relaxation and dispersion of muscular tension.

Homoeopathic Help

Type of depress-ion	General symptoms	Worse from	Better for	Remedy name
Irritable, apathetic, and indifferent with difficulty bonding with baby.	Exhausted, worn out and depressed with sensation of being unable to cope, or going out of control. Weepy and despondent with total lack of interest in sex. Mentally, emotionally and physically drained, often after two or more pregnancies close together.	Emotional demands. Rest. Skipping meals. Sympathy or affection. Touch.	Vigorous exercise in the fresh air, e.g. brisk walking. Eating small amounts often. Becoming warm in bed. After a sound sleep.	**Sepia**

Type of depress-ion	General symptoms	Worse from	Better for	Remedy name
Depression stemming from resentment, guilt or anger about birth experience.	Often needed after Caesarian section, or 'high tech' birth, where mother is left feeling violated by invasive procedures. Feels cheated out of experience of natural birth: leads to humiliation and unexpressed resentment. Physically and emotionally sensitive with terrible pains in stitches or scars.	Pressure of clothes or bed covers. Emotions. Sexual contact. Touch.	Warmth. Rest. Eating.	**Staphysagria**
Severe mood swings with involuntary bouts of weeping.	Often needed in the first few days after delivery if moods alternate quickly between euphoria and depression. Frequent sighing with a tendency to be extremely excitable. Mother may be overwhelmed by feelings of grief at having been physically separated from her baby.	Chill. Fresh air. Stimulants such as coffee. Alcohol. Strong smells, e.g. tobacco.	Being distracted. Warmth. Eating a little.	**Ignatia**
Black, deep depression with fidgetiness and jitteriness.	Withdrawn and silent, or very excitable and talkative with depression. Fears something awful will happen: that she will lose her reason or hurt the baby. Constant sighing when depressed.	Cold, chilly conditions.	Warmth. Fresh air. Motion.	**Cimic**

Type of depression	General symptoms	Worse from	Better for	Remedy name
Depression which is made much worse by sympathy or attention.	Although easily hurt, appears to others as withdrawn and reserved. Cannot weep because of depth of depression, or weeps alone because of humiliation of expressing emotions in public. Crying and receiving sympathy make things worse because they raise to the surface emotions which have been repressed.	Crying. Affection. Sympathy. Company. After eating. Making an effort. Becoming overheated.	Being left alone. Cool, fresh surroundings. Rest. Skipping meals.	**Nat mur**

If Any Of The Following Occurs, Seek Prompt Medical Advice:

■ A sense of loss of touch with reality, or separation from others.

■ Emotional numbness that alternates with outbursts of violent anger.

■ Disabling anxiety or terror about doing everyday tasks that posed no problems previously.

■ Deep, persistent or worsening depression that fails to respond to self-help measures.

■8■

The Stresses Of Modern Living: How To Cope

I
t is hard to escape the fact that we live in extremely stressful times. Advances in technology have given us the freedom to use mobile phones, fax machines, personal computers and modems which put us in instant communication with colleagues and friends. However, although these advances make life much easier in one way, they also increase our stress levels by giving us little privacy and time to ourselves. As a result, the pace of life feels faster and more demanding, with leisure time often being in short supply.

If we also consider that the little time we have in which to relax is often spent in front of the television, watching programmes that we may not be interested in but are too exhausted to switch off, we can appreciate that too stressful a lifestyle can spell disaster for our overall health and well-being.

The Nature Of Stress

The most important thing to learn about stress is that, in itself, it is neutral: it is our reaction to the stressful stimulus that makes it positive or negative. Once we have learnt techniques for stress management, we are in an excellent position to minimize the damaging effects of negative stress which feed on feelings of vulnerability and helplessness.

Because stress affects us on all levels, the general section below on stress management encompasses practical advice on techniques for relaxing the mind, calming the body and detoxifying the whole system. As a result, it is possible to benefit from a holistic approach which de-stresses mind and body, providing us with a degree of mental, emotional and physical resilience in the face of stress that we may not have thought possible.

Basic Self-Help Techniques For Stress Management

Relaxation Techniques

Pioneers in the study of deep relaxation, such as Herbert Benson, have demonstrated that achieving a relaxed state can be profoundly beneficial in combating the adverse effects of stress. By switching on the 'relaxation response' it is possible to regulate heart rate, reduce muscle tension, slow down breathing, and avoid feelings of anxiety and panic. If we learn a simple relaxation technique, we can use this in any stressful situation which may arise. By doing so, we can immediately eliminate the feeling of helplessness which is a central part of negative stress, since we have a practical tool at our disposal with which to combat the unpleasant physical and emotional symptoms that constitute a stress response.

Relaxation and Breathing

Relaxed breathing from the diaphragm (lower chest) is the the key to effective relaxation. Although it may sound obvious, learning to breathe deeply and rhythmically is a vital way of dealing with anxiety and tension.

Many of us do not realize that our breathing patterns change as soon as we begin to feel stressed, with most of the activity taking place from our upper chest. As a result, our breathing rate becomes rapid and shallow, contributing to feelings of panic and tension as the ratio between oxygen and carbon dioxide is adversely affected. However, by regulating our breathing we can break this vicious circle, and induce a feeling of calm and clear-headedness.

Diaphragmatic Breathing

When learning how to breathe from the diaphragm, it is best to lie flat on the back with knees bent and feet flat on the floor about hip width apart. This position allows us maximum opportunity for becoming aware of the movement of the diaphragm. Consciously relax, feeling the movement of air in and out of the body. Gradually change the rhythm, ensuring that as you inhale, your lungs inflate from the base to the tip, and that as you breathe out, you fully exhale from the tip to the base of the lungs.

In order to establish that this is happening, rest your hand lightly on your abdomen around the area of your navel. As you breathe in, the air should inflate the lungs fully, gently pushing your hand upwards and outwards as the maximum capacity is reached. When you breathe out, your hand should sink back to its starting position as you expel the breath from your lungs, finally exhaling from the chest. It may be helpful to visualize a balloon or bag filling with air as you breathe in, which empties and deflates as you breathe out.

It is essential not to force the pace of breathing, stopping if light-headedness or dizziness sets in. Always take things at your own pace, stopping and starting as feels appropriate. Once this technique has been mastered, it is no longer necessary to lie down, since it can be done equally effectively sitting in a chair, at a desk or in a car.

Relaxation and Meditation

Once you are at ease with using diaphragmatic breathing in stressful situations, you may also benefit from techniques that encourage top-to-toe relaxation. This may be done using progressive muscular contraction and release exercises that encourage awareness of areas of tension in the body. Many people find they are happiest to use pre-recorded audio or video tapes which take them through a guided relaxation exercise.

Alternatively, you may choose to meditate by focusing on an image, or repeating a sound to yourself over and over again. When meditating, it is best to sit in a straight-backed chair so that the spine may be kept in good alignment without causing strain or tension. The arms should be relaxed and loose, with the hands resting gently open on the knees, while the feet should feel firmly placed on the floor. Choose a room that is as quiet as possible, and well-ventilated but not chilly. Clothes should be loose, comfortable and warm, so that the mind is not distracted by feelings of discomfort or tightness.

As your eyes close, bring your attention to your breathing, observing its nature and rhythm. With each exhalation repeat a sound or word slowly to yourself, focusing your mind on each breath in and out. Continue to do this as long as you feel comfortable, stopping if you experience any dizziness or light-headedness, and starting again when you are ready.

Addictions

Although we often think of addictions within the context of a serious habit such as alcohol or drug addiction, the issue of dependence is much broader than it may seem at first. It is possible to develop a mild or serious dependence on a wide range of possible props, which may include any of the following:

- Alcohol.
- Cigarettes.
- Prescription drugs.
- 'Hard' or 'soft' recreational drugs.

189

■ Stimulants such as strong tea or coffee.

■ Painkillers.

■ Co-dependent relationships.

■ Work.

■ Punishing exercise regimes.

■ Food.

■ Dieting.

■ Falling in love.

■ Shopping.

■ Watching television.

■ Chocolate.

■ Sugar.

■ Salt.

Although this list may make sobering reading, it is obviously important to differentiate between addictive behaviour that is threatening the basic fabric of life in its broadest sense, such as severe drug or alcohol abuse, and an infrequent need for something rather less threatening, such as an occasional craving for a chocolate biscuit or cup of tea.

The way we can evaluate how dependent we are on a substance or emotional prop is to ask ourselves how we would feel if it were withdrawn for a reasonable period of time. If all we feel is mild regret or frustration, the chances are that we enjoy the pleasure-giving sensations that come from contact with the item in question, but feel we can cope without it perfectly well. However, if the thought of withdrawal provokes severe anxiety, panic, or a feeling of being unable to cope, we are likely to be addicted and need to take steps to change the situation.

Once the admission has been made that dependence is a problem, it becomes possible to come to terms with the situation by seeking help, practical information, and advice from your GP, support group or counsellor. Homoeopathic treatment has a very positive role to play in this context, since a homoeopath will be able to provide practical advice on the level of positive changes and adjustments in lifestyle that will aid coming to terms with addiction, as well as selecting the most appropriate homoeopathic remedy to encourage physical and emotional resilience during the period of withdrawal.

Because the issue of addiction is so broad-ranging, it is important to stress that professional help should be sought when coming to terms with dependence on alcohol, drugs and cigarettes so that sufficient support is made available should problems of withdrawal arise. For this reason, the homoeopathic remedies listed below for these dependencies are not mentioned in order to encourage self-prescription, they are merely included in order to give an impression of the potential range of homoeopathic treatments that may be used in situations of addiction.

Practical Self-Help

■ Many of us may find ourselves relying on a substance or activity as a way of coping with the stresses and strains that may surround us. This can be a very minor dependence such as having a single cup of coffee first thing in the morning as a way of facing the day, or watching a favourite television programme once a week in order to switch off from the cares and responsibilities of work.

However, addiction can reach serious proportions, leaving us unable to function without the 'prop' upon which we are dependent. This prop might include any of the following: alcohol, cigarettes, recreational or prescription drugs such as tranquillizers, extreme exercise regimes, food, gambling or sex. If addiction reaches a point where it is interfering with or controlling our lives, it is essential to seek professional help, such as counselling, in order to explore the factors that are leading to a state of dependency. Once we begin to comprehend the psychological issues involved, we are better placed to come to terms with our problems.

■ If you are gregarious by nature, you may derive great benefit from seeking help from a support group that has been set up with the specific aim of assisting those who are struggling with addiction.

■ Always try to keep a positive perspective on your efforts to come to terms with dependency. If you lapse, don't despair and give up, but consider your achievements and start again.

■ Make a point of 'guarding against low blood sugar levels (*hypoglycaemia*), by eating small amounts of good quality food at regular intervals, rather than going for extended periods of time without eating and drinking.

■ Concentrate on a nutritious, good quality diet, avoiding foods or drinks that may contribute to mood swings and unstable blood sugar levels. Offenders may include alcohol, coffee, strong tea, chocolate, and sugary foods and drinks. Opt instead for green, leafy vegetables, small amounts of dairy products, pulses, whole grains, nuts, and sprouted or unsprouted seeds. Drink six to eight large glasses of water daily, and drink revitalizing or soothing herbal teas, depending on your mood.

■ Snack on sunflower seeds as a way of keeping cravings at bay. They can be especially useful when giving up smoking, providing a healthy alternative to the sweets that many ex-smokers become reliant on. By substituting sunflower seeds for the latter, it is possible to avoid the tendency to dental cavities and weight gain that sugary sweets often contribute towards.

■ Find ways of congratulating and rewarding yourself as you make progress. These treats should ideally be pleasure-giving and confidence-boosting.

■ When overcoming a dependence, finding effective substitutes can help a great deal with the sense of deprivation that might otherwise occur if the addictive substance is withdrawn and nothing is put in its place. Establish the times of day and situations in which you might experience a particular craving, and substitute a more positive alternative. In other words, if your habit is to have a cigarette after meals in order to relax, drink a soothing herb tea instead, which will keep you occupied and encourage relaxation at the same time.

■ Since alcohol, cigarettes and recreational or prescription drugs leave the body deficient in certain nutrients, it can be very helpful to use vitamin and mineral supplements during withdrawal. The following should be considered: vitamins A, B complex, C, D and K. Manganese and potassium may also be helpful. Alternatively, a good quality multivitamin and multimineral should be taken.

■ Do not overlook the importance of regular, aerobic exercise when coping with the frustration or depression that can accompany facing life without an emotional or physiological prop. By taking rhythmic exercise that conditions the heart and lungs (e.g. swimming, cycling, running or rowing) we also encourage the body to produce pleasure-giving, pain-relieving chemicals called *endorphins*. These may be considered as natural antidepressants, and can do a great deal to keep us feeling positive and dynamic when the going gets tough. Ideally, we should aim to exercise on a regular basis in order to achieve this effect: three or four half-hour sessions a week would be ideal. However, it is also important to be aware that addiction to exercise itself may become a problem in certain individuals. Always make sure that exercise remains a pleasurable activity, rather than a gruelling regime that cannot be missed without feeling guilty.

■ Although it may sound obvious, admitting to the dependence is the first and most difficult thing that must be done before an addiction can be helped. Many of us who are addicted find it very difficult to face, and may be extremely resistant to any suggestion that this may be the case. However, once the vital step has been taken of admitting that a problem exists, we are at last in a position to take action to deal with the situation.

Homoeopathic Help

Type of addiction	General symptoms	Worse from	Better for	Remedy name
Reliance on caffeine, alcohol and painkillers.	Pressure of work results in symptoms of 'living in the fast lane': recurrent headaches, indigestion, insomnia, anxiety, and irritability. Relies on caffeine to keep up the pace, alcohol to unwind, sleeping pills in order to rest, and painkillers for headaches.	Coffee. Alcohol. Lack of sleep. Constipation. First thing in the morning. Stress.	Sound sleep. Warmth. As the day goes on. Peace and quiet. Regular bowel movements.	**Nux vomica**
Addiction to sugar in order to keep going.	Poor appetite with heartburn and bloated abdomen from weakness of the liver: may have a history of jaundice. Sits to a meal feeling hungry, but fills up after a few mouthfuls. Craves sugar because of persistently low energy levels.	Warmth. On waking. Afternoons. Tight clothing. High fibre foods.	Moderate temperatures. Exercise out of doors. Warm food and drinks.	**Lycopodium**
Craving for alcohol and coffee.	Creative, volatile temperament with a mind that becomes very active late at night. Feels toxic and hungover on waking. Over-reliance on alcohol may result in circulatory and/or liver problems. Cravings may be worse pre-menstrually or during the menopause.	Morning. Waking from sleep. Warmth. Tight clothes. Alcohol. Hot drinks.	Cool surroundings. Cool drinks. Fresh, cool air. Loosening clothes. Onset of a discharge.	**Lachesis**

Type of depression	General symptoms	Worse from	Better for	Remedy name
Restless anxiety with obsessive habits, e.g. workaholism or exercise addiction.	Fussy and demanding, with a tendency to criticize those who do not achieve high standards. Perfectionist at work and at home with intolerance of untidiness. Need for control leads to obsessive concerns about health, preoccupation with cleanliness and general state of anxiety. May crave alcohol and cigarettes.	At night. Contact with cold in any form. Lack of routine. Alcohol. Tobacco.	Warmth. Gentle exercise. Company.	**Arsenicum alb**
Constant exhaustion with unstable appetite and craving for alcohol.	Poor eating patterns lead to general debility and lack of energy: constantly wants to lie down and rest. Appetite is absent or voracious: craves sweets which make energy levels more unstable. May turn to alcohol when low and depressed.	Becoming overheated. After bathing. Mid-morning. Standing. Sugary foods or drinks.	Cool air. Lying down. Walking.	**Sulphur**

Professional help should be sought if dependence has developed involving any of the following:

■ **Recreational drugs.**
■ **Prescription drugs such as tranquillizers.**
■ **Alcohol.**
■ **Cigarettes.**
■ **Dieting.**
■ **Extreme exercise regimes.**

Anxiety

Anxiety is a problem that can be experienced in a variety of ways, and with differing degrees of intensity. The severity of symptoms experienced can vary from mild flutters of uneasiness to extremely distressing and disabling physical and mental sensations. These may include any combination of the following:

■ General feelings of tension, tightness and discomfort in the head, neck, shoulders and limbs.
■ Digestive problems including lack of appetite, nausea, constipation, diarrhoea or vomiting.
■ Irregular, shallow or difficult breathing leading to breathlessness, sighing or holding the breath.
■ Palpitations or rapid heart rate.
■ Dry mouth.
■ Muscle tremors or spasms.
■ Hot flushes with or without perspiration and clamminess.
■ Poor memory, lack of concentration, disorientation or temporary memory block.

Depending on the severity of the problem, it may be appropriate to use homoeopathic self-prescribing to help alleviate anxiety symptoms. If anxiety is of a short-term nature, especially if it is related to a specific stressful event, a well-selected homoeopathic remedy, combined with the self-help measures outlined below, should do a great deal to relieve immediate symptoms.

However, if anxiety has become a long-term problem, it is necessary to seek help from a homoeopath or other alternative practitioner in order to address the deeper psychological issues involved. Within this context, the appropriate homoeopathic remedy can be invaluable in aiding someone to come to terms with deep-rooted insecurity and agitation, without the problems and side effects associated with many conventional drug treatments.

Practical Self-Help

■ Learning how to induce relaxation through specific breathing techniques is one of the most practical and effective ways of combating the distress of anxiety. See section on *Relaxation and Meditation* at the beginning of this chapter for general advice on these techniques.
■ If we experience anxiety at a low-grade level over an extended period of time, taking regular exercise can provide us with an excellent way of channelling excess adrenalin, leaving us feeling calmer and less tense. Always choose a form of exercise that is enjoyable and fun to do, rather than dutifully pursuing something that is boring or uninspiring. The potential range of activities to choose from can be extremely wide, and may include any of the following: cycling, swimming, volleyball, low-impact aerobics, T'ai chi, yoga, weight training, running, skiing, trampolining, badminton or tennis. Above all, don't

be put off if you were a disaster at PE classes at school, and as a result feel exercise is something you are unsuited to. Once you find an activity that you enjoy, you may be astonished to discover how quickly your physical fitness and sense of self-esteem improve.

■ Consider the quality of your diet and eliminate any foods that may be contributing to anxious, jittery feelings. These include foods and drinks with a high sugar content, biscuits, chocolate, strong tea, coffee, alcohol, and cola-type, caffeinated drinks

■ Opt for alternatives to the drinks and beverages mentioned above. These may include caffeine-free, soothing herb teas such as chamomile. If you find herb teas which have a single, predominant flavour unpalatable, you may find some of the combinations of fruit teas more acceptable. Also experiment with grain or fig-based coffee substitutes or try decaffeinated coffee that has gone through a water-filtering process to remove the caffeine content.

■ Make sure that your diet includes a healthy supply of nutrients from fresh, whole food sources. Include regular, generous helpings of fresh fruit and vegetables (with a good proportion of these being eaten raw), wholemeal bread, pulses, small amounts of dairy products, and plenty of filtered water. Also make a point of eating foods that supply a good range of B vitamins, which play an essential role in maintaining healthy functioning of the nervous system. These include: wheatgerm, fish, eggs, yeast extract, avocados, meat, cheese, and green, leafy vegetables.

■ Add a few drops of soothing essential oils to your bathwater in order to encourage relaxation. Remember that good quality essential oils should be used very sparingly because of their degree of concentration (only two or three drops may be needed). Choose from any combination of the following soothing oils: Geranium, Neroli, Narcissus or Rose.

■ If anticipatory anxiety before a stressful event is a common occurrence, arrange things in such a way that stress can be kept to a minimum. If an important appointment is coming up, make sure that you give yourself enough time to relax the night before. Arrange to do something you find relaxing or distracting so that you have a good night's sleep. This might involve going to the cinema or on a long walk, listening to music, or spending the evening with a friend. Make sure you have a reasonably early night, avoiding caffeinated drinks, or eating a heavy meal late at night which might interrupt good quality, sound sleep. Drinking a cup of chamomile tea and soaking in a relaxing bath are also likely to help if you feel wakeful or agitated.

■ If anxiety is severe, or becoming a well-established problem, it is important to seek help from a counsellor, conventional doctor, or alternative medical practitioner.

Homoeopathic Help

Type of anxiety	General symptoms	Worse from	Better for	Remedy name
Anxiety with addictive behaviour, or dependence on stimulants.	Agitated, irritable and 'short-fused' when under pressure. Tense and stressed when anxious with a tendency to depend on caffeine to keep going, and alcohol to unwind. Palpitations and insomnia occur from excessive caffeine intake, with attendant headaches and digestive problems from dependence on alcohol.	Stimulants. Emotional or professional pressure. On waking. Cold, draughty conditions. Noisy, disruptive surroundings. Constipation.	Warmth. Peace and quiet. Sound, undisturbed sleep. Rest. As the day goes on. Regular bowel movements.	**Nux vomica**
Extreme agitation with anxiety and constant need to chatter.	Trembling and palpitations with anxiety and panic attacks. Restlessness with severe diarrhoea when under pressure. Craves sugary foods and drinks which make digestive problems worse.	At night. On waking. Eating sugar. Stuffy, airless rooms. Anticipating a stressful event.	Open air.	**Arg nit**
Anticipatory anxiety with withdrawal and self-preoccup-ation.	Chilly, weak and shaky with anxiety. Weary and apathetic with disinclination to make the slightest mental or physical effort. Indifferent, withdrawn and exhausted. Severe, painless diarrhoea with anxiety.	Becoming overheated. Thinking about coming event.	Occupation and diversion. Fresh, open air. Stimulants.	**Gelsemium**
Severe chilliness, diarrhoea and/or vomiting with anxiety.	Although exhausted, terrible physical and mental restlessness accompanies anxiety, which is especially bad at night. Anxiety in high-achievers who may become obsessive about tidiness, or convinced they are seriously ill.	Exposure to cold. Being alone. At night. Untidiness. Alcohol.	Warmth. Sips of warm drinks. Fresh air, provided body is warm. Moving about. Company.	**Arsenicum alb**

Type of anxiety	General symptoms	Worse from	Better for	Remedy name
Severe panic attacks with fear of death.	Terror-stricken and panicky in a stressful or anxious situation. Sudden, violent onset of anxiety that is so overwhelming that death seems inevitable. Specific or free-floating anxiety. Insomnia with intensification of symptoms at night leading to extreme restlessness and tossing and turning.	At night. Chill or too much heat. Noise. Bright light. Shock or stress.	Open, fresh air. Resting in peace and quiet.	**Aconite**
Anticipatory anxiety with abdominal bloating, rumbling and gurgling.	Extremely tense and nervous before an examination or speaking in public, but seems relaxed and confident to others. Anxiety causes extreme digestive problems, including severe wind after eating even a small meal. Irritable, domineering and sarcastic when threatened by anxiety.	Being unoccupied. Becoming chilled or too hot. Stuffy, airless rooms. In the afternoon or early evening.	Gentle exercise in the fresh air. Occupation and distraction. Warm food and drinks. Moderate, comfortable warmth.	**Lycopodium**
'Free-floating' anxiety with extreme sensitivity to others' feelings.	Although outgoing, sociable, and enthusiastic, quickly lapses into apathy and exhaustion. Fearful of thunderstorms, and dark, illness and being alone. Craves attention and displays of physical affection. Can be quickly reassured when anxious.	Darkness. Being alone. Overexcite-ment or stimulation. Early evening.	Reassurance. Touch. Being comforted. Massage. Warmth. Sound sleep.	**Phosphorus**

If symptoms of anxiety are severe, well-established or disabling, seek professional advice.

Depression

Although depression can occur at any time, there are certain phases in life when we may be more vulnerable to developing this condition than others. We may suffer from it at puberty, pre-menstrually (as part of pre-menstrual syndrome), after childbirth (post-natal depression) or during the menopause. We may also experience depression if we develop certain illnesses such as ME (Chronic Fatigue Syndrome), if we are under psychological strain, or experience an emotional shock such as bereavement or unexpected redundancy.

The symptoms of depression can be varied, and may differ greatly in severity from one person to another. However, the following problems are commonly experienced by those in a depressed state:

■ General feelings of sadness, despondency, despair, hopelessness or indifference, which may appear abruptly or for no obvious reason.
■ Violent, rapid or alternating swings of mood.
■ Disturbed sleep pattern with wakefulness, or light, poor-quality, unrefreshing sleep.
■ Anxiety or despondency on waking.
■ Diminished libido and sexual problems.
■ Eating disorders or disrupted eating patterns with a tendency to comfort eat or total apathy and indifference to food.
■ Alternation between constipation and diarrhoea, and/or nausea, indigestion or heartburn.
■ Hyperventilation with palpitations.
■ Poor memory and concentration.

When deciding if homoeopathic help is appropriate, it is useful to differentiate between transient, contained bouts of depression which occur in relation to a stressful, threatening or upsetting situation, and more long-term, diffused emotional problems which would suggest that depression is becoming more of an established, chronic state. While the former can benefit a great deal from self-help measures, the latter usually requires more objective help and support from a professional source.

Practical Self-Help

■ If bouts of depression are combined with anxiety, see the self-help advice in the *Anxiety* section for additional suggestions, which may be useful when combined with those given below.
■ Familiarize yourself with the foods that contribute to feelings of dynamism and well-being, and those that intensify erratic or depressive mood swings.

Examples of the former include items that provide us with optimum, high-quality nutrition such as regular and plentiful portions of fresh fruit and vegetables (ideally eaten raw or lightly steamed in order to preserve vitamin content), whole grains in the form of wholemeal bread or pasta, fish, pulses, and small quantities of dairy foods. Eat live, natural yoghurt to preserve the healthy balance of intestinal flora, drink four or five large glasses of mineral or filtered water daily in order to encourage efficient elimination of toxins, and drink soothing herbal teas such as chamomile when feeling jittery or anxious.

■ Avoid the following which tend to contribute to erratic or depressive moods: alcohol, chocolate, strong tea, coffee, sugary snacks, sweetened fizzy drinks (especially if they contain caffeine), 'junk' foods containing artificial preservatives and flavourings, and crisps and savoury snacks which are high in salt and fat content.

■ If you suspect your pattern of eating has suffered or become erratic since feeling down, a good-quality multivitamin supplement will provide the additional nutritional support which can be needed in times of stress.

■ Consider supplementing your diet with vitamin B complex, or increasing the amount of foods that are good sources of the B vitamin group. The latter have a reputation for supporting the health of the nervous system, which can be of great importance in times of emotional stress or strain. These include: fish, nuts, wholegrains, yeast extract and green, leafy vegetables.

■ Although it can be difficult to find motivation to become physically active when depressed, it is important to bear in mind that regular, rhythmic, aerobic exercise can have a profound effect in reducing the emotional distress of depression. When we are engaged in regular aerobic activity, our bodies produce chemicals that resemble natural anti-depressants. It is the secretion of these substances that is responsible for the sense of well-being often experienced after exercise which conditions the heart and lungs (sometimes referred to as 'jogger's high').

■ Aerobic exercise also encourages us to breathe more evenly and deeply, which stimulates our bodies to make maximum use of the oxygen we inhale. If we breathe correctly while we are exercising in this way, we can support our bodies in the vital processes of elimination and de-toxification. These are essential contributing factors to the sensations of vitality, alertness and overall well-being which often suffer when we are depressed.

■ Regular, absorbing, enjoyable exercise has the important effect of giving us a much-needed boost in confidence and self-esteem. By making us feel better about our bodies (especially if we have previously seen ourselves as unfit or unsuited to exercise), we can use physical activity as an essential tool in combating feelings of depression and insecurity. Once you have selected a sport that is appealing, begin slowly, avoiding making excessive demands on yourself. By not overdoing it at the outset, you are more likely to find that you feel energized and positive about continuing. Be imaginative about the possibilities open to you, aiming to find a physically stimulating activity that broadens your social circle as well. This might involve weight-training at a local gym, joining a tennis club, playing badminton, volleyball or squash.

■ When feeling down, give yourself the necessary space and conditions in which to recover. At times like this, deliberately choose to do things that are enjoyable, uplifting or relaxing. This might involve spending time with a close friend, listening to music, walking in the country, pampering yourself by taking a scented bath or watching a favourite film.

■ Make use of soothing or uplifting aromatherapy oils when depression descends. A few drops can be added to a carrier oil and massaged into the skin, or added to your bathwater. It is also possible to enjoy the benefits of essential oils by adding a sparing amount to a metal or ceramic ring which is designed to be placed on a light bulb. When the light is switched on, the ring becomes warm, diffusing the perfume of the essential oil through the room. Appropriate essential oils to consider include Jasmine, Ylang-Ylang, Rose, Geranium and Neroli.

■ When feeling low, it is best to talk feelings over with someone you are at ease with. This could be a close friend, family member or partner. Alternatively, it is sometimes easier to talk frankly about emotional problems with someone who is not directly involved, such as a counsellor or psychotherapist. A professionally trained therapist is able to take an objective stance with regard to your problems, unlike a close friend who may be unable to adopt an emotionally unbiased perspective.

Homoeopathic Help

Type of depression	General symptoms	Worse from	Better for	Remedy name
Rapid mood swings with depression.	Chattiness and euphoria may rapidly change to withdrawal and depression. Jealous, irritable and volatile when depressed. Flow of creative ideas late at night preventing sleep. Dread of sleep and depression on waking. Sense of suffocation or jerking on falling asleep.	Extreme variations of temperature. On waking. Tight clothing around neck or waist. Stuffy, overheated rooms. Pre-menstrually.	Fresh air or well-ventilated rooms. Onset of a discharge, e.g. beginning of a period. Motion. Cool drinks and food. Loosening tight clothes.	**Lachesis**

Type of depress-ion	General symptoms	Worse from	Better for	Remedy name
Depressed and fearful with anxiety about loss of control.	Restless, anxious depression that is worse at night or for being alone. Critical and unable to reach self-imposed high standards. Fussy, fidgety, obsessive and intolerant of mistakes made by others. Chilliness and digestive problems occur with depression.	Cold surroundings. At night. Alcohol. When alone. Darkness.	Warmth. Gentle movement. Sips of warm drinks. Company.	**Arsenicum alb**
Weepy depression with pre-menstrual syndrome or during pregnancy.	Despondent and depressed: bursts into floods of tears at the least provocation. Craves sympathy and attention when feeling low: crying on a sympathetic shoulder helps. Mood swings are relieved by being on the move rather than sitting still.	Resting. Evenings. Stuffy, overheated rooms. Before a period. Feeling neglected.	Gentle exercise. Fresh, cool air. Sympathetic company. Having a good cry.	**Pulsatilla**
Withdrawn depression with aversion to company.	Depression may be a reaction to long-term emotional strain or loss. Emotional problems follow a tendency to brood and bottle up feelings. Dislike of supportive or sympathetic company which is likely to bring emotions to the surface. Can't stand humiliation of crying in public: sees it as a weakness.	After crying. Displays of attention or affection. Becoming overheated. Direct sunlight. Physical exertion.	Being left alone. Cool, fresh surroundings. Gentle movement. Eating irregularly.	**Nat mur**
Depression with fear of going insane with pre-menstrual syndrome.	Gloomy, black depression alternates with euphoric state or agitated anxiety. Feels frantic, strung up and completely out of control when anxiety is at its worst. Emotional state improves with the appearance of physical symptoms.	At night. Resting. Damp, cold conditions. Pre-menstrually.	Walking. Fresh, cool air. Eating. Moderate warmth.	**Cimic**

Type of depress-ion	General symptoms	Worse from	Better for	Remedy name
Complete apathy and indifference with depression.	Moods alternate between lack of motivation, irritability, and emotional and physical exhaustion. Tense and unable to cope with domestic demands. Libido is significantly lowered or absent. Dislike of company but also fears being alone.	Sitting brooding. Going for long periods of time without eating. Emotional responsibility or demands.	Vigorous exercise in the fresh, open air. Walking in the wind. Eating small amounts often. Sound, good quality sleep. Becoming warm in bed.	**Sepia**
Extreme restlessness at night with depression.	Wakeful and uncomfortable in bed with anxious depression regarding family responsibilities, work and the future in general. Tearful and despondent for no obvious reason. Emotional and physical discomfort and uneasiness are relieved by gentle movement.	In bed. At night. Cold, damp, draughty conditions. Excessive physical effort that is continued too long. Rest.	Taking a warm bath. Gentle movement that is stopped before tiredness sets in. Warmth. Warm wraps.	**Rhus tox**

If Any Of The Following Occurs, Professional Help Should Be Sought:

■ **Persistent feelings of anxiety or uneasiness about issues that normally cause little problem.**

■ **A tendency to lose touch with reality or a feeling of separation from others. The latter may be combined with additional feelings of anger or emotional numbness.**

■ **Persistent or severe depression that does not respond to self-help measures.**

Grief and Bereavement

Bereavement and grief are experiences that we all have to cope with in the course of our lives. Although we may automatically associate grief and bereavement with the death of a close relative, partner or close friend, we may feel grief-stricken for a variety of other reasons. Those of us who have experienced the loss of a much-loved pet will understand that the death of an animal can be felt as keenly as that of a human being. We may also grieve for a relationship that has broken down, the loss of a satisfying career, or for our home if we experience homesickness after a traumatic move.

If we understand the phases we are likely to go through when we grieve, there is a good chance that we will be better able to cope with the natural emotions that surface when we experience bereavement.

The initial reaction is usually one of shock, numbness or a sense of unreality, closely followed by denial or an inability to believe that the loss has occurred. Guilt or anger may surface, with a conviction that more should have been done. It is also perfectly natural to feel temporary but overwhelming anger, for instance towards the person who has died, or with regard to the medical treatment that has failed to help.

Depression may also occur before it is possible to emerge from the most acute phase of the grieving process. Once recovery begins, the potential pleasures of living become apparent once again, although bouts of depression, sadness or wistfulness are likely to recur periodically. However, these episodes should become shorter-lived and less traumatic with the passage of time.

Homoeopathic prescribing can be immensely helpful in easing the initial shock of bereavement, as well providing extra support in the later phases of the grieving process. In the immediate hours and days after bad news has been broken, it may be necessary to repeat the indicated homoeopathic remedy every few hours in order to provide the necessary help and support.

However, once the more immediate shock has passed, it should only be necessary to repeat the indicated remedy infrequently in order to gain emotional relief. If a remedy needs to be taken frequently or routinely in order to cope, it is best to consult a homoeopathic practitioner who will be able to provide greater support through a higher potency (stronger dose) or more appropriate choice of remedy.

Practical Self-Help

■ Although there may be a great deal of emotional support offered in the early phase following bereavement, it is in the later months that support is often required but may not be so readily available. In this situation, bereavement counselling may be of great help in providing professional support and a listening ear. Having access to this important emotional sounding-board often enables us to come to terms with bereavement in a way that was not possible before counselling began.

■ It is important to pace things appropriately, so that enough emotional time and space is provided within which to grieve. Where possible, it is best to avoid rushing back to a punishing or busy schedule ahead of time, since this may have the undesirable effect of preventing the grieving process from taking its natural course. As a result, emotional responses may be suppressed, which can lead to emotional and/or physical problems later on.

■ If anxiety, panic attacks or depression occur in response to bereavement, see the advice given in the *Practical Self-Help* sections listed under the categories of *Anxiety* and *Depression*.

■ Many people find that their sleep patterns become very disrupted after the shock of bereavement. If this is the case, consider the advice given in the *Insomnia* section.

Homoeopathic Help

Type of grief	General symptoms	Worse from	Better for	Remedy name
Fearful and panic-stricken.	Needed in the early stage of bereavement, especially if bad news has been sudden or unexpected, e.g. following an accident. Agitated, restless and afraid of dying. Symptoms set in with abruptness and violence.	Touch. At night. Noise.	Cool air. Resting in moderate temperatures.	**Aconite**
Physical and emotional shock as a result of receiving bad news.	Initially reacts to shock by insisting everything is fine and no help is needed: rejects comfort and support. Physically restless and mentally morose and apathetic. Easily startled and frightened.	After sleep. Being approached. Touch.	Resting with head low.	**Arnica**
Uncontroll-able weepiness with craving for sympathy.	Constant need for comfort, company and attention which relieves symptoms. Fearful, depressed and distressed by being left alone. Frequent crying bouts provide relief and release of emotions.	Feeling neglected. Rest. In bed. Eating. At night or in the evening. Stuffy, airless rooms.	Company. Sympathy. Having a good cry. Gentle exercise in the fresh air. Cool surroundings.	**Pulsatilla**

Type of grief	General symptoms	Worse from	Better for	Remedy name
Grief with emotional instability that is not resolved by the passing of time.	Agitation and violent, spasmodic weeping bouts that may alternate with bursts of laughter. Constant sighing, with muscle twitching, hiccuping and tremors. Feels unable to cope without help.	Contact with cold, open air. Touch.	Eating. Breathing regularly and deeply. Warmth. When alone.	**Ignatia**
Established phase of grief with anger and resentment.	Suppressed emotional release: especially when anger has been denied its natural expression. Resentment felt towards the person who has died, or there may be persistent guilt and self-reproach because of not having done enough. Mentally and physically over-sensitive.	Stimulation. Chill. At night. Emotional stress.	Rest. Warmth.	**Staphysagria**
Unexpressed grief with intolerance of sympathy.	Bottles up emotions and maintains a stiff upper lip in company. Can't bear humiliation of being seen in tears in public. Avoids sympathetic company because of the risk of breaking down. Generally worse for emotional release.	Displays of affection. Touch. Sympathy. Crying. Company. Noise.	Peace and quiet. When alone. Resting. Cool surroundings.	**Nat mur**

If unresolved grief lasts longer than might be expected (more than eighteen months or two years), or if there are symptoms of depression, professional help should be sought.

■ If symptoms are severe or disabling professional advice should be sought.

Insomnia

If we have experienced the occasional frustration and misery of being unable to achieve a sound, restful, refreshing night's sleep, we are likely to be very sympathetic towards those who suffer from these problems on a recurrent basis.

Although few of us are likely to suffer from full-blown insomnia, many of us may experience sleep difficulties in response to short-term problems. In such a situation, the duration and quality of our sleep may be adversely affected, making it very difficult to initially fall asleep, or producing poor-quality, fitful rest from which we may wake far too easily.

If we need a full eight hours of refreshing, sound sleep in order to function at our optimum level, experiencing problems for an extended period of time can lead to reduced physical and mental energy. However, quality of sleep may be more important than quantity, with some of us being capable of feeling refreshed by no more than four or five hours of prime quality rest.

If we are deprived of sound sleep for long enough, the following symptoms may occur:

■ Restlessness and anxiety.
■ Poor memory and concentration.
■ Excitability.
■ Increased susceptibility to recurrent infections as the body's ability to repair damaged cells and production of antibodies that have the job of fighting illness is reduced.

We may be more at risk of developing sleep problems at certain times in our lives. These may include the following:

■ When we are subject to emotional shock or trauma such as bereavement.
■ Sleep patterns may be adversely affected if we need to be alert at regular intervals during the night. Problems of this kind may follow caring for an elderly relative for an extended period of time, coping with a young baby or small children.
■ Many women find that their sleep is very disrupted during the menopause.
■ If we are subject to anxiety, this can also contribute to poor quality or broken sleep.
■ Depression can lead to irregular sleep patterns, including a tendency to wake early, feeling low or agitated.
■ Some women find they experience periodic wakefulness for a night or two before their periods.

If sleep problems are intermittent and mild in nature, or if they arise in response to a specific event, adopting the self-help measures outlined below should do a great deal to ease the situation. In addition, occasional use of the appropriate homoeopathic remedy should also contribute to restoration of normal sleep patterns. However, it is important to remember that homoeopathic remedies are intended for short-term use only, and there should be no need to take them routinely over an extended period of time.

If you derive short-term benefit from a well-selected homoeopathic remedy, but find you need to take it frequently in order to sustain the improvement, it is important to seek advice from a homoeopathic practitioner who will be trained to evaluate your symptoms in the broadest context. When appropriate homoeopathic treatment is given in this way, it can be invaluable in helping us come to terms with deep-rooted anxiety, insecurity or grief, without the potential problems associated with orthodox drug therapy.

Practical Self-Help

■ Take time to relax and unwind for an hour or two before bedtime. Choose any way to wind down that may be helpful and appealing to you. This could include anything from having a warm (but not hot) scented bath, reading a book, listening to soothing music, listening to the radio, or going through a guided relaxation exercise.

■ Above all, avoid doing anything that is physically or mentally stimulating and reviving before you go to bed. Always avoid working until the very last minute before bedtime, since this can often lead to difficulties in mentally 'switching off' as the mind may still be preoccupied with problems which need to be solved.

■ Check that your surroundings are likely to contribute to a sound, refreshing night's sleep. The room should be well-ventilated, but not too cold or too hot. Curtains or blinds should cut out bright light, but they should not make the room so dark that it is difficult to wake up easily in the morning.

■ As a general rule, never eat a heavy meal late at night. Eating rich, heavy or large meals before bedtime can lead to indigestion and fitful or unrefreshing sleep.

■ Eliminate or drastically cut down on foods and drinks that can contribute to wakefulness or poor quality, unrefreshing sleep. These may include: fizzy, sugary, cola-type drinks with caffeine, strong teas and coffees, and regular or large helpings of chocolate. Switch to soothing drinks such as chamomile tea, barley or fig-based coffee substitutes, or warm, milky drinks with honey. However, the latter should be avoided if you suffer from bronchial problems or persistent catarrh, since dairy products appear to contribute to excess mucus production which can be especially problematic overnight.

■ Use relaxing and soothing essential oils that help induce sound sleep, such as Lavender, Neroli, Narcissus, Rose or Geranium. (However, if you are using homoeopathic remedies it is best to avoid Lavender oil, since it may interfere with the efficacy of the remedy.) A few drops of the oil may be added to your bathwater, or it may be inhaled by burning on a specially designed lamp ring or steam diffuser.

■ Taking regular exercise (ideally three or four times a week) can contribute to a sound, restful sleep pattern, especially if the activity involves spending time in the fresh, open air.

■ Consider taking up meditation or relaxation techniques which will provide you with specific exercises that can encourage you to unwind and relax.

Homoeopathic Help

Type of insomnia	General symptoms	Worse from	Better for	Remedy name
Restlessness with acute anxiety and panic attacks at night.	Sleep problems occur as a result of shock, trauma or receiving bad news. Fitful, restless sleep with nightmares and distressing dreams. Panic-stricken and intolerant of symptoms. Constant tossing and turning in an effort to get comfortable.	Night. Becoming chilled or overheated. In bed. Shock.	Moderate temperatures. Resting. Fresh air.	**Aconite**
Sleeplessness from muscular aches and pains.	Often needed after demanding physical activity resulting in tired, painful muscles. Bed feels uncomfortably hard, leading to frequent tossing and turning in an effort to find a soft spot.	Physical effort in the unfit. Touch.	Lying with head slightly lower than the body.	**Arnica**
Anxious insomnia with a tendency to wake around 2 a.m.	Terrible agitation and fear that descend at night. Symptoms are aggravated by contact with cold and eased by warmth. Hot-water bottles and sips of warm drinks are soothing. Falls asleep easily, but wakes with a start in the early hours of the morning.	Becoming chilled. After midnight. Darkness. Solitude. Excessive physical effort. Alcohol.	Warm surroundings. Sips of warm drinks. Getting up and walking about or making a hot drink. Company.	**Arsenicum alb**
Lack of sleep after too much food and alcohol.	Wakeful until the early hours, then falls into a deep sleep once it is time to get up. Difficulty relaxing and mentally switching off after stimulating work. Insomnia may be caused by caffeine addiction. Feels irritable, oversensitive and 'hangover' on waking.	Noisy surroundings. Excessive amounts of caffeine and/ or alcohol. Stress of work. Cold, draughty surroundings.	Peace and quiet. Warmth. Being left alone.	**Nux vomica**

Type of insomnia	General symptoms	Worse from	Better for	Remedy name
Disturbed sleep patterns that follow bereavement.	Inability to get to sleep with persistent, spasmodic yawning. Muscle twitching and jerking when falling asleep. Recurrent nightmares and distressing dreams. Emotional instability with violent changes of mood may be aggravated by disrupted or unsatisfactory sleep pattern.	Emotional strain. Shock. Yawning. Anxiety. Chill. Coffee. Smoking.	Being alone. Breathing regularly and deeply. Warmth. Changing position.	**Ignatia**
Difficulty falling asleep in the early part of the night from anxiety about work.	Although very drowsy, the mind cannot switch off. Persistent thoughts about business problems or domestic pressures keep sleep at bay. Once asleep, dreams work through these anxieties. Overheated surroundings make it even more difficult to relax.	Before midnight. Movement. Heat. Being disturbed.	Cool, fresh surroundings. Peace and quiet. Long, cool drinks.	**Bryonia**
Poor quality or disturbed sleep from rheumatic pains.	Terrible restlessness and discomfort at night leading to poor quality sleep or persistent wakefulness. Joint and muscle pains may be brought on by cold, damp weather. Depressed and despondent when awake during the night.	Cold, damp conditions. Keeping still. After midnight. Draughty rooms. Excessive physical exertion.	Warm bathing. Wrapping up warmly. Massage. Stretching. Changing position.	**Rhus tox**

If insomnia is becoming a well-established problem, or if sleep pattern is not substantially improved by using self-help measures, professional help should be sought.

■9■

Homoeopathy For The Over Fifties

A revolution is taking place in the way we regard the ageing process. Thirty years ago, a sixty-year-old man or woman appeared to be elderly. Today, a fit eighty year old is seen as not unusual, and a significant number of people are living well into their nineties.

However, this must be balanced against the fact that although we are faced with a larger proportion of elderly people in the overall population than ever before, the incidence of chronic illness has not been reduced. Heart disease, arthritis and cancer are still major problems, even though we are encouraged by the media and the medical profession to have ambitious expectations about enjoying a fit and active old age.

Within this context, homoeopathic medicine and other holistic therapies have a tremendous amount to offer in meeting the many expectations that have been raised but left unsatisfied by conventional medicine. Because homoeopathic medicines work by stimulating the body's own in-built capacity for self-healing, there are no risks of toxic side effects. This is of special importance when treating older patients, since their eliminatory organs (such as the liver and kidneys) do not function as efficiently as those of younger patients. As a result, highly-toxic drugs which are not being carefully monitored can cause serious side effects far more quickly.

Homoeopathy is also especially well-suited to meeting the needs of mature people who want to take an active stance with regard to managing and protecting their own health. When combined with sound nutrition, regular appropriate exercise and a well-rounded lifestyle, homoeopathic medicines can do a great deal to stimulate an extended experience of dynamic, positive health.

In this chapter you will find practical advice and information regarding a number of common health problems that we may experience as we become older. This does not mean that these conditions inevitably occur as the body ages, or that they only occur in older people. However, if any of these problems should arise, this section will provide you with advice about simple, self-help measures that may improve the disorder at a basic level.

Helpful tables are also included so that you can quickly identify which homoeopathic remedies are most likely to be indicated for each condition. Most important of all, you will find clear information about when self-prescribing is appropriate and when it is necessary to seek professional help.

See **Chapter 2**: *Homoeopathy In The Home: How To Use This Book* for more detailed information about assessing the condition to be treated, selecting and taking the indicated remedy.

Haemorrhoids

Haemorrhoids (commonly referred to as piles) are varicose veins of the anus which become swoollen, irritated or painful as a result of straining to pass a stool. The walls of the veins often become thinned, with the result that they frequently bleed during or after passage of a stool. Bleeding from haemorrhoids is characteristically bright red in colour, and may stain toilet paper or appear as streaks on the stool that has been passed.

Haemorrhoids may be internal or prolapsed (protruding). The latter may occur temporarily during the passage of a stool, or may become a long-term problem if haemorrhoids are severe. With severe haemorrhoids, bowel movements are likely to become extremely difficult and painful. There may also be a discharge of mucus or blood after passing a stool, in addition to irritation or itching around the anus.

Haemorrhoids often occur during pregnancy, after childbirth or if extra pressure is put on the veins from being overweight. However, the most common cause of haemorrhoids is stubborn constipation which results in regular, often fruitless, straining and urging to pass a stool.

If a small haemorrhoid causes little or infrequent distress, the self-help measures listed below in combination with the short-term use of a well-indicated homoeopathic remedy may be all that is needed. However, if severe or prolapsed haemorrhoids are a problem, advice should be sought from a homoeopathic practitioner.

Practical Self-Help

■ If your diet is lacking in sufficient fibre, constipation and haemorrhoids may become a problem. If you want to take an active stance to prevent these conditions from developing, or to ease an already existing haemorrhoid problem, changing poor eating habits is essential. Avoid foods that are made from white flour or sugar, or those that include a generous helping of fat, such as cream cakes, biscuits and ice cream. The proportion of fatty foods eaten should be cut down dramatically, so that they make up no more than fifteen to twenty per cent of your daily intake. Foods in this category that should be avoided include full-fat cheeses, red meat and fats that are solid at room temperature such as butter.

■ The bulk of your diet should be made up of high-fibre foods such as baked potatoes, whole grains, such as unrefined rice, raw fruit, raw, grated, or lightly-steamed vegetables, pulses, and small portions of poultry or fish if you are not vegetarian. Try to eat a generous portion of salad or fresh vegetables with each main meal, and occasionally make a large, mixed salad the main feature of lunch or dinner. Aim for four helpings of fresh fruit a day, avoiding puddings that are high in fat and sugar.

■ Drink a large glass of mineral or filtered water at regular intervals through the day. If you find it difficult to drink enough at work, keep a large bottle of mineral water near you so that you can drink at regular intervals. Remember that drinking tea and/or coffee is not a substitute, since they are beverages that have a diuretic effect, encouraging the elimination rather than the conservation of fluid in the body.

■ Take regular exercise if you have a sedentary job or lifestyle. Jogging, running or brisk walking can encourage efficient working of the bowel, while sitting during work or leisure time can do the reverse.

■ If haemorrhoids are especially painful, herbal creams are available which may ease the symptoms considerably when applied locally. These contain a combination of herbal ingredients which have a soothing, anti-inflammatory effect on irritable haemorrhoids. They are marketed by homoeopathic pharmacies such as Ainsworths or Nelsons, and may be obtained directly from the pharmacy by mail order (addresses and telephone numbers are given at the back of the book). Alternatively, health food shops or some high street chemists who stock homoeopathic remedies may stock these creams as over-the-counter products.

■ Taking a warm salt bath at regular intervals may be very effective in easing the itching and discomfort of haemorrhoids. After bathing, apply a soothing cream.

■ If haemorrhoids are extremely swollen and inflamed, soak a cotton pad in witch hazel and apply it to the sensitive area.

Homoeopathic Help

Type of haemorrhoids	General symptoms	Worse from	Better for	Remedy name
Haemorrhoids with stitching pains that radiate up spine.	Haemorrhoids with constant, fruitless urging and incomplete passage of stool. Haemorrhoids feel full and inflamed while rectum feels constricted and tight. Haemorrhoids are very sensitive to touch and bleed very readily.	Cold. Alcohol. Coffee. Habitual use of painkillers. Junk foods. Stress. Exertion. In the morning.	Warmth. Rest. Sound sleep. Later in the day.	**Nux vomica**
Haemorrhoids with pain remaining in rectum long after passage of a stool.	Well-established constipation with no desire to open bowels. When a stool eventually appears it is dark, large, hard and crumbly. Terribly painful haemorrhoids are exceptionally sensitive to slightest movement.	Movement. Warmth. Jarring. Coughing.	Keeping as still as possible. Rest. Cool drinks. Cool surroundings.	**Bryonia**
Painful haemorrhoids with itching after passing a stool.	Stinging, burning pains that shoot upwards. Constipation and haemorrhoids may be aggravated by too many starchy foods in the diet, e.g. potatoes. Lots of painful urging and straining to pass a soft stool.	Warmth of bed. Junk foods. Sitting. Every other day. Smoking. Lifting. Exertion.	Cool bathing. Fresh air. Resting.	**Alumina**
Bleeding haemorrhoids with prickling, stinging pains.	Haemorrhoids bleed profusely and frequently. Soreness of rectum with bleeding. Haemorrhoids feel tense: as though they are about to burst.	Pressure or touch. Jarring movement. Contact with cold air. Movement.		**Hamamelis**

Type of haemorr-hoids	General symptoms	Worse from	Better for	Remedy name
Bluish-tinged haemorrhoids that resemble a bunch of grapes in appearance.	Burning, bearing sensations in haemorrhoids that are relieved by movement and made more intense when sitting down. Fullness and congestion in haemorrhoids. Pulsating pains in rectum after eating.	Heat. Jarring movement. After eating or drinking. Sitting down.	Cool bathing or cool compresses locally applied. Passing wind. Contact with cool air.	**Aloe**
Prolapsed, bleeding haemorrhoids with sharp, sticking pains.	Haemorrhoids emerge during the menopause. Terrible discomfort for hours after passing a stool: rectum feels as though it is full of small, sharp sticks or splinters. Swollen, congested feeling with burning in anus.	In the morning. On waking. Movement. Stooping. Lying down. Standing.	Cool, fresh air. Bathing with cool water. Physical effort.	**Aesculus**

If Any Of The Following Occurs, Professional Help Should Be Consulted:

■ **Darkened or otherwise discoloured stools.**
■ **A marked change in bowel movement which is not attributable to any obvious change in lifestyle.**
■ **Persistent or heavy bleeding from the rectum.**

Hiatus Hernia

Although symptoms of a hiatus hernia can occur at any time, they are common in older people, especially if they are overweight. The problem is caused by stomach acid leaking into the oesophagus, through a weakened valve which normally keeps the acid in the stomach. When acid leaks out in this way, the following symptoms may occur:

■ Burning and discomfort in the chest.
■ Acidity which rises into the throat when burping.
■ Digestive discomfort which is more intense when stooping or bending.

Because the symptoms of hiatus hernia usually occur on a chronic basis, i.e. they are subject to repeated flare-ups over an extended period of time, this is a condition that should be treated by a homoeopathic practitioner. Although the self-help measures suggested below will be useful in generally improving the condition, and the occasional dose of a well-indicated homoeopathic remedy may do a lot to ease immediate digestive discomfort, deeper-acting treatment is likely to be needed from a trained homoeopath in order to deal with the underlying problem.

Practical Self-Help

■ Eat small amounts frequently rather than leaving long gaps between large, heavy meals. Always avoid eating a large quantity of food late at night, since this is likely to cause great discomfort which can prevent sleep.

■ If you do not suffer from swollen ankles, propping up the head of the bed by approximately 10 centimetres (4 inches) may make you more comfortable at night. Alternatively, sleep in a semi-sitting position by using a couple of square, continental pillows, or three conventional pillows.

■ Where possible, avoid stooping after eating which encourages acid to travel into the gullet.

■ Avoid gulping food, making sure that each mouthful is chewed thoroughly. By taking time to enjoy your meals, there is less of a tendency to bolt when eating, which can lead to an excess of air being swallowed.

■ Many people who suffer from hiatus hernia are also overweight. If you feel that excess pounds are contributing to your problem, it is essential to take positive steps to bring your weight to its optimum level.

■ Smoking, coffee and alcohol are best avoided if you suffer from digestive problems, because they are major irritants of the stomach lining. As a result, they can contribute to acidity, discomfort and nausea.

■ If you suffer from distension and swelling of the stomach and/or abdomen after meals, it may be helpful to wear loose clothes or those that have an elasticated waistband.

Homoeopathic Help

Type of digestive discomfort	General symptoms	Worse from	Better for	Remedy name
Digestive problems come on soon after eating.	Nausea and sense of weight in the stomach set in quickly after eating. Acidity and heartburn, with rush of bitter-tasting saliva in the mouth. Thirsty with desire for long, cold drinks of water. Irritable and withdrawn with digestive discomfort.	Movement. Becoming overheated. Sitting up. Eating. Touch or pressure.	Cool surroundings. Keeping as still as possible. Lying down. Warm drinks.	**Bryonia**
Digestive discomfort that follows eating an excessive amount of rich food or drinking too much alcohol.	Terrible nausea and tension in stomach with constipation and headache. 'Morning after' syndrome with coated tongue and bad taste in the mouth. Stomach pains come on an hour after eating, with heartburn and sensitivity to constricting clothing around the waist.	Eating. Drinking coffee. Overuse of painkillers. Touch. Lack of sleep. Stress. Cold conditions.	Lying down. Resting. Sound sleep. Warmth. Peace and quiet.	**Nux vomica**
Digestive problems that come on in the early hours of the morning.	Burning pains that are relieved by warmth: acidity in stomach is soothed by frequent sips of warm drinks. Extreme restlessness, chilliness and anxiety during the first part of the night.	At night. Becoming chilled. Cold drinks or cold food. Being alone.	Warmth. Frequent sips of warm drinks. Gentle movement. Company.	**Arsenicum alb**
Digestive discomfort that comes on after eating too much fatty food.	Heavy sensations, acidity and wind in stomach follow eating too much red meat, cheese or rich dishes with creamy sauces. 'Repeating' of food eaten much earlier. Nausea and discomfort begin a couple of hours after eating, or in the evening. Restless, weepy and in need of sympathy when feeling sick.	Hot, stuffy rooms. Lying down. Warm food or drinks. Heavy, restricting clothes.	Cool, fresh air. Cool drinks. Gentle movement. Uncovering, or loosening clothes. Sympathy and attention.	**Pulsatilla**

217

Type of digestive discomfort	General symptoms	Worse from	Better for	Remedy name
Extreme belching brought on by eating sweet foods.	Nausea is eased by eating nutritious light foods. Violent belching does not relieve digestive discomfort. Stomach pain comes on soon after eating with flatulence and bloating. Symptoms arise due to anxiety, stress or mental strain.	Warmth. Stuffy rooms. Sugary diet. At night. On waking.	Fresh air. Light clothing. Walking in the fresh air.	**Arg nit**
Heaviness and excessive gas in stomach relieved by burping.	Stomach is so disordered that even plain, light foods feel heavy and indigestible. Burning in stomach extends to the back. Sensation of food being digested slowly and with difficulty. Craves fresh air and feels much better for being fanned.	Stuffy, overheated rooms. Humidity. Movement. Walking outside. After eating.	Fresh air. Being fanned. Belching. After sleep.	**Carbo veg**
Digestive problems with bloating, and noisy rumbling and gurgling.	Stomach fills up very quickly: sits down to a meal feeling hungry but can't finish it. An hour later, wants to eat again. Acidity and burning in the stomach that rises into the gullet. Frequent belches do nothing to relieve digestive uneasiness.	Cold drinks. Cold surroundings. Stuffy, overheated rooms. Pressure of waistband. Emotional stress. Physical or mental effort.	Warm drinks. Moderate warmth. Loosening clothes. Fresh air. Being distracted.	**Lycopodium**

Seek Prompt Medical Help If Any Of The Following Occurs:

■ **Right-sided, severe pains that radiate from front to between the shoulder blades, that do not improve within a couple of hours.**
■ **Severe or persistent nausea and vomiting accompanied by abdominal pain.**

■ Vomit that contains traces of blood that look dark red, or resemble coffee grounds.

■ Unexplained weight loss or loss of appetite.

■ Persistent and severe belching with distended stomach.

Hot Flushes

Although hot flushes may sound a minor problem, a large percentage of menopausal women find them extremely distressing. The severity of hot flushes can vary enormously, with some women experiencing tremendous uneasiness and distress, while others are hardly bothered at all. Common symptoms experienced during a hot flush or night sweat include the following:

■ Violent and abrupt onset of waves of heat which may be restricted to the torso, head and face, or may affect the whole body. The skin becomes deeply flushed and pink, especially in stuffy, overheated rooms where fresh, cool air is in short supply.

■ A vague sense of anxiety or foreboding often precedes a flush. This can commonly occur at night, when some women find they wake seconds before the onset of a night sweat. This may happen once or twice a night, adversely affecting sleep quality so that we feel unrefreshed and exhausted on waking.

■ Heavy, drenching perspiration may occur during or soon after a hot flush. This can be one of the most unpleasant symptoms because of the clammy, chilly, exhausted feelings that are left behind after the flush has gone.

■ Hot flushes are frequently accompanied by panic attacks and anxiety, often linked to embarrassment or fear that the flush has been noticed by others. Other possible symptoms may include physical and emotional weariness, headaches and dizziness.

If hot flushes are mild or happen on an irregular basis, the self-help measures outlined below, in addition to occasional use of a well-selected homoeopathic remedy, may be all that is needed to substantially improve symptoms. However, if hot flushes occur within the overall context of additional distressing or severe menopausal symptoms, it is more appropriate to consult a homoeopathic practitioner for help and advice.

Practical Self-Help

■ Adopt eating patterns that help guard against erratic or low blood sugar levels developing since a tendency to hypoglycaemia may aggravate hot flushes. It is important to eat small amounts regularly, rather than large meals with long intervals in between. Foods which stabilize blood sugar levels include fresh fruit, chopped, raw vegetables, rice cakes topped with cheese or savoury spreads, live, natural yoghurt or fromage frais. Avoid alcohol and strong, frequent cups of tea and coffee. Choose herb teas, grain coffees, fresh, unsweetened fruit juices or filtered water instead. Foods to avoid where possible include any products made from white (refined) sugar or flour, e.g. cakes and biscuits, those that are high in saturated fat, e.g. cream cakes, full-fat cheeses, or red meat and bacon. Chocolate and carbonated, sugary drinks should also be kept to a minimum, since they tend to play havoc with blood sugar levels. If you are unsure about symptoms which suggest that low blood sugar levels may be a problem, these include:

- Fuzzy-headedness, confusion and poor concentration.
- Drowsiness after meals.
- Severe mood swings.
- Abrupt, short-lived bursts of energy after eating, followed by exhaustion.

- Regular, aerobic, rhythmic exercise can do a great deal to stimulate circulation, ease hot flushes and improve energy levels. Beneficial activities should be brisk enough to produce a sweat, but not so demanding that they cause breathlessness. If you are working at an optimum level it should be possible to conduct a conversation without breathing becoming laboured, difficult or strained. Ideal activities include brisk walking, dancing, cycling or low-impact aerobics. However, avoid jogging or jarring movements if you have any joint problems or weakness in the ankles or knees.
- Relaxation and meditation techniques can be invaluable in easing the stress and anxiety that often accompany a hot flush. Once you have found a technique which works for you, it is worth making it a regular feature of each day.
- Learning how to breathe from the abdomen (diaphgramatic breathing) can provide us with an essential tool that can be used at any time to calm the mind and relax the muscles of the upper body. Since hot flushes can leave us feeling out of control and anxious, learning how to focus on our breathing technique can put us rapidly and effectively back in an empowered position. See **Chapter 8**: *The Stresses of Modern Living: How to Cope* for information on diaphragmatic breathing and other relaxation techniques.
- Wear loose, layered clothing made of natural fibres such as cotton or linen, rather than polyester blends. By wearing items that can be easily and discreetly removed, you are far more likely to feel relaxed and comfortable in surroundings where you cannot control the temperature to suit your needs.
- If you suffer from night sweats, wear light nightwear such as a cotton T-shirt, rather than choosing nightdresses made from man-made fabrics like nylon. Keep a towel, dry T-shirt, sponge and a bowl of tepid water by the bed. If you feel flushed and drenched with perspiration during the night, remove your damp T-

shirt, sponge yourself with the cool water, and put on the fresh shirt once you feel cool. This is much less disturbing than getting up in the middle of the night to look for dry clothes and sponging down in the bathroom.

Homoeopathic Help

Type of flush	General symptoms	Worse from	Better for	Remedy name
Hot flushes and night sweats that come on in stuffy, badly-ventilated rooms.	Sick, faint sensations precede or occur during a flush. Easily overheated at night with a marked dislike of heavy bedclothes. Tearful and emotional with menopausal symptoms: craves sympathy which helps a great deal.	Heat. Lack of fresh air. Heavy or warm clothes. Humidity. Becoming warm in bed. Resting or lying down. Evenings or at night.	Cool surroundings. Cool bathing. Fresh, open air. Cool food or drinks. Uncovering, or loosening clothes. Gentle exercise in the open air.	**Pulsatilla**
Upward moving flushes that rush from chest to head.	Palpitations, panic and pulsations with hot flushes. Disorientation and confusion may accompany anxiety. Sensitive to heat around the head or movement which exaggerates the distress of hot flushes. Dizziness, nausea and sensation of pressure in the head.	Warmth. Motion. Becoming chilled. Alcohol. Bending the head backward.	Fresh air to the head and face. Keeping as motionless as possible.	**Glonoin**
Hot flushes that are much worse for constricting clothes around the neck.	Hot and flushes through the day, cold and clammy at night. Flushes feel like waves of heat coursing through the body. Contact with heat is intolerable. Often wakes from sleep with symptoms. Talkative, anxious and subject to violent mood swings with menopausal symptoms.	Warmth. Hot drinks. Lack of fresh air. Constriction around the neck. On waking. At night.	Cool, fresh surroundings. Cool drinks. Eating small amounts. Onset of a discharge, e.g. beginning of a period. Gentle movement.	**Lachesis**

Type of flush	General symptoms	Worse from	Better for	Remedy name
Patchy flushes of heat localized in face, neck, ears, hands or feet.	Red, rosy patches appear on cheeks during a flush. Pulsating sensations of heat which rapidly shift from one part of the body to another. Persistent right-sided headaches during the menopause.	At night. Humid conditions. Physical effort. Chill. Touch.	Rest. Sound sleep.	**Sanguinaria**
Terrible heat sensitivity with marked aggravation of symptoms after bathing.	Rapidly overheated or chilled. Flushes are likely to be much worse at night in bed: has to push feet out of covers in order to get comfortable. Symptoms are intensified by physical effort or standing: instinctively wants to lie down in order to recover.	Overheated rooms. Becoming warm in bed. Damp, cold conditions. After washing. Stimulation. On waking.	Lying down. Resting. Moderate temperatures.	**Sulphur**

When hot flushes are persistent, severe, frequent or well-established, professional help should be sought rather than relying on self-medication.

Osteoarthritis

The onset of osteoarthritis has traditionally been regarded as an inevitable part of the ageing process, with the affected joints becoming stiff and painful through a general process of wear and tear. The areas most usually affected include the weight-bearing joints of the hip, knee and spine. These become distorted as the cartilage that provides a smooth covering for the ends of bones is worn down. When this happens, the underlying bony tissue becomes thickened and mis-shapen, resulting in restricted movement in the affected joint, as well as pain and discomfort.

Although it has been estimated that some degree of osteoarthritic degeneration has usually occured in ninety per cent of people over forty years of age, it is also becoming clear that there are positive steps we can take at an early age to protect the quality and mobility of our skeletal systems. The advice included in the *Practical Self-Help* section gives a general idea of the steps we can take to protect the health of our joints from middle age onwards.

Practical Self-Help

■ Being overweight can aggravate problems with arthritis in the weight-bearing joints of the hips and knees. If we carry excess pounds, following a sensible, gentle, weight-loss plan can do a great deal to improve our overall sense of health and well-being once we reach middle age.

■ Certain foods have a reputation for aggravating osteoarthritis. These include: foods made from refined (white) flour and sugar, red meat, dairy foods, citrus fruit (including oranges), tomatoes, peppers, potatoes, tea, coffee, alcohol, and convenience foods that include a large amount of artificial preservatives, colourings and flavourings. Where possible, eliminate these from your diet for a month and concentrate instead on white fish, pulses (beans, lentils, etc.), infrequent helpings of chicken or eggs, brown rice, rye bread, home-made muesli, non-citrus fruit, unroasted, unsalted nuts, freshly-pressed fruit juices (avoiding citrus), herb teas, coffee substitutes, home-made soups, mineral or filtered water, and sugar-free oatcakes. In order to isolate the foods that may be aggravating your joint problems, introduce the foods included in the first list one at a time. If you have a flare up of your joint pains, eliminate the offending food, and try introducing the item again once your joints have settled down. If you experience the problem a second time, the chances are that you have a sensitivity to this food, and should avoid it whenever possible.

■ Persistent, severe constipation may aggravate joint problems. Instead of relying on laxatives to deal in the short-term with irregular or unsatisfactory bowel movements, it is better to address the problem by rectifying any imbalances that may exist in the diet. Increase the amount of mineral or filtered water drunk on a daily basis (aim for approximately four or five large glasses each day), keep fatty, rich foods to a minimum, eat eggs in moderation, and increase the ratio of high-fibre foods such as wholemeal bread, raw vegetables and fruit (excluding citrus fruit), lentils, beans and peas.

■ Stay as mobile as possible in order to keep muscles flexible and strong. Choose any activity that you find enjoyable and fun, avoiding any physical exercise that involves pounding, jarring movements such as jogging. Swimming is an excellent choice, because the buoyancy of the water provides support for the joints while they are being moved. Additional activities to consider include walking, cycling and yoga.

■ The following supplements can also play a part in alleviating joint pain, stiffness and degeneration: vitamins A, B complex, C and E. Although vitamins C and B complex are water-soluble and readily flushed out of the body, it is important to bear in mind that vitamins A and E are fat-soluble. As a result, if too much is taken, potentially toxic side effects may develop. In order to avoid this problem, always stay well within the recommended daily allowance for these vitamins. It can also be beneficial to have regular breaks from using supplements, rather than relying on them on a long-term basis. Extract of green lipped muscle and devil's claw are also thought to relieve joint problems. These may be obtained from a health food shop.

■ If joint and/or muscle pains occur on a regular basis it may be helpful to seek treatment from an osteopath or chiropractor. Alternatively, if aches and pains seem to spring from muscular tension, a regular massage may be very helpful in easing stiffness of the neck, shoulders and back.

Homoeopathic Help

Type of osteo-arthritis	General symptoms	Worse from	Better for	Remedy name
Pain and stiffness in joints eased by gentle exercise.	Joints feel worse in bed or on waking: once up and about, they feel much more comfortable. Pain and stiffness are much worse in cold, damp weather. Restless, depressed and despondent with pain: especially in bed at night.	Keeping still. At night. Cold, damp weather. Becoming chilled after overheating. Initial movement. Jarring or jolting.	Warmth. Hot bathing. Continued movement (provided it is not exhausting). Support to painful joint. Stretching. Massage.	**Rhus tox**
Joint pain and stiffness eased by resting and keeping as still as possible.	Painful joints look red, swollen and hot. Stiffness and discomfort set in as the day goes on: on waking, joints are more comfortable. Persistent constipation and headaches may accompany joint problems. Arthritis following injury to the affected joints. Irritable and bad-tempered with pains.	Movement. Getting up from a sitting position. Stooping. Jarring movements or coughing. Touch.	Bandaging painful joint. Keeping still. Warmth locally applied. Lying on painful side.	**Bryonia**

Type of osteo-arthritis	General symptoms	Worse from	Better for	Remedy name
Swollen joints that react very badly to heat in any form.	Painful, stiff, rosy-red, puffy joints that are subject to stinging, prickling pains. Tendency to swollen, puffy ankles. Acute attacks of pain flare up very quickly and violently. Fidgety and restless with discomfort.	Contact with warm air. Warm bathing. Touch. Keeping still. After sleep.	Contact with cool air. Cool bathing. Gentle movement. Uncovering.	**Apis**
Stiffness and pain in joints that feel cold.	Although affected joints feel cold to the touch, they become less stiff and painful from bathing with cool water. Pains may begin in the joints of the feet and move upwards. May be indicated for lingering after-pains following a steroid injection.	Heat. Warm covering. Movement. At night. Alcohol. Eating eggs.	Cool bathing. Cool compresses. Rest.	**Ledum**
Joint and muscle pain following a fall or injury.	Aching, bruised pain and stiffness in joints that feel worse for the slightest touch or movement. Difficult walking because of aching in hip bones or because of weakness in knee joints. Exhausted and prostrated by pains.	Old injuries. Jarring. Touch. After sleep. Overexertion. Cold, damp weather. Movement.	Lying with head lower than the body.	**Arnica**
Stiff, painful joints that are worse for resting.	Red, swollen joints with desire to stretch muscles in order to get comfortable. Acute joint problems may be aggravated by rich, heavy diet including red meat and dairy foods. Although chilly, contact with warmth aggravates the pains. Weepy and depressed with joint problems.	Heat. Heavy clothes or bed covers. Rest. At night. Getting feet damp.	Cool, fresh air. Uncovering. Gentle movement. Pressure. Massage. Cool bathing or cool compresses. Having a good cry.	**Pulsatilla**

225

Type of osteo-arthritis	General symptoms	Worse from	Better for	Remedy name
Joint pains in poor quality bones that get worse in cold weather.	Chilly sensation in painful, stiff joints. Weakness in affected limbs made worse by climbing stairs. Lack of strength and pain in hip joints. Tendency to easy fractures because of poor-quality, weakened bones. Pains are intensified in cold, damp weather.	Change of weather. Exposure to cold draughts. Dehydration. Movement. Lifting. Stress. Climbing stairs.	Warm, dry conditions. Resting. During the summer.	**Calc phos**

If Any Of The Following Occurs, Professional Help Should Be Sought:

■ **Persistent and/or severe pains with increasing lack of mobility in the affected joint or joints.**

■ **Redness, heat and swelling of the small joints of the fingers or toes, and/or the knee and ankle joints.**

■ **General feeling of unwellness, feverishness or malaise with joint pains.**

Osteoporosis

The symptoms of osteoporosis (a tendency to thin or brittle bones) may include any of the following:

■ A tendency to easy fractures from jolting, jarring or minor falls. If the bones of the wrist break readily as a result of minor trauma, this would suggest that bone density needs to be examined. Other bones that may be extra vulnerable include those of the hip, spine and neck.

■ Extreme pain or discomfort in the weight-bearing joints of the back, hips and knees.

■ Restricted movement or immobility of the spine and chest.

■ Weakness or muscular spasms of the pelvic floor muscles.

■ In advanced osteoporosis, height loss and a 'dowager's hump' may develop, which gives a characteristic stooped appearance in advanced age.

There is currently a debate concerning the treatment of this condition by using hormone replacement therapy. Although many conventional physicians advocate HRT as the treatment of choice for those at risk of developing osteoporosis, there is a growing body of opinion which argues that there are alternative ways of addressing this problem and that the potential risks associated with HRT outweigh the benefits of this controversial approach to treating menopausal symptoms.

Although osteoporosis can affect men, women are generally more at risk of developing this condition in the post-menopausal years. It has been suggested that the onset of osteoporosis is linked to dwindling oestrogen supplies, as the fertile period of a woman's life comes to its close. If a woman experiences a menopause at an average age of fifty, thinning or weakening of the bones can begin at any stage after the mid-thirties, when it is estimated that peak bone mass should be reached. However, bone density may suffer earlier in those who have an increased risk of developing osteoporosis. Factors which may influence a predisposition to this problem include the following:

■ Surgically-induced or very early menopause (in rare instances, this may happen in one's twenties or early thirties). If both ovaries are removed during a hysterectomy, we stand a greater chance of developing osteoporosis than if one or both ovaries are left in place.

■ Chemotherapy or radiotherapy may also result in an early menopause in a young woman, with the same drawbacks as outlined above.

■ A tendency to develop osteoporosis may be inherited if we have close female relatives who suffer from this problem.

■ Steroid use may increase a predisposition to osteoporosis.

■ A poor-quality diet, with deficient amounts of calcium and magnesium, combined with regular or heavy consumption of caffeine, alcohol and strong tea, can increase the risk of osteoporosis. Smoking also has the effect of lowering oestrogen levels, which can may also aggravate a tendency to this condition.

■ A sedentary lifestyle with little or no weight-bearing exercise increases the risk of developing poor quality, de-calcified bones, especially when combined with other factors mentioned above.

■ Low body weight with absence of periods, that is associated with eating disorders such as anorexia or bulimia nervosa in adolescence, leaves us open to developing osteoporosis in later life. Because the teenage years are a vital time when bone mass is being established, adhering to starvation diets at this age can have a devastating effect on the quality of our skeletal systems.

From a holistic perspective, alternative approaches to healing such as homoeopathy, herbalism and acupuncture have a great deal to offer those who suffer from menopausal problems, including osteoporosis. However, because of the potential seriousness of the condition and its complications, this is a situation that must be dealt with by a trained practitioner rather than the self-prescriber. Although the self-help measures suggested below can be extremely valuable for those of us who are keen to take preventative action at any early stage against developing osteoporosis, those who have this condition should seek professional help.

Practical Self-Help

■ Exercise plays an extremely important role in protecting the quality of our bones from middle age onwards, by stimulating the production of small amounts of oestrogen. It is important to become fit and active as early as possible, since we reach our maximum bone mass in our mid-thirties. As a result, if we take regular exercise before we reach our middle years, we have a better chance of preserving strong, healthy bones in the later phase of our lives. Ideally, we should concentrate on rhythmic, weight-bearing activities in order to protect and encourage healthy bone density. Good examples of this kind of exercise include weight training, cycling, low-impact aerobics, or walking at a brisk pace. Additional forms of exercise that encourage muscular strength and stamina, which also benefit the heart and lungs, include swimming, tennis, badminton and yoga. However, it is best to avoid physical activities that put added strain on the vulnerable joints of the knee, ankle and hip, such as jogging on hard surfaces, or playing a fast game of squash.

■ If you are considering supplementing your daily intake of calcium, bear in mind that it is most beneficial to take a combined formula of calcium plus magnesium. These two minerals complement each other, and need to be obtained by the body in a specific ratio for maximum absorption to take place.

■ Strive to include healthy portions of calcium-rich foods in your diet, avoiding an excessive reliance on the obvious dairy foods such as milk, cheese and milk-based products. In addition to modest portions of dairy foods, eat regular helpings of the following: spinach, tofu, kale, broccoli, wild greens, whole grains, chick peas, soya beans, almonds, hazelnuts, molasses and sea vegetables such as kelp.

■ Include magnesium-rich foods in your diet, such as: almonds, whole grains, pulses, eggs, liver, green, leafy vegetables, and black-eyed peas.

■ Eat sparing quantities of foods that contain phosphorus. Although this mineral can stimulate increased calcium absorption, an excessive amount will have the opposite effect, encouraging calcium to leach out of our skeletal systems. It is best to avoid the following foods, or to strictly restrict the amount that is eaten if osteoporosis is a potential problem. They include 'instant', dehydrated snacks such as packet soups, powdered desserts and dried noodles. Soft drinks, processed cheeses and meats should also be avoided or kept to a minimum.

■ Although basic protein requirements must be met for building and repair of body tissues to take place, including an excessive amount of animal protein such as red meat in the diet can aggravate osteoporosis.

■ Alcohol, caffeine and cigarettes should also be treated with respect if we are concerned about the risk of osteoporosis, since all three can encourage the de-mineralization of our bones, leaving them brittle and vulnerable to fracture. Smoking has the additional drawback of reducing oestrogen production, as well as being associated with a host of additional health hazards such as heart and lung disease.

■ Additional supplements that may play a role in promoting healthy bone density include vitamins D, C and E, zinc, silicon and boron.

If Any Of The Following Occurs, Professional Help Should Be Sought:

■ **Severe or recurrent pain in the back, neck or hip.**
■ **A tendency to weakness of the joints or stress fractures.**

Sciatica

Sciatica is a painful condition that is caused by pressure or compression of the sciatic nerve. This can be the result of osteoarthritis, a protruding (prolapsed) disc, or a consequence of fusion of the vertebrae. Symptoms include shooting pains in the buttock and leg, which may become more intense when sitting, sneezing, coughing or bending. Pains may sometimes be eased by standing.

Because a tendency to sciatica can be a chronic (recurring) problem, this is a condition that is best treated by a trained practitioner. The following table of homoeopathic remedies is included in order to give some idea of the potential choice that is available for the acute treatment of sciatic pain. If one remedy stands out as fitting your symptoms very well, it is worth using it for short-term relief until professional advice is obtained. In addition to homoeopathic prescribing, it is also appropriate to consider one of the following therapies which can do a great deal to ease the distress of sciatica: acupuncture, osteopathy or chiropractic.

Practical Self-Help

■ Warm compresses can be soothing when applied to the painful area. A commercially-produced electrical heat pad may be useful, or a hot-water bottle wrapped in a soft cloth or cover.

■ Avoid wearing high heels or using shoulder bags that can encourage twisting or poor alignment of the spine.

■ Check that your mattress is comfortable and not too hard or too soft. If it sags in the middle, place a board beneath it.

■ If you suspect that recurring bouts of sciatica are linked to poor postural habits, consider consulting an Alexander Technique teacher for preventative advice, once an osteopath or chiropractor has been given the opportunity to deal with the immediate problem.

■ Since being overweight can aggravate back pain, a sensible weight-loss plan should be followed if you feel that this may be a factor that applies to you.

Homoeopathic Help

Type of sciatic pain	General symptoms	Worse from	Better for	Remedy name
Sciatica with heaviness and trembling of legs.	Legs feel weak and unsteady with sciatic pain. Discomfort is especially severe at night, preventing sleep. Initial movement after rest is difficult, as well as the first few steps when walking.	Initial movement. Cold, damp conditions. Becoming heated.	Continued movement. Resting propped-up. Bending forwards.	**Gelsemium**
Sciatic pain that is severe when sitting down.	Left-sided sciatica that may occur after a fall or injury involving the coccyx (base of the spine). Pains are violent, shooting and sharp. Tingling, burning, numb sensations in affected limb.	Jarring. Injuries or falls. Exertion. Cold, damp conditions. Change of weather.	Massage. Lying face down.	**Hypericum**
Sciatica that is aggravated by rest.	Terrible discomfort and restlessness in bed at night. Pains are relieved by warm compresses and hot bathing. Feels generally improved by gentle movement, provided it does not become too demanding.	Contact with cold, damp air. Uncovering. Initial movement. Rest. Overexertion. Jarring.	Hot bathing. Warmth. Massage. Warm wraps to painful area. Support to painful part. Stretching. Changing position. Warm, dry conditions.	**Rhus tox**

Type of sciatic pain	General symptoms	Worse from	Better for	Remedy name
Sciatica that is eased by flexing legs towards abdomen.	Severe sciatic pain that alternates with sensation of numbness or cramp. Lying down, jarring and motion make discomfort more intense.	Movement. Cold, damp air. Lying down.	Flexing legs. Sitting in a chair.	**Gnaphalium**
Contracted, band-like sensations with sciatica that react well to firm pressure.	Terrible pain with sciatica that leads the patient to twist and turn, and cry out in distress. Cutting, pinching, gnawing pains are closely followed by numbness which is eased by pressure. Shooting pain extends from top of leg to foot.	Cold, draughty conditions. At night. In bed. Becoming chilled. Lying on painless side.	Gentle movement. Firm pressure. Warmth. Resting. Bending double.	**Colocynthis**
Sciatica with shooting pains that rapidly dart about from place to place.	Severe, unbearable, cutting, twisting, griping pains that cause anxiety, shuddering and trembling. Right-sided, burning, sciatic pain that shoots down the thigh, relieved by lying still.	Bending double. Evening. At night. Movement. Sitting up.	Stretching. Bending backward. Firm pressure. Standing.	**Dioscorea**
Sciatica with pains in lower legs and feet.	Intense, radiating, lightning-like pains that lead to restlessness or prostration. Attacks of sciatica may be brought on by becoming chilled and wet. Pains are made more intense by coughing or jarring movements.	Cold, damp air. Uncovering. Touch. At night. Exhaustion.	Hot bathing. Warmth. Bending double. Massage. Firm pressure.	**Mag phos**
Sciatica with tearing pains in the thighs.	Pains extend from hip to knee on the affected side, with weakness in the legs and jerking, spasmodic movements of the muscles. Affected limb feels cold and weak, compelling rest. Pains are sharp, stabbing or throbbing when lying on the painful side.	Cold draughts. Becoming overheated. Exertion. In winter. Stooping. Change of weather. Touch. Movement.	Heat.	**Kali carb**

Type of sciatic pain	General symptoms	Worse from	Better for	Remedy name
Sciatica which is relieved by lying down.	Left-sided sciatic pain that is intensified by sitting down. Tension and contracted feeling in leg muscles, especially in the tendons of the hamstring muscles, which cause pain on walking. Sciatica may be aggravated by being severely overweight.	Evening. Walking. At night.	Lying down.	**Ammonium mur**

If sciatic pain is severe, persistent or recurring, professional help should be sought.

Varicose Veins

Problems with varicose veins are very common, especially in women. A tendency to develop varicose veins may be inherited, or certain factors can result in an increased risk of developing this condition. These may include the following:

■ A job which involves standing for lengthy periods of time.
■ Being overweight.
■ Being pregnant.

The characteristic knobbly, distended appearance of varicose veins results from excess blood draining into the superficial veins of the legs. The valves in these veins normally prevent this back-flow occurring when they work efficiently. However, when they become less effective at this job, the superficial veins become enlarged and twisted in response to the increased pressure of the back-flow of blood.

Common symptoms of varicose veins include the following:

■ Swollen, bluish, prominent-looking veins that are especially visible when standing. These are most likely to affect the calf, ankle, thigh or groin.
■ The discomfort associated with varicose veins may alternate from aching to itching of the skin covering the affected vein.
■ Swelling and aching may affect the whole of the leg, with ankles and feet

becoming especially swollen at night.

■ Women may find that discomfort from varicose veins is worse before and during their periods.

■ If varicose veins are severe, the skin around the affected vein may break down, resulting in a varicose ulcer.

If problems with varicose veins are minor or intermittent in nature, the practical advice given below, combined with the occasional use of a well-indicated homoeopathic remedy, may help a great deal in easing pain and itching.

However, if there is any suggestion of ulceration, or if varicose veins are combined with general circulatory problems, professional help should be obtained from a homoeopathic practitioner.

Practical Self-Help

■ Make time for a regular walk every day, avoiding standing, or sitting with legs crossed whenever possible.

■ When resting, elevate the legs higher than the body in order to ease distended, aching veins.

■ If a varicose ulcer occurs, keep the ulcerated skin clean and covered by a sterile dressing to which **Calendula** cream should be added. Because of its healing, soothing, antiseptic qualities, **Calendula** cream can be very helpful in promoting efficient and speedy healing of ulcerated skin. Although **Arnica** may be taken internally for symptoms of varicose veins, ***never*** apply **Arnica** cream to broken or ulcerated skin, since it can aggravate inflammation and discomfort.

■ Being overweight can increase problems with varicose veins. Adopt a high fibre diet that is low in fat, sugar, refined foods and alcohol, while also taking up a regular, enjoyable form of exercise.

■ Constipation can aggravate symptoms, so protect against it by eating a high-fibre diet which is rich in wholefoods such as whole grains, pulses, fresh fruit and vegetables. Drink a minimum of five glasses of filtered water daily, avoiding regular consumption of drinks that have a diuretic effect such as strong coffee or tea. Also avoid foods that have been refined or processed, such as white flour, sugar, or 'instant' convenience foods, or those that contain a high proportion of saturated fat. These include cheese, cream, red meat and butter.

■ Use support stockings or tights where necessary, avoiding clothes or hold-up stockings that are very tight around the hips or thighs.

■ Certain nutrients have a reputation for improving circulation, and may help with the management of symptoms of varicose veins. These include vitamins C, B3 (part of the B complex group), and E. Rutin may also help by strengthening the walls of the affected veins. Rutin can be obtained through eating buckwheat, or it can be taken in supplement form.

Homoeopathic Help

Type of varicose veins	General symptoms	Worse from	Better for	Remedy name
Varicose veins with extreme restlessness and chilliness.	Burning pains in varicose veins are relieved greatly by warmth. Sensation as though waves of ice-cold or burning liquid is surging through veins. Constantly chilly because of inefficient circulation. Anxious and mentally and physically restless when in pain.	Cold in any form. Becoming chilled. Late at night. Keeping still.	Warmth. Warm compresses. Warm bathing. Resting propped-up in bed. Gentle movement.	**Arsenicum alb**
Severe pains with constricted feeling in veins.	Poor circulation with history of problems with chilblains. Legs feel bruised and prickly. If individualizing symptoms are absent, or difficult to spot, this is the first remedy to consider.	Pressure. Contact with open air. Chill. Movement. During the day. Touch or contact. Jarring. Bruising.	At night.	**Hamamelis**
Poor circulation with varicose veins that are painful when sitting or standing.	Symptoms may be restricted to the right leg, or more severe on the right side. Changeable, shifting, flitting pains with varicose veins prone to ulceration. Circulatory problems lead to persistently cold hands and feet and a tendency to chilblains. Depressed and weepy with discomfort.	Resting. Becoming overheated. Warm bathing. Heavy clothes or bed covers. Chill or damp.	Cool bathing. Contact with cool, fresh air. Gentle exercise. Uncovering. Firm support or pressure.	**Pulsatilla**

Type of varicose veins	General symptoms	Worse from	Better for	Remedy name
Ulcerated varicose veins with burning, itching pains.	Widespread problems with varicose veins affecting the arms, legs and genital area. Pulsating, cramping pains in calves at night. Burning sensations in veins are improved by contact with cool air. Easy-bleeding varicose ulcers that heal and break out again.	Heat. Humidity. Motion. Becoming chilled. Stuffy conditions.	Contact with cool air. Fanning painful area. After sleep.	**Carbo veg**
Stiff, aching legs that bruise easily.	Swollen feet with terribly restless legs: tosses about constantly in bed trying to find a comfortable position. Bruised pains with varicose veins that feel sensitive to the slightest touch or movement. Tired and exhausted with pains.	Jarring movement. Physical effort. Touch. After sleep. Motion. Cold, damp conditions.	Resting with head lower than the body.	**Arnica**
Varicose veins that are very heat-sensitive.	Purple-coloured, distended veins that affect the left leg, or begin on the left side and move to the right. Movement makes discomfort in veins less distressing. Pounding, bursting pains are made more intense by contact with heat.	Tight, restricting clothing. Heat. After sleep. Keeping still. During the menopause.	Contact with cool air. Cool compresses locally applied. Onset of a discharge. Gentle exercise.	**Lachesis**

If Any Of The Following Occurs, Professional Help Should Be Sought:

■ **Severe varicose veins with ulceration.**
■ **A knock or blow to the skin covering a varicose vein can result in a severe loss of blood which requires swift medical attention.**
■ **Persistent or very severe pain in a varicose vein.**
■ **Brownish discolouration of the skin affecting areas where circulation is poor.**

■10■

Remedy Information: Essential Aspects

I n this section you will find an expanded picture of most of the homoeopathic remedies mentioned in the self-help tables. The way in which the
information is presented is designed to provide an overview of the central or
essential features of each remedy. As familiarity with the remedies and their
application grows, it should become increasingly easy to differentiate between
each one with confidence. However, it is worth noting that not every remedy
mentioned in the tables is given an expanded treatment in this section, since the
information given about smaller remedies within the table format should be
detailed enough to lead to a confident prescription.

Aconite (Monkshood)

Often Indicated For:
■ Anxiety and panic attacks
■ Breathlessness
■ Chill
■ Chickenpox
■ Colds
■ Croup
■ Dizziness
■ Earache
■ Eye injuries
■ Flu
■ Grief
■ German measles
■ Insomnia
■ Labour
■ Measles

- Mumps
- Neuralgia
- Palpitations
- Sore throats
- Shock
- Teething

Essential Features

- Most often needed in the early stages (the first 24–48 hours) of a quickly-developing problem with violent or severe symptoms.
- Problems often follow becoming chilled, exposure to dry, cold winds, or severe emotional trauma.
- Terrible anxiety, fever and restlessness with preoccupation with death.
- Extreme sensitivity to, and intolerance of, pain with strong aversion and fear of being touched.
- Extreme chilliness with muscle twitching and tension.
- Symptoms may subside as rapidly as they set in.

Emotional State

- Fear and panic in stressful situations, such as admission to hospital for surgery, especially if there is a strong conviction that something will go wrong.
- Terrible anxiety and panic with a conviction that death will occur.
- Frequent, overwhelming panic attacks with specific fear of crowds, open spaces and the dark.
- Severe emotional reactions may follow general shock or trauma, such as witnessing an accident.
- Awful sensitivity on mental, emotional and physical levels.

Head Symptoms

- Sudden, severe headaches with fever and trembling.
- An upsetting or frightening experience may bring on bouts of giddiness or headache.
- Headache is generally improved by contact with fresh air and made worse from stuffy, airless rooms.
- Lying down and resting relieves dizziness and headache, although it aggravates most other symptoms.

Eye Symptoms

- Rapid-developing, violent symptoms.
- Eye injuries with swelling and burning.
- Burning, watering, red eyes with over-sensitivity to light.
- Painful sensitivity to the reflection of sunlight from snow.

Ear, Nose and Throat Symptoms
■ Earache from leaving the ears exposed in cold winds.
■ Runny nose quickly follows exposure to chill, or cold, east winds.
■ Clear, fluent, hot nasal discharge with head cold.
■ Headache with blocked nose is eased by being out of doors, and from contact with fresh air.
■ Hoarse, dry, tingling throat with difficulty swallowing.
■ Tight, narrowed, dry sensation in throat on swallowing.
■ Deep red, inflamed throat with burning and prickling sensations.

Chest Symptoms
■ Exposure to chill, or dry, cold winds brings on dry, barking cough.
■ Anxious breathlessness during sleep, and on getting up.
■ Dry cough is aggravated by being upset, during the night, talking, eating or drinking.
■ Frequent waking at night with choking fits and violent cough.
■ Palpitations with terrible anxiety and flushes of heat.
■ Shortness of breath when rushing, or climbing stairs.

Digestive Symptoms
■ Sudden onset of digestive upsets after emotional trauma or shock.
■ Very thirsty for water, which is the only thing that does not taste bitter.
■ Severe tenderness in stomach that is aggravated by moving.
■ Very restless and distressed with stomach pains.
■ Rapidly-developing diarrhoea after shock or trauma.

Urinary Symptoms
■ Urination problems such as retention of urine in new-born babies.
■ Sudden onset of violent, cutting, tearing pains with cystitis.
■ Constant desire to pass water with anxiety, distress and pain.
■ Concentrated, dark, and/or bloody urine which feels hot to pass.

Gynaecological Symptoms
■ Period problems may originate from a time of stress, fear or shock.
■ Hot flushes, numb, or tingling sensations with pains.
■ Severe, cutting, stabbing or tearing pains.
■ Becomes frantic with pains, which feel unbearable.
■ Panic with heavy bleeding.
■ Gushing, bright menstrual flow.

Flushes And Fever
■ Violent, rapidly-developing fever and inflammation follows exposure to dry, cold winds or becoming chilled.
■ Sudden onset of high temperature, anxiety, and flushes of heat with hot head and cold body.

Sleep
- Disrupted sleep pattern may follow being involved in, or witnessing an accident, or any other emotional shock or trauma.
- Sleepless and restless at night, and drowsy during the day.
- Fitful sleep, with tossing and turning.
- Anxious, disturbed sleep with terrors and nightmares.

Skin Symptoms
- Extra-sensitive skin with extreme sensitivity to, and discomfort from, slightest touch.

Aggravated By
- Contact with dry, cold winds, or chill.
- Exposure to extreme hot or cold surroundings.
- Fright, shock or emotional trauma.
- During the night.
- Overheated, stuffy rooms.
- Lying on painful areas.

Improved By:
- Sound sleep.
- Fresh air.
- Perspiring.

Agnus Castus (Chaste tree)

Often Indicated For:
- Pre-menstrual tension
- Menopausal problems
- Headache
- Cystitis
- Colic
- Pains in joints from old injuries, strains, or sprains that have not completely healed.

Essential Features
- Lowered libido as an expression of diminished energy and vitality.
- Alternating chills with flushes of heat anywhere in the body.
- Heavy, bruised sensations.
- Weak muscles.
- Total apathy and indifference.

Emotional State
- Rapid changes of mood between euphoria and depression.
- Fragile self-esteem: alternates between over-confidence and lack of self-worth.
- Lack of libido in its broadest sense: diminished pleasure and enjoyment in life.

- Depression with a belief that the best years are in the past, and that there is nothing in the future to anticipate with excitement or pleasure.
- Weary and despondent as a result of general exhaustion.
- Broods on illness and fear of dying.
- Poor memory with a tendency to lose the thread of conversation.

Head Symptoms
- Headaches affect the crown of the head, the right temple, or above the right eye.
- General movement makes the headache worse, as well as specifically moving the eyes when reading.
- Heavy, pressured feeling in the head.

Digestive Symptoms
- Standing makes queasiness and nausea more pronounced.
- Hunger pangs which are not satisfied by eating.
- Colicky abdominal pains that are more intense from pressure of sitting.
- Constipation with dragging sensation in the bowels: wants to support affected area with hands.
- Noisy flatulence during sleep.
- Sore abdomen that is sensitive to the touch.

Urinary Symptoms
- Cystitis with frequent need to pass copious amounts of discoloured, dark urine.
- Pain and discomfort after passing water.

Gynaecological Symptoms
- Heavy, lengthy periods that may continue for a couple of weeks.
- Drooping, weak sensations with prolapse of womb.
- Transparent, or yellow-coloured, vaginal discharge.
- Aversion to sex as a result of general weariness and exhaustion or indifference.

Joint And Muscle Symptoms
- Generalized inflammation and swelling of the joints.
- Easily-dislocated joints with residual pains, and lack of flexibility from old injuries that have not fully healed.

Aggravated By:
- Effort.
- Motion.

Improved By:
- Keeping still.
- Rest.

Anacardium (Marking nut)

Often Indicated For:

- Anxiety
- Constipation
- Cough
- Depression
- Headache
- Morning sickness
- Painful periods
- Palpitations
- Rheumatism

Essential Features

- Extreme fidgeting, restlessness or exhaustion.
- Constricted feelings occur anywhere in the body like a lump, hoop or plug.
- Emotional distress is directly linked to hormonal fluctuations (e.g. pre-menstrual or menopausal problems).

Emotional State

- Feels body and mind are separated, leading to sensation of being in a dream with general sense of unreality.
- Strong sense of being two people, or having two wills which pull in opposite directions.
- Compelled to do things against natural inclination or will.
- Obsessive or fixed ideas: strong sense of being followed or watched.
- Depression, anxiety and despondency with fear of death.
- Contradictory behaviour: laughs uncontrollably at serious things, and becomes serious when something amusing happens.
- Compulsion to curse and swear.

Head Symptoms

- Headaches with dizziness and confusion as a result of exhaustion.
- Headache is eased by eating, and made more intense by bending the head backwards, noise and movement.
- Tension headaches from mental strain with pressing pain in the forehead.

Chest Symptoms

- Tickling in the throat with choking cough.
- Coughing and gagging after eating.
- Coughing spasms are aggravated at night and after food.
- Flushes of heat and headache with coughing bouts.

Digestive Symptoms
- Unpleasant taste in the mouth when not eating.
- Nausea on waking.
- Eats regularly in an effort to relieve hunger pangs.
- Cold drinks make stomach pains worse, but they are relieved by warm food.
- Discomfort in stomach after eating, or when under mental stress or strain.
- Constipation with sensation of a plug in the rectum.
- Difficulty passing even a soft stool with urgent desire to open bowels.

Urinary Symptoms
- Frequent need to pass water at night.

Gynaecological Symptoms
- Frequent, scanty periods.
- 'Spotting' between periods.
- Itching, irritation or burning around vaginal entrance with vaginal discharge.

Joint And Muscle Symptoms
- Frequent episodes of cramp or pain that occur when walking or resting at night.
- Sense of weakness or 'giving' in the knee joints when walking.
- Constricted feeling in the knees: as though they had been wound with a firm bandage.
- Sensation of numbness or 'going to sleep' in limbs when resting.

Sleep
- Goes to sleep early with a tendency to disturbed or poor quality sleep.
- Cramps in limbs prevent sound sleep.
- Wakes with headache after nightmares or anxious dreams.

Aggravated By:
- Mornings.
- Initial movement.
- Mental strain.
- Exposure to cold draughts.
- Having an empty stomach.

Improved By:
- Rest.
- Eating.
- Warmth.

Apis (Honey bee)

Often Indicated For:
- Allergic reactions

- Bites
- Cystitis
- Hayfever
- Laryngitis
- Measles
- Mumps
- Nappy rash
- Osteoarthritis
- Prickly heat
- Shock
- Sore throats
- Stings
- Wounds

Essential Features

- Extreme allergic reactions involving rapid swelling, inflammation and accumulation of fluid in the tissues.
- Terrific heat sensitivity with severe, burning, stinging pains that are soothed by cool bathing and contact with cool air.
- Symptoms set in with violence and rapidity, causing fast-advancing swellings that look rosy-pink, puffy and water-logged.
- General state of fluid-retention with 'water bag' swellings anywhere in the body that 'pit' on pressure (a dent is left in the swelling after pressure is applied, and removed).
- Marked sensitivity to touch and pressure, especially to the abdomen.

Emotional State

- Problems occur after a period of stress, trauma or emotional upset.
- Extreme sensitivity, and aversion to slightest touch or physical contact.
- Fidgety, irritable and fussy with discomfort.
- Very tearful with inability to stop crying.
- Cries out during sleep from pain.
- Agitated, busy and restless when ill.
- Demands company and attention, but rejects affection when unwell.

Head Symptoms

- Hot head with throbbing headache.
- Headaches are aggravated by jarring movements and warm surroundings.
- Thick, fuzzy sensation in head is relieved by pressure.
- Dizzy sensation with headache is intensified by resting, lying down, and closing the eyes, and eased by moving about.

Eye Symptoms

- Severe swelling underneath the eyes.

- Watery eyes with light sensitivity.
- Discomfort and swelling are temporarily eased by cool bathing.

Ear, Nose And Throat Symptoms

- Redness and swelling of both ears.
- Violent sneezing fits with allergic reactions
- Permanently blocked nostrils and/or scanty nasal discharge.
- Water-logged, 'glossy' appearance to the throat.
- Inflamed throat with puffy, swollen uvula.
- Throat feels tight and narrowed, leading to difficulty in swallowing: even sips of water go down with difficulty.

Chest Symptoms

- Breathing problems are intensified when leaning forwards or backwards.
- Breathlessness is worse in warm, stuffy surroundings.
- Croupy cough at night which is eased by coughing until mucus is raised.
- Harsh, dry cough which begins with constricted sensation in the throat.

Digestive Symptoms

- Burning pains in stomach are aggravated by sneezing bouts.
- Distended, tense stomach that is extremely sensitive to touch or slightest contact.
- Residual raw, burning sensations following attacks of diarrhoea which are soothed by cool bathing and cool compresses.

Urinary Symptoms

- Generalized aching, soreness and discomfort with bladder and kidney disorders.
- Kidney problems cause fluid retention, with puffiness being especially pronounced around the eyes.
- Reduced, concentrated, scalding urine that causes great discomfort when it needs to be passed frequently.
- Lack of or reduced thirst with urinary problems.

Gynaecological Symptoms

- Burning, stinging pains and discomfort in the pelvic area.
- Severe right-sided ovarian pains which spread to the left.

Joint And Muscle Symptoms

- Swollen, rosy-pink, taut, inflamed joints that are soothed by cool bathing and cool compresses.
- Stinging, burning pains in affected joints.
- Cold hands and feet with red, inflamed fingers and toes.
- Severe swelling of the finger and toe joints.

Flushes and Fever

- High temperature with marked absence of thirst.

■ Once fever subsides, thirst sets in.

■ Very much worse for contact with heat in any form when feverish, and made much more comfortable for cool applications and fresh air.

Sleep

■ Very uncomfortable and distressed if overheated in bed.

■ Cries out in restless sleep.

■ Tosses and turns, and throws covers off in order to cool down.

Skin

■ Often indicated for treating hives that come on after overheating.

■ Stinging, itching skin that is relieved by cool bathing and contact with cool air, and made much worse by becoming heated.

■ Blotchy, pink, puffy, raised eruptions that look water-logged.

Aggravated By:

■ Slight touch or contact.

■ Heat in any form.

■ Warm drinks.

■ Keeping still.

■ Lying down.

■ After sleep.

■ Night.

Improved By:

■ Cool air.

■ Cool compresses.

■ Cool bathing.

■ Uncovering.

■ Gentle movement in fresh, cool air.

■ Sitting up.

Arg nit (Silver nitrate)

Often Indicated For:

■ Acidity in the stomach

■ Anticipatory anxiety

■ Diarrhoea

■ Disturbed sleep pattern linked to anxiety

■ Extreme reactions to stress

■ Headache

■ Heartburn

■ Wind and flatulence

Essential Features

- Extreme anxiety linked to a coming event.
- Digestive problems such as diarrhoea are sparked off by anxiety and tension.
- Squeezing, constricted sensations can occur anywhere in the body.
- Marked cravings for sugary or salty foods which aggravate the general situation.

Emotional State

- Extremely agitated, anxious and restless when thinking about a coming stressful event.
- Anxiety about heights, small spaces, bridges, high buildings or being in a crowded place.
- Very restless when agitated; hurries from one thing to the next as a way of coping with agitation and distress.
- Constantly hurried and fearful of being late or missing appointments.
- Talkative and chatty when anxious.

Head Symptoms

- Throbbing headache is intensified by warmth and eased by contact with cool things.
- Expanded or enlarged feelings in the head which are eased by tight pressure.

Digestive Symptoms

- Nausea that may be initially relieved by eating.
- Nervous diarrhoea that is aggravated by eating sweet things.
- Nausea and bloating may come on a little while after eating: passing wind and belching don't help.

Urinary Symptoms

- Blood-streaked urine with discomfort on passing water, that may be brought on by nervous upsets.
- Scalding feelings occur during and after passing small amounts of concentrated urine.

Gynaecological Symptoms

- Irritation and inflammation around vaginal entrance with sharp, sticking pains.
- Intermittent yellow-coloured discharge from vagina.
- Painful, irregular periods with all symptoms being aggravated pre-menstrually and during period.
- Tender ovaries with pains radiating from base of spine to thighs.

Sleep

- Exhausted and achy on waking.
- Restless, anxious and unable to get to sleep when thinking about a coming event.

■ Unable to get comfortable in bed because of feeling chilled or too hot.

Joint And Muscle Symptoms

■ Severe back pain when getting up after sitting down that is relieved when standing or walking.

■ Pains in the small joints of the wrists, hands and feet.

■ Cramping pains in calves at night.

Aggravated By:

■ Sugar.

■ Stress.

■ Anticipation.

■ Stuffy rooms.

■ Warmth.

■ Night.

Improved By:

■ Firm pressure.

■ Fresh, cool air.

Arnica (Mountain daisy)

Often indicated For:

■ Abscesses

■ Bruising, shock, accident or trauma of any kind. Its effective action aids in reducing blood loss, encourages re-absorption of blood from bruised tissues, and encourages healing of wounds.

■ Dental work trauma

■ Grief

■ Immediate pain and shock of fractures

■ Insomnia

■ Muscle aching after overexercising

■ Muscle cramps

■ Osteoarthritis

■ Pre, and post dental work trauma (helps ease anxiety and emotional stress as well as physical trauma)

■ Strains and sprains

■ Vaginal bruising and shock following childbirth

■ Varicose veins

■ Whooping cough

Essential Features

■ Bruised, aching, sore pains.

■ Extreme restlessness from discomfort.

247

■ Oversensitivity to touch.

■ A tendency to easy bruising.

■ General sensations of stiffness and weariness.

■ Pains and discomfort are worse at night and for exposure to cold, damp conditions.

Emotional State

■ Restless, agitated and bad-tempered with pain.

■ Intolerant of company, or people who try to help: pushes them away during the immediate shock following an accident or fall.

■ Marked dislike of anyone approaching because of aversion to being touched.

■ Insists on being left alone.

■ Extreme mental and physical oversensitivity with aching pains.

■ Withdrawn and morose.

■ Difficulty concentrating with tendency to forgetfulness.

Head Symptoms

■ Dizziness on waking or moving which is made more intense when closing the eyes.

■ One-sided headache with nausea.

■ Sharp pains with headache, as though the skull were being pierced with a nail.

Eye Symptoms

■ Conjunctivitis or eye strain with burning sensations.

■ General trauma, bleeding or bruising following an eye injury.

■ Swollen eyelids from bruising.

Ear, Nose And Throat Symptoms

■ Shooting pains in and behind the ears.

■ Nosebleeds with tingling in nose, following injury.

■ Aching, bruised sensations in the throat.

Chest Symptoms

■ Burning, raw, bruised sensations in the chest.

■ Dry, tickly cough that is worse in the mornings.

■ Stitching pains in the chest, and soreness of the ribs that are aggravated by moving and coughing.

■ Whooping cough in children with tendency for child to become distressed before coughing spasms.

Digestive Symptoms

■ Nausea with excessive amounts of salivation.

■ Extreme or total absence of thirst.

■ Nausea is increased by the thought of food or eating.

■ Colicky pains in the abdomen with wind.

■ Diarrhoea is passed involuntarily.

Urinary Symptoms

■ Frequent urge to pass urine, which is voided with great difficulty.

■ Waits for a while before flow of urine starts.

■ Urine may be retained after an excessive amount of exercise.

■ Blood-stained urine.

Gynaecological Symptoms

■ Severe after-pains following long or traumatic labour.

■ Bruised pains which may be especially distressing at night.

■ Exhaustion during the menopause with hot flushes to head, cold body and palpitations.

Sleep

■ Extremely restless in bed: the surface feels too hard to rest on.

■ Difficulty falling sleep before the early hours of the morning.

■ Fitful sleep with tendency to wake from bad dreams.

■ Aches all over with tiredness.

Skin Symptoms

■ Indicated for boils or abscesses that are very painful, but do not come to a head.

■ Aching, soreness and tenderness after bruising and injury.

Joint And Muscle Symptoms

■ General aching, throbbing and burning pains with exhaustion after over-exertion.

■ Aching, heavy feelings in arms and legs with general weariness and tiredness.

■ Sore, bruised feelings in swollen hands or feet.

■ Muscle and joint pains feel much worse for exposure to cold, damp conditions.

Aggravated By:

■ Over-exposure to heat or sunlight.

■ Too much exercise.

■ Alcohol.

■ Movement.

■ Being touched.

■ Being approached.

■ Damp.

■ Cold.

Improved By:

■ Resting with head lower than body.

Arsenicum alb (White oxide of metallic arsenic)

Often Indicated For:

- Addiction
- Anxiety
- Chickenpox
- Colds
- Coughs
- Cystitis
- Depression
- Diarrhoea
- Digestive disorders
- Hayfever
- Headaches
- Heartburn
- Indigestion
- Influenza
- Insomnia
- Mastitis
- Morning sickness
- Nappy rash
- Painful periods
- Vomiting
- Varicose Veins

Essential Features

- Extreme physical and mental restlessness, chilliness and anxiety.
- All symptoms set in or become more intense with the onset of night: especially after midnight.
- Great sensitivity to cold and chills, with a marked improvement of symptoms from contact with warmth.
- Extreme physical and mental weariness and exhaustion with symptoms.
- Strongly indicated where vomiting and diarrhoea occur simultaneously.
- Burning pains are soothed and eased by contact with warmth.
- Very chilly and pale.

Emotional State

- Oversensitive and fussy about surroundings when ill.
- Although mentally, emotionally and physically exhausted, cannot relax if surroundings are untidy or in need of cleaning.
- Terribly physically and mentally restless with exhaustion.
- Awful anxiety, building to a state of panic that gets steadily worse as the night goes on.

- Much worse for being alone, especially at night.
- Specific fears of the dark, death, germs and serious illness.
- Paces around the room in order to try and keep control.
- Obsessional behaviour may develop as a result of anxieties about hygiene and cleanliness.
- Despairing when ill, believing that the situation is beyond hope or help.
- Self-critical and highly-competitive, often demanding unrealistically high standards from others.

Eye Symptoms
- Swollen, red eyes with burning pains that are aggravated by bright light.
- Inflammation and swelling of the eyelids.
- Watery, burning eyes with extreme light sensitivity.
- Discomfort in eyes is relieved by warmth.

Head Symptoms
- The head is the only part of the body that is relieved by exposure to cool, fresh air; everything else is better for contact with warmth and warm applications.
- Headaches develop in the afternoon and get steadily worse as the night goes on.
- Vomiting and nausea with headache.
- Headaches are intensified by movement, noise and bright lights.
- Pains come on as a result of anxiety, becoming overheated or too much excitement.

Ear, Nose And Throat Symptoms
- Maddening itching, burning and/or tingling in the ears.
- Burning nasal discharge leaves the nostrils and upper lip red, burning and sensitive.
- Violent sneezing with scanty, burning, clear nasal discharge.
- Burning pains in the throat are soothed by sips of warm drinks.
- Difficulty swallowing from constricted, burning sensation in throat.

Chest Symptoms
- Anxious and wheezy with dry cough.
- Coughing spasms are aggravated by lying flat or becoming chilled.
- Wheezing may be brought on by a reaction to stress and anxiety.
- Dry, persistent cough becomes worse at night, and is relieved by sitting propped-up in bed in a warm room.

Digestive Symptoms
- Cannot bear the thought, sight or smell of food.
- General state of restless exhaustion occurs as a result of vomiting and diarrhoea happening simultaneously.
- Discomfort and burning pains in stomach are relieved by warm drinks.

■ Despite the fact that the stomach is very sensitive to touch, it feels more comfortable for warm compresses applied locally.

■ Sips of warm drinks are soothing, although long, cold drinks are vomited back immediately.

Urinary Symptoms

■ Generally chilly, feverish, restless, nauseated and anxious with kidney or bladder disorders.

■ Kidney problems may be related to a general state of dehydration, which occurs as a result of vomiting and diarrhoea happening together.

■ Distressing burning sensations occur on passing urine.

Gynaecological Symptoms

■ Very distressed and restless with period pains leading to an extreme state of prostration and exhaustion.

■ Severe period pains cause diarrhoea and/or vomiting.

■ Pains feel better from warmth in general, and also from heat locally applied to the painful area.

■ Sensitivity with irritation, and burning, watery discharge from the vagina.

Flushes And Fever

■ Burning sensations with high temperature are eased from warmth or heat locally applied.

■ Extremely chilly with feverishness: waves of ice-cold water seem to surge through the body.

■ Desire for frequent sips of warm drinks, rather than large gulps of cool liquids when feverish.

Sleep

■ Extremely mentally and physically restless at night, when symptoms develop or become more apparent.

■ Wanders about at night as a result of restlessness, may sit up and read, or have a cup of tea in order to try to relax.

■ Feels drowsy by day and sleepless at night.

■ Wakes with anxiety thinking about the things that have to be organized for the following day.

■ Wakes after midnight (around 1 a.m.) feeling worried and sweaty.

Skin Symptoms

■ Repeated, compulsive scratching that causes weeping and bleeding of the skin, leaving the skin raw.

■ Itchy, burning skin that feels more irritated and uncomfortable after scratching.

■ The irritation is eased temporarily by rubbing, but burning sensation remains.

■ Skin eruptions are soothed by contact with warmth.

Joint And Muscle Symptoms
- Restlessness and difficulty sleeping from pain and discomfort in legs at night.
- Pains in the upper back are relieved by lying down and resting.

Aggravated By:
- Becoming cold or chilled.
- Cold draughts.
- At night: especially after midnight.
- Being alone.
- Lying flat in bed.
- Cold food or drinks.
- Alcoholic drinks.

Improved By:
- Warmth.
- Frequent sips of warm drinks.
- Warmth applied to the painful area.
- Company and distractions.
- Gentle movement.
- Headache is specifically improved by fresh air.
- Perspiring.

Belladonna (Deadly Nightshade)

Often Indicated For:
- Abscesses
- Boils
- Bleeding
- Chickenpox
- Colds
- Croup
- Cystitis
- Earache
- German measles
- Headache
- High fever
- Influenza
- Mastitis
- Measles
- Migraines
- Mumps
- Nappy rash
- Sore throats

- Sunstroke
- Teething

Essential Features

- Rapidly developing inflammation or fever with high temperature, and hot, dry, bright red skin which is burning when touched.
- Extreme irritability, restlessness and bad-temper in those who are normally mild and placid.
- Marked oversensitivity and acuteness of the senses, including overreaction to light, noise and touch.
- Throbbing, pulsating, pounding pains.
- Symptoms may affect the right side of the body, or be worse on the right than the left side.
- Although extremely hot, becomes very easily chilled, with a resulting aversion to the slightest draught of cold air.
- Feels generally worse after sleep.

Emotional State

- Intolerant, irritable and bad-tempered with onset of symptoms.
- Alternates between overexcitability and drowsiness or lethargy.
- Someone who has a normally placid and easy-going nature becomes rapidly aggressive and difficult to please when they enter a state that requires **Belladonna**.
- Becomes semi-delirious with rapid onset of very high temperature.
- Very sensitive to stimuli with a tendency to become easily startled or overexcited.
- Restless and agitated, but not as terrified or anxious as someone needing **Aconite** (the other main remedy that is often required in rapidly, developing, initial stages of fever and illness).
- Becomes apathetic and indifferent, just wanting to be left alone in peace.
- May speak very quickly or become totally disinclined to talk.
- More aggressive and irritable than anxious, fearful or panicky.

Head Symptoms

- Violent, throbbing headaches with extremely sensitive scalp.
- Aversion to having hair touched because of sensitivity of the scalp.
- Head symptoms are relieved by bending the head backwards.
- Headaches specifically feel better from cool applications and exposure to open, fresh air (although most symptoms feel worse for exposure to cold).
- Headache is aggravated by lying flat, bending forwards, bright light, noise and jarring movements.
- Headaches are frequently right-sided with accompanying dizziness that is made more intense for movement and turning over in bed.

Eye Symptoms

- Eyes feel hot and gritty, and look inflamed and red.
- Aching pains in the eye sockets spread to the head in general.
- Twitching, spasmodic movements of muscles of eyelids.
- Tendency for capillaries of the eyes to burst, leading to easy bleeding.
- High temperature causes glassiness of the eyes with dilated pupils.

Ear, Nose And Throat Symptoms

- Piercing, sharp, aching pains with earache.
- Earache is often right-sided or worse in the right than the left ear.
- Oversensitivity to noise with earache.
- Red, hot, flushed face with red, swollen tip to nose.
- Very acute sense of smell with unpleasant odour in nasal passages.
- Extremely sensitive, dry, throbbing pains in throat that make swallowing liquid very difficult: drinks may be forced into nose in an effort to swallow.
- Tonsils become rapidly swollen, bright red and inflamed, especially on the right side.
- Rapidly-developing hoarseness with complete loss of voice.

Chest Symptoms

- Coughing fits are preceded by tickling and irritation in the throat.
- Dry, harsh, barking, croupy cough that is aggravated by lying flat at night.
- Cough is temporarily broken and eased by bringing up mucus.

Digestive Symptoms

- Although thirsty for sharp drinks (such as lemonade), drinking is distressing if pain or swelling is present in the throat.
- Oversensitive, or overly-acute sense of taste.
- Cramping, colicky pains are eased by bending forwards or backwards.
- Hyper-sensitivity of stomach and abdomen: even the light touch of bed covers and clothing cause distress and discomfort.
- Diarrhoea with constant urge to pass a stool.

Urinary Symptoms

- Concentrated, dark, bloody or cloudy urine, with kidney or bladder disorders.
- Frequent or constant urge to pass water, which is distressing to pass because of burning, cutting sensations.
- Constricted feeling and spasms in bladder after passing water.
- Great difficulty and effort in voiding urine, or there may be constant dribbling or trickling of urine, and loss of bladder control.
- Stress incontinence may be aggravated by walking, or standing for lengthy periods of time.

Gynaecological Symptoms

- Right-sided pain in ovary.
- Irregular or early periods with flooding and cramping pains.

- Heavy bleeding with strong, painful contractions.
- Gushing, hot, clotted, bright-coloured flow of blood with period.
- Bearing down sensations with or without actual prolapse of the womb.
- Feels as though contents of pelvis are about to fall out.

Flushes And Fever

- Although burning hot, feels very sensitive to exposure to cold draughts of air or uncovering.
- Hot head with cold extremities.
- Tendency for parts of the body that are covered to perspire.
- Rapid, violent onset of high temperature with very hot, bright red, dry skin.
- Uneven circulation with a tendency to easily feel boiling hot.
- Skin flushes bright red, leaving it dry, hot and burning to the touch.
- High temperature with very rapid, bounding pulse.

Skin Symptoms

- Intensely flushed, hot, dry, bright red skin that radiates burning heat.
- Extremely painful and hypersensitive skin.
- Sunburnt, sensitive skin.

Joint And Muscle Symptoms

- Marked restlessness with joint pain: must keep constantly on the move.
- Exposure to cold draught or damp conditions causes a stiff, painful neck.
- Joints are generally swollen, hot and bright-red looking.
- Joint pains are worse from exposure to cold, and feel eased by keeping still and warmth.

Aggravated By:

- Draughts of cold air.
- Cold in general.
- Lying on painful, inflamed parts.
- Noise.
- Bright light.
- Jarring
- Movement.

Improved By:

- Resting.
- Peace and quiet.
- Resting propped-up in a darkened room.
- Warm surroundings.
- Bending the head backwards.
- Wrapping up snuggly.

Bryonia (White bryony)

Often Indicated For:

- Constipation
- Coughs
- Croup
- Digestive Disorders
- Fractures
- Headaches
- Haemorrhoids
- Indigestion
- Influenza
- Insomnia
- Joint pains
- Mastitis
- Measles
- Mumps
- Muscle over-exertion
- Osteoarthritis
- Whooping cough

Often needed in conditions that develop in a slow, insidious way: e.g. coughs and colds that appear after a few days of feeling off-colour, or joint pains that build up slowly.

Essential Features

- Slow-developing problems that are brought on by becoming chilled after being overheated, exposure to cold, east winds, or in response to fright, resentment or anger.
- Dry, sensitive skin and mucus membranes, leading to painful dryness of bodily openings such as the vagina.
- Marked intolerance of heat and warmth.
- General tendency towards dryness leads to problems with stubborn constipation, with attendant complications of headache and nausea.
- All symptoms are worse from the slightest movement and relieved considerably by keeping as still as possible.

Emotional State

- Extremely irritable, bad-tempered and cross if disturbed.
- Wants to lie as still as possible in a quiet, cool room.
- Marked disinclination for any kind of physical effort or making conversation.
- Frustrated and angry about being unwell: wants to get back to normal.
- Becomes angry and abusive when crossed or contradicted.

257

■ General state of anxiety about finances, work and overall lack of security.

■ Discontented and difficult to please: asks for something and then rejects it.

Head Symptoms

■ Headaches occur as a result of constipation.

■ When in pain, instinctively wants to hold the head firmly to keep it as still as possible.

■ Headache is worse from heat and better for cool in any form.

■ Severe frontal headache with bursting or throbbing pains, which are made worse by the slightest movement, eating and stooping.

■ Headache may be present on waking which is located above the eyes or at the back of the head.

Eye Symptoms

■ Hot, burning, gritty sensation in eyes.

■ Red, sore, inflamed eyes and eyelids that feel worse for the slightest movement.

■ Discomfort in the eyes feels worse for heat.

Ear, Nose And Throat Symptoms

■ Shooting pains in the ears when walking in the fresh air, which persist afterwards.

■ Sensitivity to noise, or a feeling as though ears are stopped up.

■ General dryness of nasal passages, with irritation extending to the throat and upper chest.

■ Pains in forehead with nasal discharge.

■ Red, sore swelling of nose.

Chest Symptoms

■ Scanty mucus which is raised with great difficulty.

■ Dry, tickling, irritating cough with gagging.

■ Coughing bouts are brought on by entering or staying in a warm room.

■ Wants to take a deep breath, but this makes the cough worse.

■ Chest pain is relieved by firm pressure, so hand is pressed instinctively to the painful area in the chest or head when coughing.

Digestive Symptoms

■ Awful indigestion with heavy, nauseated feeling in stomach.

■ Dry, parched mouth with marked thirst for long, cool drinks.

■ Nausea is aggravated by eating and movement, and temporarily relieved by bringing up wind.

■ Sore, tender, painful stomach.

■ Exhausting diarrhoea that is made much worse by the slightest movement.

■ Diarrhoea that is brought on by eating too much acid fruit.

■ Constipation with dry, large, hard, dark stools that are very difficult to pass.

Urinary Symptoms

■ Urgent desire to pass dark coloured, reddish, hot urine.
■ Cutting pains when urinating.
■ Burning sensations and discomfort before urinating.
■ Stress incontinence is aggravated by lifting heavy weights or moving.

Gynaecological Symptoms

■ General symptoms of pre-menstrual syndrome with extremely painful, enlarged breasts.
■ Mastitis with heavy, hot, painful breasts.
■ Delayed periods from stress or overexertion which occur before the period is due.
■ Pain in groin before period begins.
■ Burning pains when the flow starts.

Flushes And Fever

■ Marked dislike of being wrapped-up warmly, or to being in warm surroundings.
■ Feverish with marked thirst for long drinks of cold water.
■ Perspires with fever at night.

Sleep

■ Unrefreshing sleep with a tendency to wake feeling anxious when dropping off to sleep.
■ Very drowsy during the day with great difficulty sleeping at night.
■ May be subject to nightmares or sleepwalking.

Joint And Muscle Symptoms

■ Pale red, taut, swollen, painful joints.
■ Sharp, tearing, stitching pains that are aggravated by the least movement.
■ Although keeping still eases joint pains, discomfort may be so intense that the patient becomes very restless, thus making the pains worse.
■ Difficulty walking because of sore, aching feet, or weakness in the thigh muscles.

Aggravated By:

■ Initial movement after resting.
■ Physical or mental exertion.
■ Sitting up after lying down.
■ The slightest movement.
■ Warmth.

Improved By:
- Firm pressure to painful parts.
- Cool in general.
- Lying as still as possible.
- Perspiring.
- Resting.

Calc carb (Calcium carbonate)

Often Indicated For:
- Chapped skin
- Chilblains
- Cradle cap
- Insomnia
- Nappy rash
- Pre-menstrual syndrome
- Teething
- Thrush

It is worth noting that this remedy is seldom indicated for short-lived, acute problems, and is most often used for long-term, far-reaching, constitutional treatment. Therefore, it must be stressed that it is a remedy that does not require frequent repetition.

Essential Features
- Slowed-down vital processes with inefficient circulation, poor digestion and constipation.
- Permanently poor energy levels and stamina with a tendency to become breathless and sweaty on the slightest exertion.
- Slow, sluggish metabolism with persistent problems with weight gain.
- Insufficient muscle tone and strength, leading to recurrent problems with strains and sprains.
- Repeated pattern of constant infections in winter such as colds, sore throats, ear infections and swollen glands which linger from one bout to the next.
- Strange, rare and characteristic symptom of feeling perfectly well when constipated.
- Children who need **Calc carb** experience developmental milestones later than expected (closure of fontanelles, teething, walking and talking).
- Discharges tend to smell sour (e.g. sweat, breath or stools).

Emotional State
- Sensitive and fearful by nature: specific fears of the dark, being alone and general lack of confidence.
- Insecurity and poor self-esteem dates from childhood when he or she may

have been noticed as being overweight and/or unfit. Consequently, there may be a lingering dislike or fear of being singled out for unpleasant attention, or being the butt of a joke.

■ Extremely poor emotional and mental stamina: complete exhaustion sets in rapidly when stressed.

■ Unable to think clearly, with a tendency to become confused when stressed.

■ Strong-willed, obstinate personalities who approach tasks with dogged determination at their own slow pace.

■ Very sensitive to criticism.

■ Becomes withdrawn, uncommunicative or lacking in responsiveness as a defence mechanism for coping with feelings of inadequacy.

■ Strong element of self-consciousness with fear of other people seeing their confusion, insecurity or distress.

■ Extreme dislike of being rushed or hurried.

■ Sluggish and slow physical and mental reactions.

Head Symptoms

■ Headaches are generally improved by resting and taking it easy.

■ Queasy feelings with headache that are improved by warmth, and made more intense by contact with cold in general, or draughts of cold air.

■ Dizziness and headache are brought on by exhaustion following physical effort.

■ Headaches may be brought on by exposure to bright light, the effort of talking or loud noise. They are eased by resting in a warm, darkened room.

Eye Symptoms

■ Veiled or filmy sensation over eyes with eye strain.

■ Eyes become strained and tire quickly from reading or watching television.

Ear, Nose And Throat Symptoms

■ Shooting, pulsating pains in the ears.

■ Humming, buzzing or cracking noises in the ears.

■ Thick nasal discharge with soreness of the nose.

■ Painless hoarseness or loss of voice on waking.

■ Persistent and/or recurrent winter sore throats with swollen glands.

Chest Symptoms

■ Tickly, irritating, nocturnal cough.

■ Rattling, productive, coughing spasms, with large amounts of sweet-tasting, thick, yellow mucus.

■ Pressure in the stomach and/or pains in the head when coughing.

Digestive Symptoms

■ Averse to hot foods, or those with a milky, slimy texture such as milk puddings.

■ Peculiar cravings for indigestible foods such chalk or coal. Others include pasta, eggs, bread, sweets and salt.

■ Slow, sluggish digestion with stubborn constipation or alternation between diarrhoea and constipation.

■ Sluggish digestion leads to nausea and sour belching.

■ Generally feels better when constipated.

Urinary Symptoms

■ Recurrent cystitis with concentrated, dark, brown-tinged urine.

■ Sour, unpleasant-smelling urine.

Gynaecological Symptoms

■ Right-sided pain in the ovary which extends to the thigh on the same side.

■ Irregular or early periods following a time of stress or over exertion.

■ Cramping period pains that adversely affect the stomach.

■ Thick, itchy, burning, sour-smelling vaginal discharge with itching, smarting thrush.

■ Pre-menstrual syndrome with enlarged, tender breasts before and during the period.

Flushes And Fever

■ Easily overheated and flushed, but hands and feet constantly feel ice-cold, damp and excessively clammy.

■ Tendency to sweat suddenly from exertion when feverish.

■ Strong tendency to sweatiness and sudden flushes of heat, especially on scalp and feet when under bed covers at night.

■ Burning, hot flushes quickly turn into cold, clammy sweats.

■ Frequent night sweats, or sweats that come on as a result of overexcitement, fear or anxiety.

Sleep

■ Sleep problems emerge in childhood with a tendency to nightmares, screaming, grinding teeth or sleepwalking.

■ Fitful, disturbed sleep with a tendency to recurrent bad dreams.

■ Wakes very anxious and agitated after sleep, so that it takes a long time to calm down.

■ Recurrent pattern of difficulty in initially getting to sleep, with a tendency to wake between 2 and 3 a.m.

■ Drenching night sweats which make the scalp and feet especially clammy.

■ Pushes feet out of the bedclothes because of hot, burning sensation on the soles.

Skin

■ Chronic skin problems date from childhood, including eczema, nappy rash, urticaria, warts and cradle cap.

■ Dry, cracked or chapped skin during the winter months.

Joint And Muscle Symptoms

■ Hot, inflamed, swollen joints that develop nodules or bony outgrowths.

■ Stiffness and pain are made worse by cold, damp conditions.

■ Persistent cramping pains in calf muscles at night.

■ Lax ligaments lead to a tendency to repeated or easy sprains and strains.

■ The ankle joints are especially vulnerable, with a tendency to 'turn over' very easily.

■ Poor quality or brittle bones are a result of poor metabolism of calcium.

■ Curvature of the upper spine occurs as a result of poor muscle tone.

Aggravated By:

■ Cold, damp conditions.

■ Draughts of cold air.

■ Bathing in cold water.

■ Changes from warm to cold weather.

■ Before and after a period.

■ Standing for any length of time.

■ Being observed when under pressure.

■ Criticism.

Improved By:

■ Dry warmth and fine weather.

■ Rest.

■ Moderate temperatures.

■ When constipated.

Calendula (Marigold)

Although mainly used as an external application in the form of lotion, cream, ointment or diluted tincture, this remedy can also be given internally in tablet form in order to encourage speedy, clean healing of cuts, grazes and wounds.

The antiseptic properties of this remedy make it an ideal skin salve for wounds and abrasions, since it:

■ Promotes healing of tissue.

■ Slows down blood loss.

■ Helps inhibit infection.

Cantharis (Spanish fly)

Often Indicated For:
- Bladder infections
- Burns
- Conjunctivitis
- Gastritis
- Midge bites
- Kidney infections
- Nappy rash
- Scalds
- Sunburn

Essential Features
- One of the main remedies to consider in cases of cystitis where there are very few differentiating symptoms.
- Violent, rapidly-developing symptoms that occur with very little warning.
- Externally chilly and shivering with a strong sense of internal burning and irritation.

Emotional State
- Extreme sensitivity to any sensory stimulation including bright light or slight touch.
- Irritability and bad-temper when ill.
- Confused thought patterns to the point of seeming stupefied.
- Hyper-excitability or delirium.
- Drowsiness and lethargy with raised temperature.

Head Symptoms
- Tension headaches which extend from the nape of the neck that feel better for walking.
- Headache with violent, throbbing, stabbing pains.

Eye Symptoms
- Conjunctivitis with smarting, burning sensations.
- Eyes develop a yellowish tinge.

Ear, Nose And Throat Symptoms
- Burning heat and inflammation of the ears.
- Nose is burning hot, red and swollen with extended cold.
- Difficulty swallowing fluid because of burning and rawness in the throat.
- Tight, constricted feeling when drinking.

Chest Symptoms
- Inflammation of the larynx.
- Burning in chest with abundant, ropy mucus that is difficult to raise.

Digestive Symptoms
- Violent burning in stomach with possible vomiting.
- Tender, swollen abdomen with watery diarrhoea.
- Bends double in order to gain relief.
- Urging for a bowel movement when urinating.

Urinary Symptoms
- Acute distress with frequent urge to pass water.
- Rapidly-developing, burning and cutting pains before, during, and after passing water.
- Similar sensations in the kidneys with accompanying tenderness.
- Discomfort and irritation in the bladder which extends through the whole urinary tract.

Gynaecological Symptoms
- Burning pains in ovaries.
- Heightened sensitivity of genital area leads to increased libido and desire.
- Burning vaginal discharge.

Flushes And Fever
- Although the skin is cold to the touch, there is a strong sense of burning-up inside.
- Shivery and cold, with clammy sweat on extremities and genital area.

Sleep
- Drowsy by day but unable to sleep at night due to intense discomfort from symptoms.

Skin
- Large blister formation with intense burning.
- Itching blisters with burning pains.

Aggravated By:
- Touch.
- Drinking.
- Movement.
- Coffee.

Improved By:
- Warmth.
- Passing wind.
- At night.

Carbo veg (Vegetable charcoal)

Often Indicated For:
- Acid stomach
- Blood loss
- Bronchitis
- Collapse
- Diarrhoea
- Exhaustion
- Flatulence
- Headache
- Influenza
- Laryngitis
- Loss of voice
- Nosebleeds
- Shock
- Sunstroke
- Wheezing
- Whooping cough
- Varicose veins

Essential Features
- Extreme faintness and weakness with pale, clammy skin and 'air hunger' (craving for fresh air).
- Frequent stretching, yawning and tiredness as a result of poor circulation and inability to make effective use of oxygen.
- Burning pains may occur anywhere in the body.
- Marked exhaustion on making the least effort.
- Very pale with bluish tinge to the skin.
- Reacts badly to extreme changes in temperature.

Emotional State
- General anxiety with specific fear of the dark.
- Confused and withdrawn, or irritable.
- Apathetic and indifferent to surroundings when ill.
- Depressed with confusion and poor memory.

Flushes And Fever
- Although cold to touch, feels burning-up inside.
- Sweaty, clammy and chilly with craving for fresh air: wants to be fanned.
- Burning heat can be rapidly followed by drenching, clammy sweat and chilled feeling.
- Sleep is interrupted by profuse, frequent night sweats which especially affect the limbs and face.

■ Flushes of heat are brought on after eating spicy food or drinking wine.

Head Symptoms

■ Headache with throbbing pain in temples and dizziness.
■ Sensation of a tight band around the head.
■ Headaches are made more intense by the least movement and effort.
■ 'Morning after' headache with heavy feeling in the head.

Eye Symptoms

■ Itchy feeling in margins of eyelids.
■ Burning eyes with heavy feeling in eyelids.

Ear, Nose And Throat Symptoms

■ Right-sided pain and redness of the ear with swollen glands.
■ Sneezing with frequent nosebleeds.
■ General unwell feeling with mucus in nasal passages.
■ Sore, red, cold nose that looks inflamed at the tip.
■ Burning sensations in throat, with hoarseness and loss of voice.
■ Sore throat is worse from exposure to damp air, talking and clearing the throat.

Chest Symptoms

■ Great distress from feeling of burning and weakness in chest.
■ Breathlessness and suffocative feelings come on after lying down and are eased by contact with fresh air.
■ Lots of rattling mucus in the chest which is brought up with great difficulty and effort.
■ Coughing spasms end in gagging or vomiting of mucus, with flushing of the face.

Digestive Symptoms

■ Burning sensations in the stomach.
■ Persistent, constant belching which gives only short-lived relief.
■ General queasiness and nausea from overindulgence.
■ Rumbling and diarrhoea with colicky pains and incarcerated wind.

Urinary Symptoms

■ Persistent, urgent, anxious desire to urinate day and night.
■ Urine is scanty, concentrated, deep-coloured, cloudy and reddish in colour.
■ Difficulty urinating after a night's sleep.
■ Smarting on passing water.

Gynaecological Symptoms

■ Headaches with cramping pain before the period begins.
■ Thick, white or yellowy-green discharge before periods.

- Burning, itching discharge with general sensitivity of genital area.
- Early or very heavy periods with pale menstrual flow.
- Exhaustion in breast-feeding mothers with milk that is slow to develop.

Sleep

- Wakes from sleep feeling clammy and drenched in perspiration.
- Light sleep with twitching and jerking.

Skin

- Ulcers form and develop rapidly.
- Easy bruising with burning sensations on the skin.

Joint And Muscle Symptoms

- Poor circulation with a tendency for the limbs to become rapidly numb.
- Restlessness with aching, bruised discomfort in arms, back, wrists and small joints of the hand.
- Pain and sensitivity at the base of the spine which is intensified by sitting down.

Aggravated By:

- Warm, stuffy surroundings.
- Alcohol.
- Humidity.
- Movement.
- After eating.
- Severe cold.

Improved By.

- Fresh, cool, open air.
- Being fanned.
- Sleep.
- Breaking wind.

Causticum (Potassium hydrate)

Often indicated For:

- Bladder infections
- Bronchitis
- Burns
- Eye infections

Essential Features

- Slow, insidiously-developing symptoms following a period of stress, emotional strain and/or generally becoming 'run down'.
- General state of debility and growing exhaustion when ill, with an overwhelming need to rest and take it easy.

■ Characteristically raw, burning, sore and cramping pains occur anywhere in the body.

■ Problems especially affect the tendons and small joints in the hands and feet, leading to stiffness, deformities and cramping pains.

■ Gradual, progressive paralysis may accompany joint problems such as arthritis, or may occur in the face (*Bell's Palsy*).

■ Symptoms are aggravated or brought on by contact with sharp, east winds, or raw, cold weather.

Emotional State

■ Often indicated in cases of long-continued emotional stress, grief or worry which has slowly undermined the health. This may occur after the strain of domestic worries, nursing or caring for a sick relative, experiencing financial problems, or having to cope with too little sleep.

■ Intense sympathy with the sufferings of others and hatred of injustice.

■ Defends others against unfair treatment or behaviour by becoming actively involved in charities or caring organizations.

■ Hypersensitive to noise, touch or excitement.

■ Poor memory with absent-mindedness.

■ May become critical, suspicious or irritable when unwell.

■ Timid, anxious and nervous, with a tendency to obsessive behaviour such as repeatedly checking that locked doors have been secured correctly, or that domestic appliances have been switched off.

■ Long-term fear of the dark, with a dread of going to bed, may have continued from childhood.

■ Covers up feelings of insecurity or lack of confidence by a veneer of sarcasm.

Head Symptoms

■ Tight, constricted feeling in scalp which is relieved by warmth.

■ Headaches with facial neuralgia or numbness (*Bell's Palsy*).

■ Pains in the head are worse in a warm room.

■ Nausea with headache.

■ Dizziness with lack of co-ordination.

Eye Symptoms

■ Heavy sensations in eyelids.

■ Grittiness of the eyes with a need to close them.

Ear, Nose And Throat Symptoms

■ Burning pains in the ears with difficulty hearing.

■ Itching in the nasal passages and at tip of nose.

■ Dry, stuffed-up nose.

■ Thick, yellowy-green mucus at the back of the throat.

■ Raw, burning, sore throat with hoarseness or complete loss of voice.

■ Discomfort in the throat is worse in the mornings.

Chest Symptoms

■ Irritating dry, hollow cough from tickling in the throat.
■ Tight chest and constant breathlessness with cough.
■ Coughing bouts are eased by sips of cold drinks, and made more intense by getting warm in bed.
■ Burning in the throat and chest with cough.
■ Wheezing when sitting or lying down.
■ Leaking of urine when coughing.

Digestive Symptoms

■ Raw, burning feeling in the stomach, with acid that rises into the gullet.
■ Nausea and acidity in stomach.
■ Burning thirst for cold drinks.
■ Colicky pains that are eased by lying down and by bending double.
■ Haemorrhoids and/or anal fissure with itching, raw, sharp pains.
■ Stools may be passed involuntarily.

Urinary Symptoms

■ Cystitis with acute sensitivity to cold.
■ Stress incontinence is aggravated by coughing, sneezing, excitement or laughing.
■ Frequent urge to pass large quantities of urine, with a tendency to involuntary passage of urine when asleep.
■ Urine is passed slowly or with difficulty: this is eased by drinking cold drinks.
■ Irritation and itching around entrance of urethra.

Gynaecological Symptoms

■ Heavy, clotted flow with delayed periods.
■ Bleeding stops temporarily when resting or lying down.
■ Depressed, dizzy and pale before a period.
■ Weary and exhausted with lack of sexual drive.
■ Vaginal discharge at night, but stops during the day.
■ Breast-feeding problems with reduced milk supply and cracked, sore nipples.

Sleep

■ Restless legs with severe insomnia.
■ Wakes with a start from anxious sleep.
■ Sees frightening images on falling asleep.
■ Anxiety at night due to fear of the dark, which may have been present since childhood.

Skin

■ Poor-healing skin with sensitivity in old scars which refuse to heal completely.
■ Easily-bleeding warts on the eyelids, face, and hands.

■ Spots and eruptions behind the ears.

■ Persistent acne on the forehead and cheeks.

■ Severe itching on the back and calves of the legs, which is especially distressing at night.

Joint And Muscle Symptoms

■ Pains in muscles as a result of too much exercise.

■ Weakness and trembling of the hands with drawing pains in the fingers.

■ Stiff, swollen joints that are much worse when getting up from a chair.

■ Raw, tearing joint pains that especially affect the knees. They are worse for windy, cold weather and improved by warm, humid conditions.

■ Cramping pains especially affect the leg muscles and the feet.

Aggravated By:

■ After bathing.

■ The onset of cold weather.

■ Dry, cold, east winds.

■ Cold draughts.

■ Violent or abrupt changes of temperature.

■ Coffee.

■ At night.

■ On waking.

■ Travelling in a car.

Improved By:

■ Becoming warm in bed (except for chest symptoms).

■ Cold drinks.

■ Warm, damp weather.

Chamomilla (Chamomile)

Often Indicated For:

■ Burping

■ Croup

■ Diarrhoea

■ Earache

■ Headache

■ Labour pains

■ Mastitis

■ Mumps

■ Neuralgia

■ Painful periods

■ Sciatica

- Teething
- Toothache
- Vertigo
- Whooping cough

Essential Features

- Extreme sensitivity to and intolerance of pain, which drives to desperation.
- Great mental and physical irritability with a tendency to become hot and bothered.
- Becomes flushed with pain and anger.
- All symptoms get worse at night when lying in bed.
- Great weakness with pains.
- Muscular spasms and twitching.

Emotional State

- Extreme physical and emotional oversensitivity.
- Becomes impatient and extremely frustrated with pain, leading to feelings of being out of control and violence: may become verbally abusive.
- Throws things about in anger and frustration.
- Strong aversion to being touched.
- Shouts and screams with pain.
- Paces the floor in an effort to calm down.
- Offended easily: refuses to answer questions.
- Children howl and scream in pain and frustration.
- Children can only be pacified by being rocked or carried.

Flushes And Fever

- Moist, hot head with perspiration.
- General hot and flushed appearance: one cheek may be red and the other pale.
- Thirsty for cold drinks.
- Feet feel hot and are constantly moved about the bed in the search for a cool spot.

Head Symptoms

- Head feels more comfortable for being wrapped up, and from warmth in general.
- Headache is brought on or aggravated by feeling angry.

Eye Symptoms

- Swollen eyes on waking with eyelids that stick together.

Ear, Nose And Throat Symptoms

- Earache with swelling and pain of glands in the face and neck.
- Shooting pains in the ears when stooping.
- Sneezing with dry, irritated nose.
- Obstructed, blocked nostrils with hot, watery discharge.

- Sore throat with swollen tonsils and glands.
- Roof of mouth and throat look inflamed and dark red.
- Feeling of a plug in the throat with difficulty swallowing food.

Chest Symptoms

- Coughing fits in children are brought on by anger and frustration.
- Disturbed sleep from coughing which leads to bad temper on waking.
- Dry, hacking cough at night that is set off by talking.
- Breathlessness with a feeling of tension in the chest and larynx.

Digestive Symptoms

- Pains in stomach are eased by drawing knees up to chest when lying down.
- Colicky pains that feel better from heat locally applied, but are not improved by passing wind.
- Stomach pains with greenish-coloured, watery diarrhoea.
- Diarrhoea accompanies teething problems in children.

Urinary Symptoms

- Yellowish, cloudy, hot urine.
- Discomfort, itching and burning when passing urine.

Gynaecological Symptoms

- Pre-menstrual syndrome with extreme mood swings and irritability.
- Unbearable cramps with period that resemble labour pains.
- Deep-red, clotted, heavy menstrual flow with breakthrough bleeding between periods.
- Unbearable, ineffective labour pains that drive to distraction and fury: mother becomes abusive with pain.
- Enlarged, extremely tender breasts with sensitive, sore nipples.

Sleep

- Moans, tosses and turns, and starts in sleep.
- Disturbed, restless, poor-quality sleep with frequent bad dreams.

Aggravated By:

- Anger and frustration.
- Lying in bed.
- Damp.
- Exposure to wind and draughts.
- Being covered.
- Windy weather.
- Before or during periods.
- Coffee or sedatives.

Improved by:
- Being rocked or carried.
- Warm, moist conditions.
- Car travel.

China (Peruvian bark)

Often Indicated For:
- Anaemia
- Bleeding
- Catarrh
- Constipation
- Diarrhoea
- Exhaustion
- Gallstone colic
- Influenza
- Labour pains
- Neuralgia
- Period problems
- Tinnitus
- Varicose veins

Essential Features
- Extreme mental and physical exhaustion, which may develop after an extended time of physical or emotional strain.
- A tendency to become weak from an underlying problem with anaemia.
- Debility may also follow fluid loss such as diarrhoea, vomiting, sweating or loss of blood.
- Sharp, tearing, cutting pains.
- Overall tendency to fluid retention.
- Extreme sensory sensitivity, with aversion to even light touch, or briefest contact with cold draughts.

Emotional State
- General state of weakness leads to intolerance of and hypersensitivity to noise.
- Irritability and touchiness with a need to be left in peace.
- Fear and general anxiety becomes marked at night, with specific fear of animals and dogs.

Flushes and Fever
- Drenching, frequent night sweats.
- Marked thirst with sweating and hot flushes.

■ Unstable circulation with flushes of heat, and hot sweats alternating with chills and shivers.

Head Symptoms
■ Throbbing pains in the sides of the head with painful, tender scalp.
■ Headaches are generally eased by warmth and firm pressure, while they are made more severe from contact with cold draughts, jarring, touch, and movement in general.

Digestive Symptoms
■ Unpleasant heavy feeling in the stomach after eating, with distension and flatulence.
■ Little or no appetite with constantly full sensation in the stomach.
■ Bitter or acid taste to wind that is raised from the stomach.
■ Cold feeling in the stomach, with a craving for spicy foods.
■ Queasiness with gall-bladder problems or jaundice.
■ Painless, profuse, offensive, watery diarrhoea which is more intense at night.

Gynaecological Symptoms
■ Early, extremely heavy, dark, clotted flow with periods.
■ Severe flooding with periods approaching the menopause, leading to extreme weakness and possible anaemia as a result of blood loss.

Joint And Muscle Symptoms
■ Discomfort in joints is much worse for movement.
■ Rapid-developing numbness in limbs when any pressure is applied to them.
■ Weak, trembling legs from making the least physical effort.

Aggravated By:
■ Cold in general.
■ Movement.
■ Light touch.
■ Draughts of cold air.
■ At night.
■ Acid foods and fruit.
■ Eating.

Improved By:
■ Warm drinks.
■ Rest.
■ Firm pressure.

Cimic (Black snake root)

Often Indicated For:

- Back pains
- Depression
- Neuralgia
- Period problems
- Post-natal depression
- Pre-menstrual syndrome
- Tinnitus

Essential Features

- Symptoms shift between emotional and physical problems.
- Changeable symptoms which flit from one part of the body to another.
- Extreme restlessness with constant changing of position.
- Constantly chilly, with problems getting warm.
- Problems often affect the left side of the body.
- Weak, trembling, bruised feeling in the muscles.
- Pains shoot through the body like electric shocks.
- All symptoms are more intense during a period.

Emotional State

- Problems with health follow a time of great emotional stress or strain.
- When emotional problems are severe, physical symptoms are less troublesome, and vice-versa.
- Deep depression alternates with exhilaration, euphoria or talkativeness.
- Gloomy and depressed: feels as though a black cloud is looming over them.
- Strong fear of losing reason or of dying.
- Overtalkative, fidgety and on edge: constantly changes topics.
- Suspicious about everyone and everything, including doctors and medical treatment.
- Often indicated after childbirth when black moods and depression may be very marked.

Head Symptoms

- Headaches are improved by pressure, and contact with cool, fresh air, while they feel worse for noise, during a period, or movement.
- Neuralgia in the cheekbones is eased at night, but builds up by the following morning.

Eye Symptoms

- Aching pains in the eyeballs that are worse for the slightest movement, and eased by pressure.
- Pains over the eyes extend to the nape of the neck.

Digestive Symptoms

■ Nausea and burping with severe headache.

■ Sick, sinking feelings in the stomach and vomiting are related to gynaecological disorders such as painful periods.

■ Colicky cramps in the stomach are eased by bowel movements and firm pressure from bending double.

■ Alternating diarrhoea and constipation.

Urinary Symptoms

■ Frequent desire to pass increased quantity of urine.

■ Pressing pains in the small of the back and the kidneys.

Gynaecological Symptoms

■ Problems develop or get worse during the menopause, such as heavy periods, depression, headaches, migraines or hot flushes.

■ Well-established problems with irregular periods that are either too frequent or too early.

■ Heavy, dark, clotted bleeding during periods that causes great distress.

■ Cramping, bearing down pains become more intense as the menstrual flow increases.

■ Burning pains in breasts with periods.

■ Shooting pains shift from side to side during labour.

Joint And Muscle Symptoms

■ Sore, shooting muscle pains that lodge in the back of the neck, shoulders and heels.

■ Muscle pains are eased by continued movement, and aggravated by damp, cold conditions.

■ Well-established back pain and stiffness that is sparked off or made worse by physical strain or effort, or becoming cold or damp.

■ Back pains are soothed by lying flat, and feel more severe for initial movement after resting or keeping still.

■ Back pain extends into the thighs.

■ Rheumatic pains are worse at night and during a period.

Aggravated By:

■ Touch.

■ Damp.

■ Cold.

■ Night.

■ During a period.

■ Initial movement after resting.

Improved By:
- Pressure.
- Warmth.
- Eating.
- Movement.
- Fresh air.

Gelsemium (Yellow jasmine)

Often Indicated for:
- Anticipatory anxiety
- Diarrhoea
- Headaches
- Influenza
- Labour pains
- Measles
- Neuralgia
- Sciatica
- Vertigo

Essential Features
- Symptoms develop insidiously and progressively over a period of time, rather than with speed or with violence.
- Flu-like state with generalized aching, shivering and chills running up and down the spine.
- Profound sense of physical and mental weakness, and exhaustion.
- Trembling and heaviness of the limbs when making an effort of any kind.

Emotional State
- Symptoms may be brought on by hearing bad news, shock, excitement or a sudden fright.
- Mental and physical weariness, fatigue and exhaustion.
- Indifferent and apathetic: can't be bothered with anything, just wants to be left alone in peace.
- Unable to motivate themselves to get involved in any activity that calls for effort or enthusiasm.
- Specific fear of the dark and anxiety about death when feeling depressed.
- Confused, withdrawn and untalkative when stressed or anxious.
- Withdrawn and brooding with anxiety rather than chatty and talkative.

Head Symptoms
- Dizziness, giddiness and lack of co-ordination when walking before the onset of a headache.

■ Severe headache with specific feeling of the head being compressed by a tight band that rests above the eyes.

■ Headaches are worse for exposure to warmth, and better for resting and keeping still, ideally propped-up in bed. Some headaches are eased by passing copious amounts of urine.

■ Headaches occur during the menopause with drowsiness, giddiness and problems focusing the eyes.

■ Pains begin at the base of the neck and extend to the forehead.

Eye Symptoms

■ Heavy, droopy, sagging eyelids as a result of illness or tiredness.

■ Dizziness and blurred vision, with tiredness, that is aggravated by motion.

Ear, Nose And Throat Symptoms

■ Blocked ears with shooting pains that travel from the throat into the ear on swallowing.

■ Puffy, red, swollen sore throat.

■ Swallowing is difficult and uncomfortable from sensation of lump in the throat.

■ Slow developing cold or flu symptoms that begin with severe sneezing, and hot nasal discharge.

■ Complete blockage of nose with red, inflamed nostrils.

Chest Symptoms

■ Violent coughing spasms with sore chest.

■ Sudden bouts of breathlessness with shallow breathing.

Digestive Symptoms

■ Frequent, painless diarrhoea as a result of nervous tension or anticipatory anxiety.

■ Unusual symptoms of dry mouth and lips without thirst.

Urinary Symptoms

■ Dribbling of urine due to weakness of the bladder, or lack of control over sphincter muscle of the bladder.

Gynaecological Symptoms

■ Giddiness and faintness before periods.

■ Period pains extend into the back and down the thighs.

■ Heavy, contracted feeling in womb with pains.

■ Threatened miscarriage from fear or anxiety.

■ Unfruitful labour pains with very slow dilation of cervix, or 'backache' labour.

Sleep

■ Jerks awake from sleep with a start.

■ General restlessness and fitful, disturbed sleep from aches and pains.

Flushes and Fever

- Flushed, hot head and face with cold extremities.
- Although feeling shivery, averse to being in warm room.
- Trembling and shivery, with chills running up and down spine.
- When perspiration breaks, it does little to relieve the general sense of discomfort.
- Muscular trembling and weakness with unsteady, wobbly legs.

Joint and Muscle Symptoms

- Weak, heavy, aching sensations in arms and legs.

Aggravated By:

- Overheated rooms.
- Humidity.
- Exposure to cold draughts.
- Bright sunlight.
- Brooding on symptoms.
- Mid-morning.

Improved By:

- Fresh air.
- Moderate warmth.
- Headaches are relieved by passing large quantities of urine.
- Continued, gentle movement.

Hepar sulph (Sulphide of calcium)

Often Indicated For:

- Abscesses
- Boils
- Chilblains
- Cough
- Croup
- Earache
- Laryngitis
- Sinusitus
- Sore throat
- Styes
- Swollen glands
- Wheezing
- Whooping cough

Essential Features

- Extreme sensitivity on mental, emotional and physical levels.

■ Slow-healing skin with poor-healing wounds that leave a scar or become easily infected.

■ Infections set in quickly with production of thick, yellowish pus or mucus.

■ Offensive-smelling discharges.

■ Characteristic sharp, splinter-like, bruised pains.

■ Generally chilly with a terrific sensitivity to cold draughts of air.

Emotional State

■ Terrific physical and mental sensitivity with frequent outbursts of irritability and bad temper.

■ Hypersensitive to and intolerant of slightest physical pain or discomfort.

■ Easily angered and generally difficult to get on with when ill.

■ Becomes violent with frustration and temper.

■ Dissatisfied and generally hard to please when unwell.

Eye Symptoms

■ Conjunctivitis or recurrent styes with thick, sticky, yellow discharge.

■ Extreme light-sensitivity.

Ear, Nose And Throat Symptoms

■ The slightest contact with cold air leads to immediate sneezing.

■ Sinus pain and inflammation with thick, yellow, nasty-smelling mucus.

■ Pressure and pain at the root of the nose with sinus problems.

■ Painful sore throat with sensation as though a fish bone or sharp object were sticking in sides of throat.

■ Right-sided pains in the throat that extend to the ear with swollen glands.

■ Severely inflamed or septic tonsils with yellow-coloured ulcers.

■ Laryngitis which is much worse for exposure to cold.

Chest Symptoms

■ Throat and chest feel better for drinking warm drinks.

■ Productive, rattling cough with copious, thick, yellow mucus that is very difficult to raise or dislodge.

■ Severe coughing bouts which may be set off, or made worse by slightest contact with cold draughts of air or uncovering.

■ Becomes sick and sweaty in the effort of bringing up phlegm.

Digestive Symptoms

■ Severe burping with distension and swelling of stomach.

■ Painless diarrhoea occurs immediately after eating.

■ Swelling of the glands in the abdomen with shooting pains.

Sleep

■ Wakes with a start from sleep, feeling agitated.

■ Drowsy and sleepy during the day, and restless and sweaty at night.

Skin

■ Especially indicated for boils and abscesses that are slow to come to a head or resolve themselves, provided the general symptoms agree.

■ Slow-healing skin with cuts that quickly become infected.

■ Wounds and skin eruptions are extra sensitive to contact with cold air.

Flushes and Fever

■ Nasty, offensive odour to perspiration.

■ Hypersensitive to cold draughts of air: has to be kept warm and snug or symptoms feel much worse. Even putting a hand or foot out of the bed covers causes great distress.

■ Perspires easily and profusely after making the slightest physical effort.

Joint and Muscle Symptoms

■ Easily dislocated joints that feel weak and trembly when walking.

■ The knee joints are especially vulnerable to dislocation.

■ Stiff, swollen, painful joints feel worse for contact with cold, draughty weather conditions.

■ Cramps in the calf and thigh muscles are especially severe at night.

Aggravated By:

■ Cold, draughty surroundings.

■ Cold drinks and food.

■ Light touch.

■ Lying on the painful part.

■ Morning.

■ Evening.

■ Winter.

Improved By:

■ Humid, warm conditions.

■ Warmth.

■ Eating.

Hypericum (St John's wort)

Often Indicated For:

■ After-pains of labour

■ Bites and stings

■ Bruises

■ Cough

■ Injuries to nerves

■ Neuralgia

■ Pains in scar tissue
■ Puncture wounds
■ Sciatica

Essential Features
■ Special affinity for injured areas that are rich in nerve supply, e.g. crushed fingers or toes.
■ Pains are more severe than the extent of the injury would seem to merit.
■ All symptoms are worse from being touched.

Emotional State
■ Distress, depression or drowsiness following an accident or wound.

Head Symptoms
■ Headaches that follow falls which involve the base of the spine.

Muscle And Joint Symptoms
■ Crushing pains in fingers, toes or base of the spine following an accident.
■ Sharp, cutting, intermittent pains shoot away from injured spot.
■ Damaged parts are extremely sensitive to touch.
■ Injured areas are so sensitive that the slightest movement causes great distress and weeping.
■ Pains are especially severe on rising from a sitting position.

Aggravated By:
■ Touch.
■ Contact with damp, cold air.
■ Movement

Improved By:
■ Keeping as still as possible.

Ignatia (St Ignatius' bean)

Often Indicated For:
■ Back pain
■ Exhaustion
■ Fainting
■ Grief
■ Hiccoughs
■ Indigestion
■ Insomnia
■ Lack of appetite
■ Post-natal depression
■ Sore throat

Essential Features

■ Contradictory symptoms such as nausea or indigestion that are relieved by eating, painful sore throat that is eased by swallowing solid food, or tickling in the throat that is made more intense when coughing.

■ Trembling, shaking, with muscle spasms and twitching.

■ Hiccups and sighing are common features of the **Ignatia** state.

■ Symptoms of emotional shock, trauma and grief often require **Ignatia**.

Emotional State

■ Those who are in need of **Ignatia** are often in an excitable, nervous or extra-sensitive state.

■ Eases the symptoms of homesickness where there is an excessive amount of disorientation and distress.

■ Violent, rapid mood swings with alternation between uncontrollable tears and hysterical laughter.

■ Although upset, bottles up emotions until they explode in hysterical trembling and crying.

■ Contradictory moods: laughter alternates with tears, or anger with guilt and remorse.

■ Hypersensitive to noise, criticism, pain, or strong odours.

■ Resentful and misunderstood with constant sighing.

Head Symptoms

■ Headaches develop in response to stress, grief, emotional shock or strong smells.

■ Sharp, spasmodic pain with headache as though a nail were sticking into the side or back of the head.

■ Dizziness and unsteadiness with hot, heavy sensation in the head.

■ Migraines with problems focusing the eyes, and visual aura of bright zig-zags before the eyes.

Ear, Nose And Throat Symptoms

■ Inflammation and burning heat in the ears.

■ Oversensitivity of hearing or hearing loss occur as a result of stress or worry.

■ Dry head cold with dull headache.

■ Persistent loss of voice and/or sore throat which develop in response to emotional strain, trauma or upset.

■ Characteristic sensation of a lump in the throat which makes swallowing very difficult.

Digestive Symptoms

■ Lots of bitter-tasting saliva in the mouth.

■ Burping and hiccoughing that are aggravated by eating, with the taste of undigested food rising into the throat from the stomach.

■ Sinking sensation in the stomach with an instinctive desire to take a deep breath in order to feel relief.

- Unpleasant, empty, hungry sensation in the stomach that is related to anxiety.
- Hunger pangs and empty feelings are not eased by eating.
- Craving for indigestible things such as heavy foods, or acidic flavours.
- Constipation with spasmodic, cramping pains.
- Painless diarrhoea that is triggered by emotional stress.
- Contradictory symptom of soft stools being harder to pass than hard ones.

Gynaecological Symptoms
- Menstrual problems that are related to hormonal disturbances and imbalances, often following emotional shock or trauma.
- Cramping, colicky period pains which feel better when resting, from firm pressure or from change of position.
- Heavy, clotted, dark, offensive menstrual flow.
- Often needed for post-natal depression or unpredictable mood swings following childbirth.

Sleep
- Moans and whimpers in sleep.
- Wakes easily from light, fitful sleep.
- Twitches, jerks and jolts in limbs on falling asleep.

Muscle And Joint Symptoms
- Intermittent sciatic pain, which is worse during the night and in cold weather.
- Tingling, cramping pains radiate from the back down the legs.

Aggravated By:
- Yawning.
- Suppressed emotion.
- Emotional trauma or shock.
- Bereavement.
- Fear or anxiety.
- Strong odours such as cigarette smoke.
- Sugary foods.
- Pressure on non-painful areas.
- Exposure to cold.

Improved By:
- Eating.
- Warmth.
- Distraction.
- Pressure to painful parts.

Ipecac (Dried root of ipecacuanha)

Often Indicated For:
- Bleeding
- Catarrh
- Morning sickness
- Nausea
- Painful periods
- Vomiting
- Wheezing
- Whooping cough

Essential Features
- Awful sensitivity to movement which makes everything feel generally much worse.
- Severe, constant nausea is characteristic of the **Ipecac** state.
- Breathlessness with weariness and exhaustion.
- Tendency to easy, frequent bleeding.

Emotional State
- Irritable from the least provocation.
- Extremely sensitive to noise, especially to loud music.
- Very dissatisfied, impatient and bad-tempered.
- Anxiety and fear of death.

Flushes And Fever
- Sudden onset of feverishness with shivering and trembling.
- Lack of thirst with high temperature.
- Very chilly with sensitivity to the least draught of cold air.

Head Symptoms
- Sick headache involving the whole head.
- Awful, severe nausea with headache, making the patient look deathly pale and ill.

Eye Symptoms
- Watering, painful eyes with light sensitivity.

Ear, Nose And Throat Symptoms
- Coldness of the ears when feverish.
- Nosebleeds with blocked nostrils.
- Running nose with blood-stained mucus.
- Sore, painful throat which feels tight and constricted.
- Rough, stinging pains in the throat.

Chest Symptoms

- Chest problems make it difficult to lie flat: must sit up to breathe.
- Sudden coughing bouts with rattling and wheezing in chest.
- Gagging and vomiting at the end of coughing spasms.
- Dry, irritating cough from tickling and irritation in air passages.

Digestive Symptoms

- Terrible, persistent nausea, with excess of saliva in the mouth accompanies all symptoms.
- Sick feeling is not relieved by anything, including vomiting, and is made much more intense by the slightest movement.
- Swollen, bloated abdomen with constant desire to pass a stool.
- Copious, watery, greenish-coloured diarrhoea.
- Painful, loose stools follow eating too many sweet things or unripened fruit.

Urinary Symptoms

- Extreme nausea and/or vomiting with kidney or bladder infections.
- Urinary problems with shooting pains in the sides.
- Red-tinged urine from streaks of blood or reddish sediment.

Gynaecological Symptoms

- Irregular bleeding or 'spotting' between heavy periods.
- Nausea and faintness with heavy bleeding.
- Flooding, gushing, bright red menstrual flow.
- Awful morning sickness in pregnancy which is worse for the slightest movement.
- Excessively heavy bleeding during and after childbirth.

Aggravated By:

- Being overheated or too cold.
- Eating.
- The slightest movement.
- Touch.
- Dry, humid weather.
- Eating red meat.

Improved By:

- Firm pressure.
- Rest.
- Keeping the eyes closed.
- Keeping still.
- Fresh air.

Kali bich (Bichromate of potash)

Often Indicated For:

- Bronchitis
- Catarrh
- Cough
- Croup
- Flatulence
- German measles
- Headache
- Post-nasal drip (This refers to mucus that drips from the back of the nose to the throat)
- Sinusitis
- Wheezing

Essential Features

- Extreme weariness and lethargy with marked sensitivity to cold.
- Discharges and catarrh that are characteristically stringy, ropy, yellow-coloured and stubborn to move.
- Pain occurs in small spots or flits from place to place.
- Alternating conditions (e.g. stomach disorders alternate with rheumatic aches and pains, or headaches alternate with visual disturbance).
- Recurrent or rapidly-forming ulcers.
- Symptoms are much worse from contact with cold draughts or becoming chilled.

Emotional State

- Exhausted and listless.
- Total aversion to the idea of mental or physical effort.
- Anxiety rises from or is lodged in the chest.
- Difficulty in concentrating or thinking clearly.
- Anxious when meeting new people.

Head Symptoms

- Vertigo with nausea and/or vomiting.
- Migraines with nausea and vomiting that are worse at night.
- Sinus headache with discomfort and tenderness at the root of the nose.
- One-sided headaches that lodge over the eye, which are better for firm pressure and made more intense by stooping.
- Aching sensations in the bones of the head and face.

Eye Symptoms

- Dry, sensitive eyes that burn and itch.
- Recurrent conjunctivitis with heat and redness of the eyeball.

■ Inflamed eyes with eyelids that are red and swollen at the edges.

Ears, Nose And Throat Symptoms

■ Recurrent or severe earache with offensive-smelling, yellow discharge and swollen glands.

■ Severe tickling and itching in the ears.

■ Painfully dry, blocked nose from sticky, yellow discharge.

■ Discomfort in the nose is worse for warm, stuffy rooms, and eased by contact with cool air.

■ Profuse nasal discharge burns the nostrils and upper lip.

■ Unpleasant smell in the nose.

■ Catarrh at back of throat which is stringy, stubborn and difficult to raise.

■ Irritating sensation as though a hair is resting on the tongue.

■ Sore throat with water-logged, enlarged uvula.

■ Inflamed throat is soothed by warm drinks.

Chest Symptoms

■ Croupy cough with breathlessness and gagging when attempting to raise mucus from chest.

■ Heavy feeling like a weight on chest on waking, which is relieved by coughing up mucus.

■ Cough is worse on waking in the morning, and is often accompanied by back pain.

■ Coughing spasms are relieved by lying down and by warmth.

■ Food is vomited back up if coughing bouts occur soon after eating.

■ Stitching pains extend from below the breast bone to the back.

Digestive Symptoms

■ Uneasy, anxious feeling in the stomach.

■ Belching eases stomach upsets.

■ Headaches with stomach upsets that are worse from eating.

■ Lethargy and headache with persistent constipation.

■ Pale stools are passed involuntarily.

■ Bloated, swollen abdomen comes on after eating.

■ Colicky pains are relieved by warmth and firm pressure.

Urinary Symptoms

■ Burning sensation during and after urinating.

■ Constant urge to pass water through the day and night.

■ Fluid retention that is connected to kidney problems.

■ Low back pain or stitching pains.

Sleep

■ Drowsy, unrefreshing sleep.

■ Exhausted and listless as a result of poor sleep quality.

■ Wakes abruptly around 2 a.m. with breathlessness, nausea or feeling hot and sweaty.

■ Disturbed sleep from upsetting dreams.

Joint And Muscle Symptoms

■ Pains in hip and knee joints that are increased by movement or standing.

■ Sciatic pain shoots from buttock to calf muscle, and is made more intense by movement.

■ Sore heels when walking.

■ Aches and pains in shoulders that are worse at night.

Aggravated By:

■ Becoming chilled or exposed to cold winds.

■ Uncovering.

■ In winter.

■ Stooping.

■ Touch.

■ Waking from sleep.

■ Hunger.

■ Being alone.

■ Becoming overheated.

■ 2–5 a.m.

Improved By:

■ Summer weather.

■ Firm pressure to painful parts.

■ During the day.

■ Movement.

■ Warmth.

■ Wrapping up.

■ Being in bed.

Kali carb (Potassium carbonate)

Often Indicated For:

■ Anaemia

■ Back pain

■ Bronchitis

■ Catarrh

■ Labour pains

■ PMS

■ Sciatica

■ Thrush

- Wheezing
- Whooping cough

Essential Features

- Extreme sensitivity to cold and liability to become easily chilled.
- Weakness may be related to underlying problems of anaemia.
- General tendency to fluid-retention and swelling.
- Burning pains in parts that feel cold to the touch.
- Flitting pains that are soothed temporarily by warmth.
- Wherever they occur, pains are characteristically stabbing, stitching, sharp or cutting.
- Problems are often restricted to the right side of the body.

Emotional State

- Crotchety and full of complaints: feels at odds with everyone and everything.
- Jumpy and nervous, with an inclination to be oversensitive to noise or shocks of any kind.
- Overtired, highly-strung, edgy and irritable.
- Feels unable to cope with stress, and severe mood swings.
- Lots of fears and anxieties, including a specific fear of being alone, anxiety about the future, or fear of death. In addition, may be afraid of the supernatural.
- Although dislikes being alone and wants company, sympathy is rejected.

Head Symptoms

- Burning pains in scalp, sinuses above eyes, or in cheekbones.
- Recurrent headaches occur as a consequence of chronic sinus pain.
- Headaches are made much worse for contact with cold air, and relieved by being wrapped up warmly and firm pressure.
- Wraps up the head well in order to avoid inhaling cold air.

Eye Symptoms

- Puffy eyelids with sharp pains in the eyes.

Ear, Nose And Throat Symptoms

- Shooting pains in the ears, with swollen glands and yellow discharge.
- Nose blocks up in a warm atmosphere, which eases headache.
- Uncomfortably dry nasal passages with very red, inflamed and swollen nose.
- Recurrent colds with loss of voice.
- Profuse amount of saliva in the mouth and throat.
- Coughs up catarrh into throat with difficulty.
- Sticking, sharp pains in throat with a feeling of swallowing over a ball or lump in larynx.
- Persistent, chronic, unpleasant-tasting catarrh hangs on from a previous cold that has not fully cleared up.

Chest Symptoms

- Dry, hacking cough with swollen upper eyelids.
- Wheezing and vomiting with chilly feeling in chest.
- Wheezing cough is eased by sitting up and bending forwards.
- Yellowish-green, lumpy mucus that is very difficult to raise.
- Pressure, shooting and burning pains in chest when breathing.

Digestive Symptoms

- Weak, sinking feelings in the stomach that are made worse by eating.
- Heavy, unpleasant sensation in the stomach after a meal.
- Burning in the stomach and heartburn are aggravated by cold drinks.
- Marked distension and swelling in abdomen that comes on after eating.
- Severe burping and flatulence, with distension that develops soon after eating.
- Colicky pains that are eased by warmth, hot drinks and hot water bottles. Bends double with pains.
- Alternating constipation and diarrhoea, with burning sensations in rectum and anus that are soothed by bathing with cool water (unlike burning pains that occur anywhere else in the body).

Urinary Symptoms

- Frequent need to pass water, with burning pains that occur during and after urination.
- Flow of urine takes a while to start.
- General problems with puffiness and fluid retention as a result of inefficient or sluggish kidneys.

Gynaecological Problems

- Extremely chilly with cramping pains before a period starts.
- Constipation with period pains.
- Very heavy flow with periods that may not respond to any conventional medical measures (e.g. surgical techniques such as dilatation and curettage).
- Exhaustion after intercourse.
- Tendency to miscarriage in pregnancy.
- Low back pain in pregnancy or 'backache labour'.

Sleep

- Wakes in the early hours of the morning with horrible nightmares, with great difficulty in getting back to sleep again.

Joint and Muscle Symptoms

- Legs 'give way' without warning as a result of extreme muscular weakness.
- Pain and weakness in the back that extends to the thigh muscles.
- Back pain and muscle weakness may be worse before a period, and when walking. It is relieved by lying down, and by firm pressure applied to the painful area.

Aggravated By:
- Cold air or draughts.
- Change in weather.
- Light touch.
- Overheating.
- Coffee.
- In the early morning.

Improved By:
- During the day.
- Leaning forwards.
- Moist, warm weather.

Lachesis (Surukuku snake venom)

Often Indicated For:
- Addiction
- After pains in childbirth
- Croup
- Depression
- Earache
- Headaches
- Hot flushes
- Laryngitis
- Migraines
- Mumps
- Periods
- Pre-menstrual syndrome
- Sore throats
- Ulcers
- Varicose veins

Essential Features
- There is a characteristic mottled, purple appearance to the skin from poor circulation leading to a tendency to develop varicose veins, or to bruise extremely easily.
- Symptoms tend to be left-sided or to develop on the left and move to the right.
- Symptoms are generally at their worst on waking, from contact with heat in any form, or for any sense of constriction (e.g. tight clothes around the neck or waist).
- Sleep generally makes everything worse, resulting in a marked dread of going to bed or falling asleep.
- Menopausal problems tend to respond well to **Lachesis** provided the general symptoms agree. Possible conditions that may benefit from this remedy often

include the following: menopausal depression, hot flushes, circulatory disorders including high blood pressure and phlebitis.

■ Extreme mental and physical sensitivity with a marked fear of, and aversion to, being touched (especially around the throat).

Emotional State

■ Rapid and severe mood swings that alternate between euphoria and depression.

■ Chatty with a tendency to talk very quickly, constantly switching from one topic to another.

■ Many problems stem from unsatisfying or disturbed sleep patterns. As a result, most symptoms are worse on waking from sleep.

■ Nocturnal by nature: works best at night, feeling full of energy and bright ideas when it's time to go to bed.

■ Averse to falling asleep because of a fear of dying before waking.

■ Mental and physical exhaustion and extreme fatigue are not improved by sleep.

■ Severe anxiety and depression on waking.

■ Bursts of confidence and high self-esteem alternate with extreme troughs of depression, inadequacy and lack of self-worth.

Head Symptoms

■ Headaches may be triggered or made much worse by bright lights.

■ Headaches or migraines characteristically develop when waking from sleep, and usually affect the left side or move from left to right.

■ Headaches are eased by lying down, the onset of a nasal discharge, or warmth.

■ Migraines or headaches characteristically appear, or are made much worse, before a period, while they are eased as soon as the flow begins.

■ Distressing dizziness with migraine-type headaches that are made more intense by closing the eyes.

Eye Symptoms

■ Painful, itching, stinging, sensitive eyes that feel worse for being touched, although there is a strong instinct to rub them constantly in search of relief.

■ Oversensitivity to light with redness and burning pains.

Ear, Nose And Throat Symptoms

■ Earache with sore throat.

■ Sneezing with blocked nose on waking.

■ Nose feels more comfortable for the onset of a discharge such as a nosebleed.

■ Hoarseness with sharp pain in the throat that is worse on waking from sleep.

■ Choking sensation and irritation in throat.

■ All throat problems are made worse by swallowing saliva, but feel soothed by swallowing solid food.

■ Cool drinks soothe the throat, while warm drinks make pain and discomfort worse.

■ The throat is extra-sensitive to touch and pressure, so that a polo-neck jumper or a scarf tied around the neck cause great distress.

■ Sore throats are often left-sided, or begin on the left and move to the right.

Digestive Symptoms

■ Severe pain from chronic gall-bladder problems.

■ Bloating, wind and distension are relieved by passing a stool, and made much worse for pressure of tight or restrictive clothing.

■ Stools are difficult to pass because of throbbing pains in rectum or bleeding haemorrhoids.

■ Persistent constipation with purple-coloured haemorrhoids that bleed very readily.

Gynaecological Problems

■ Especially indicated for menopausal conditions such as severe hot flushes, heavy periods with severe clotting, or violent mood swings, provided the general symptoms fit.

■ Severe pre-menstrual syndrome with left-sided ovarian pain, irritability to the point of frenzy, and extreme, violent mood swings.

■ All symptoms are relieved and obviously improved as soon as the period begins.

■ Menstrual flow is dark, clotted and extremely heavy.

Flushes And Fever

■ Disturbing sensation of waves or flushes of heat flowing through the body.

■ The head becomes extremely overheated, while the hands and feet remain icy cold during a hot flush.

■ Hot flushes are made much more distressing and uncomfortable when wearing tight clothing around the neck.

■ Rapid volatile changes of temperature with constant fluctuations between heat and cold.

■ Awful sensitivity to becoming overheated with a complete intolerance of warm, airless rooms and a preference for cool, fresh conditions.

Sleep

■ Starts awake with falling sensation on going to sleep.

■ Awful sleep problems including night sweats, feelings of panic and suffocation, anxiety and panic attacks.

■ Marked fear of falling asleep because all symptoms are worse on waking.

■ Horrific dreams promoting confusion and disorientation on waking.

Skin

■ Skin flushes readily with a tendency to broken capillaries, varicose veins and a general blotchy, purple tinge.

■ Reddish-purple boils or abscesses form easily and bleed copiously.

Aggravated By:
■ Sleep.
■ Heat.
■ Stuffy rooms.
■ At night.
■ Cold draughts.
■ Hot sunlight.
■ Alcohol.
■ Constriction.
■ Before a period.

Improved By:
■ Fresh, cool air.
■ Cool drinks.
■ Cool bathing.
■ Onset of a discharge.
■ Movement.
■ Eating solid food.
■ As the day goes on.

Ledum (Wild rosemary)

Often Indicated For:
■ Black eyes/bruises
■ Boils
■ Joint pains
■ Osteoarthritis
■ Prickly heat
■ Puncture wounds
■ Sprains
■ Stings
■ Strains

Essential Features:
■ Pains are characteristically sharp and stabbing. They shift about, often moving from lower limbs to upper areas of the body.
■ Affected areas become swollen and taut, often with fluid retention.
■ Skin tends to become septic and infected very easily and quickly.
■ **Ledum** has an unusual, characteristic symptom of chilly, painful, stiff areas being soothed by cool bathing or cold compresses.
■ Bruised, aching pains through the whole body.

- Although swollen and hot, joints do not look red.
- Hard, painful swellings with tearing pains.

Emotional State
- Withdrawn, cross and irritable.
- Sighs between bouts of crying when low and depressed.

Head Symptoms
- Pressing pains with headache are relieved by cool air, and made more intense by keeping the head covered.

Digestive Symptoms
- Excess of saliva in the mouth with nausea.
- Nausea is made more intense when walking in the open air or when perspiring.

Urinary Symptoms
- Red deposits or sediment in urine.
- Joint pains are associated with passing copious amounts of colourless, clear urine.
- Frequent urge to pass water with irregular, interrupted flow.
- Residual discomfort and burning sensations after passing water.

Gynaecological Symptoms
- Generally better for fresh, cool air during periods, despite feeling chilly.
- Menstrual flow is bright red and heavy.

Flushes and Fever
- Although feeling generally chilly, finds the warmth of the bed unbearable, and flings off covers in an effort to cool down.
- Marked thirst for cool drinks.

Joint and Muscle Symptoms
- Swollen, hot, stiff joints which respond well to cool bathing. However, they are made more uncomfortable from warm bathing, or the heat of the bed.
- Knobbly, distorted outgrowths of the small joints of the fingers and toes.
- Joint pains move in an upward direction through the body.
- Stiffness and pain of the lower back is made more intense by sitting in one position for too long.

Skin
- Itchy eruptions are worse for warmth in general, and specifically on covered parts of the body.
- Itching and discomfort are made more intense by becoming heated in bed, but feel immediately eased by cool air or bathing with cool water.
- Crusty eruptions around the nose and mouth.

■ Puncture wounds feel cold to the touch.

Aggravated By:
■ Warmth.
■ At night.
■ Being well wrapped up.
■ Heat of the bed.
■ Walking.
■ Alcohol.

Improved By
■ Cool bathing.
■ Cool compresses.
■ Contact with cool air.
■ Resting.

Lycopodium (Club moss)

Often Indicated For
■ Addiction
■ Anxiety
■ Constipation
■ Diarrhoea
■ Digestive disorders
■ Flatulence
■ Gallstone colic
■ Heartburn
■ Indigestion
■ Pre-menstrual syndrome
■ Sore throat
■ Wheezing
■ Whooping cough

Essential Features
■ Digestive symptoms are especially characteristic and prominent, with a strong tendency to production and accumulation of excess wind, as well as rumbling, gurgling and distension.
■ Symptoms generally develop or get much worse in the afternoons and early evenings. They improve as the evening progresses.
■ Problems characteristically affect the right side of the body initially, and move to the left.
■ Poor physical stamina, with a tendency to become rapidly worn out after moderate physical effort.

■ Although chilly as a rule, becoming overheated causes as much distress as being chilled.

Emotional State

■ Extremely anxious and insecure about speaking in public: such as contributing to a seminar or business presentation. However, although lacking confidence when anticipating the event, when it occurs, it goes very well.

■ Dislikes feeling crowded, but also fears being totally alone. Prefers to have someone within calling distance if needed.

■ Very easily made irritable and sensitive to criticism: flies off the handle when corrected.

■ Specific fears of the dark, ghosts and strangers. Also very unhappy at feeling hemmed in, or having constricting clothing around the neck or waist.

■ Constantly preoccupied with or worried about financial problems, and fear of losing a grip on daily affairs. This is linked to a fundamental anxiety about fear of failure and losing control.

■ Adopts a veneer of abrasiveness and sarcasm, as a way of covering up anxiety and lack of confidence.

■ Can appear unemotional and detached, with intellectual abilities being developed at the expense of emotional expression.

■ Sensitive to pain, noise and music.

■ Hurried in movement, speech and eating habits. Speaks so quickly that words get jumbled up.

■ Tendency to forgetfulness and confusion when overtired.

Flushes And Fever

■ Although extremely chilly, aversion to being overheated or spending time in stuffy, airless rooms.

■ Sudden hot flushes are a result of emotional stress or anxiety.

■ Flushes of heat leave an unpleasant clammy feeling in their wake.

■ Flushes are aggravated by tight clothes, or feeling hemmed in by company or confined surroundings.

Head Symptoms

■ Crushing, violent headaches that are made worse by warmth, becoming overheated and lying down.

■ Headaches may be brought on by low blood sugar levels as a result of delayed meals.

■ Pains are eased by cool, fresh air and gentle movement.

■ Dizziness that is intensified by walking, eating, drinking or talking.

Eye Symptoms

■ Recurrent styes and/or eye infections, with sticky, pussy discharges.

■ Dry, smarting eyes and eyelids, with a tendency to become swollen.

Ear, Nose And Throat Symptoms

■ Singing, tinkling, buzzing sounds in the ears.

■ Recurrent colds with sinus problems and blocked up nose.

■ Productive, thick, yellowy-green catarrh which settles at the back of the throat.

■ Choking and burning sensations in the throat.

■ Ulcerated throat which is relieved by warm and worse for cold drinks.

Chest Symptoms

■ Severe headache from persistent coughing spasms.

■ Episodes of coughing come on when breathing deeply or by swallowing saliva.

■ Shallow breathing when sleeping or making a physical effort.

■ Raw, bruised, pressured feeling in the chest.

■ Pain and discomfort in the chest is made worse after speaking.

Digestive Symptoms

■ Digestive uneasiness is often caused by 'nerves' or anticipatory anxiety (such as worrying about an exam or stressful event to come). Common digestive reactions to stress include lots of rumbling, gurgling, 'butterflies' in the stomach, diarrhoea or very loose stools, or alternating diarrhoea and constipation.

■ Begins a meal feeling hungry, but can't eat very much without the stomach becoming rapidly overfull.

■ Incomplete, sour-tasting belches that leave a burning sensation in the gullet.

■ Nausea is relieved by fresh air, and made worse for being in a stuffy room.

■ Hunger develops within an hour or two of eating.

■ Discomfort and acidity come on immediately after eating, and are eased by warm drinks but aggravated by cold.

■ Pressure or constriction from a waistband or tight belt make digestive uneasiness and discomfort worse.

■ Heartburn and indigestion from production of excess acid in stomach and accumulation of wind in the abdomen.

Urinary Symptoms

■ Cloudy, dark and strong-smelling urine.

■ Frequent urge to pass water at night.

■ Aches and pains in the sides are severe before urinating, and relieved afterwards.

■ Flow of urine may be slow to start.

Gynaecological Symptoms

■ Very severe period pains with cramps in the lower back that extend to the front of the thighs.

■ Period pains are relieved by drawing knees into the abdomen.

■ Intense vaginal itching with, or without, fishy-smelling, abundant discharge.

■ Strange sensation as though wind was passing through the vagina.

■ Depression, headaches and severe abdominal bloating with pre-menstrual syndrome.

■ Dark, clotted, flooding flow approaching the menopause.

Skin

■ Dry, irritated skin which burns and itches violently.

■ Skin problems are much worse for becoming warm in bed, and are eased by contact with cool applications.

■ Intensely itchy, scaly scalp with a tendency to severe or stubborn dandruff.

■ Dry, brittle, easily-broken hair and nails.

Aggravated By:

■ Mornings.

■ Afternoons.

■ Early evening.

■ Waking.

■ Warm, stuffy rooms.

■ Becoming overheated.

■ Draughts of cold air.

■ Touch or constricting clothing.

■ Weight of bedclothes.

■ Becoming overtired.

Improved By:

■ Fresh air.

■ Moderate warmth.

■ Uncovering.

■ Warm drinks.

■ Loosening tight clothing.

■ Gentle exercise.

Mercurius (Quicksilver)

Often Indicated For:

■ Abscesses

■ Bronchitis

■ Catarrh

■ Chickenpox

■ Earache

■ Influenza

■ Mastitis

■ Mouth ulcers

■ Mumps

■ Sinusitus
■ Sore throat
■ Swollen glands

Essential Features

■ Awful mental and physical restlessness that is much worse at night.
■ Extreme debility and weariness with a tendency to anaemia.
■ Adverse reaction to extreme heat or cold resulting in restlessness, uneasiness and general discomfort.
■ Recurrent or persistent pain and swelling of the glands in the neck, armpits or groin.
■ Discharges such as saliva, mucus or sweat are increased, and may smell offensive.
■ Puffiness of the face, fingers, ankles or feet from a tendency to fluid retention.

Emotional State

■ Very anxious, fearful and restless for no obvious reason: finds it impossible to stay in one position for long.
■ Emotional unease and discomfort are much worse at night.
■ Severe panic attacks with a need to escape or run away.
■ Easily flustered and hurried, or completely indifferent and apathetic.
■ Poor memory with depression and distorted sense of time.

Head Symptoms

■ Headaches that are worse at night and on waking, and better for being up and about.
■ Headaches are often left-sided, or more intense on the left than the right side.

Eye Symptoms

■ Extreme light sensitivity with blurred vision or black 'floaters' (spots) in front of the eyes.
■ Discomfort in the eyes is made worse from warmth and during the night.

Ear, Nose And Throat Symptoms

■ Earache is especially severe at night.
■ Sharp pains in the ears with thick, offensive discharge.
■ Sore, raw nostrils with thick, offensive, green mucus.
■ Although swallowing is difficult due to the degree of dryness and soreness in the throat, there is a compulsion to do so frequently because of the increased amount of saliva in the mouth.
■ Large, painful, recurrent ulcers in the mouth and throat.
■ Recurrent or persistently swollen glands.

Chest Symptoms

■ Coughing spasms with nausea that are increased at night, from lying on the right side, and from lying down.

Digestive Symptoms

- Unpleasant, metallic, sweet taste with increased amount of saliva in the mouth and nausea in the stomach.
- Swollen, enlarged tongue that takes the imprint of teeth around the edges.
- Cramping pains and diarrhoea are made more intense by stooping or bending forwards.
- Stomach upsets follow eating too many sweet foods.
- Burning, watery diarrhoea that gets more severe as night approaches.

Gynaecological Symptoms

- Stinging, burning pains when ovulating (at mid-cycle).
- Maddeningly itchy, green-tinged, vaginal discharge with extreme irritation that is worse during the night and when urinating.
- Vaginal itching and irritation are soothed by cool bathing.

Sleep

- Drowsy by day with severe insomnia at night.
- Overpowering restlessness and physical unease when warm in bed at night.
- Heavy, offensive-smelling night sweats.
- Frequent waking from night sweats, anxiety and palpitations.

Flushes And Fever

- Alternating hot flushes with shivering bouts of extreme chilliness.
- Hot flushes on the head and face, while the body remains very chilly.
- Extremely heavy, offensive-smelling perspiration that is especially marked at night.
- Extreme thirst with perspiration.

Joint And Muscle Symptoms

- Painful, stiff neck and back muscles with low, burning back pain that radiates to the thigh muscles.
- Terrible aching and restlessness in the limbs that is particularly marked at night.
- Legs constantly move at night in an effort to get comfortable when warm in bed.
- Painful joints look swollen and pale, and feel more uncomfortable for contact with extreme heat or cold.
- Stiffness and cramping pains in the small joints of the hand and fingers.

Aggravated By:

- Becoming warm in bed.
- Night and evenings.
- Extremes of heat or cold.
- Draughts of cold air.
- Eating.
- Perspiring.

303

- Touch.
- Lying on the right side.

Improved By:
- Moderate temperatures.
- Resting.

Nat mur (Common salt)

Often Indicated For:
- Allergic rhinitis
- Catarrh
- Cold sores
- Cracked, chapped skin
- Depression
- Eye strain
- Grief
- Hayfever
- Headaches
- Hives
- Migraines
- Morning sickness
- Prickly heat
- PMS
- Post-natal depression
- Thrush

Essential Features
- Often well-indicated for symptoms arising from hormone imbalance such as mood swings, pre-menstrual or menopausal headaches or migraines, and fluid retention.
- A marked tendency to allergic reactions such as allergic rhinitis, hives, prickly heat, stress-related skin reactions and hayfever.
- Dryness and sensitivity of the skin and mucus membranes leading to cracked lips and dryness of the vagina.
- Aggravation and intensification of symptoms such as headaches, rashes or hot flushes, from warmth and exposure to hot sunlight.
- Depression, withdrawal and dislike of sympathy are central features of the **Nat mur** emotional picture.
- Exhaustion and weariness are marked, especially in the morning.

Emotional State
- Extreme introversion and difficulty in freely expressing emotion, with a tendency to bottle up and repress feelings.

■ Crying does not provide a release from distress, but tends to make things generally worse. This is especially the case if tears are shed in public, since it leads to feelings of humiliation and embarrassment.

■ Symptoms of illness often set in after bereavement, grief or break up of a close relationship, where emotional release has been blocked up or denied.

■ Although miserable and depressed, sympathy and displays of physical affection are strongly disliked.

■ Alternating, shifting moods between excitability, euphoria and sadness.

■ Fear of small, closed spaces or of being robbed.

■ Easily made to feel lonely and neglected if overlooked or not included.

■ Cries in private when upset, bottles up anger and resentment.

■ Emotional symptoms aggravated and intensified at times of hormonal change, e.g. at puberty, pre-menstrually or at the menopause.

Head Symptoms

■ Headaches are associated with fluctuating hormone levels, and may be much worse before, during or after a period, or during the menopause.

■ Delayed meals also trigger headaches: face may go pale and pinched with pain, nausea and possible vomiting.

■ Pains are worse for movement in general, and are eased by lying down and sleeping.

■ Headaches occur with giddiness and nausea of travel sickness.

■ Migraines with numb, tingling lips, nose and tongue, and visual disturbance with zig-zag patterns appearing before the eyes.

Eye Symptoms

■ Dry, gritty eyes that water easily: especially when walking in strong, cold winds.

■ Sensitive, itchy, swollen eyes with hayfever.

Ear, Nose And Throat Symptoms

■ Painful cracking sensation in the ears when swallowing.

■ Shooting, pulsating pains in ears with possible offensive discharge.

■ Recurrent colds, allergic rhinitis or hayfever symptoms that start with bouts of persistent, repeated sneezing.

■ Recurrent cold sores that break out around the mouth and nose. They may be triggered by emotional stress, colds or exposure to sunlight.

■ Copious, clear, watery nasal discharge that feels as though a hot tap has been turned on. This may alternate with very dry, uncomfortable stuffed up feeling in the nose, and nasal discharge that looks like egg white.

■ Nose runs like a tap or drips persistently when stopping or bending forwards.

■ Dry mouth and lips with characteristic crack in the middle of lips, or in the corners of the mouth.

■ Hoarse, irritated, tickly throat.

Digestive Symptoms

■ Discomfort in the stomach with 'repeating' of food eaten earlier.

■ Unpleasant sinking sensation in the stomach with nausea.

■ Craving for, or marked aversion to, salty foods.

■ Upset stomach with 'mapped' tongue (shiny areas that look as though the surface of the tongue has been partially removed).

■ Uncomfortable, heavy feeling in the stomach with slow or sluggish digestion.

■ Well-established constipation with severe straining to pass hard, dry stools.

■ Nausea and colicky pains are eased by passing wind.

Urinary Symptoms

■ Very uneasy and self-conscious about passing water in public lavatories; must wait for a long time before the flow will start.

■ Passes copious quantities of pale urine.

■ Stress incontinence with leakage of urine when walking, sneezing or coughing

Gynaecological Symptoms

■ Poor tone of pelvic organs with a tendency to prolapse of the womb and bladder.

■ Persistent painful dryness of the vagina leads to an aversion to intercourse because of the burning, smarting sensations that ensue.

■ Severe nausea and morning sickness in pregnancy with vomiting of watery, frothy phlegm.

■ Early, heavy periods, or delayed menses with scanty flow.

■ Low back pains with or without actual prolapse of the womb. These are relieved by sitting or lying with firm pressure at the hollow of the back.

■ Fluid retention before periods leading to breast swelling and tenderness, and discomfort around the waist.

Skin

■ Dry skin with a tendency to crack easily, especially during the winter months.

■ Generally itchy, irritated, blotchy skin from exposure to strong sunlight or warm conditions.

■ Skin is made more sensitive from contact with warmth, and feels soothed by cold bathing and exposure to cool, open air.

Sleep

■ Night sweats occur in the second half of the night.

■ Problems initially getting to sleep, or once asleep, wakes at frequent intervals brooding on distressing thoughts.

Flushes and Fever

■ Palpitations accompany feeling flushed, and hot and bothered.

■ Flushes ascend rapidly and without warning to the chest and head, while the lower half of the body remains cool.

Aggravated By:
- Emotional stress and strain.
- Sympathy and consolation.
- Displays of physical affection.
- Overexcitement.
- Crying.
- After sleep.
- Extreme temperatures.
- Sunlight.
- Becoming heated.
- Stuffy rooms.
- Physical exertion.
- Touch or pressure.
- During or at the end of a period.

Improved By:
- Peace and quiet.
- Being alone.
- Cool air.
- Skipping meals.
- Gentle movement.
- Cool bathing.
- Sea air may improve or aggravate symptoms.
- Tight clothing.

Nux vomica (Poison nut)

Often Indicated For:
- Addiction
- Anxiety
- Cold
- Colic
- Constipation
- Cough
- Cramp
- Croup
- Cystitis
- Digestive disorders
- Gallstones
- Haemorrhoids
- Hangovers
- Headaches

- Heartburn
- Indigestion
- Insomnia
- Labour
- Migraines
- Nausea
- Over-indulgence
- Painful periods
- PMS
- Vomiting
- Wheezing

Essential Features

- This is one of the first remedies to consider in a 'hangover' situation, or if feeling generally 'out of sorts' following over-indulgence in food, alcohol and cigarettes
- **Nux vomica** is also frequently indicated when side effects arise following a course of conventional medication. These may include constipation that follows frequent or overuse of painkillers, or general digestive upsets that may occur after regular use of anti-inflammatories.
- Illness may follow a lifestyle that is excessively stressful with a resulting reliance on alcohol and cigarettes to unwind and relax, caffeine and other stimulants to keep alert, and a poor diet that is high in 'junk' foods and lacking in essential nutrients. Common symptoms that arise from this pace of life and that respond well to **Nux vomica** include headaches, indigestion, nausea, constipation and insomnia, provided the characteristic symptoms of the remedy are present.
- Physical and mental oversensitivity leads to extreme irritability with a tendency to 'fly off the handle' at the least provocation. Physical oversensitivity leads to severe discomfort when exposed to noisy, cold, draughty conditions, with a marked tendency to feel soothed by warm, quiet surroundings.
- All symptoms have a tendency to be worse on waking first thing in the morning, and improve steadily as the day goes on.
- Pains tend to be spasmodic, constrictive and cramping in nature.

Emotional State

- Extreme sensitivity on emotional, mental and physical levels with severe or persistent problems with sleep disturbance.
- Touchy, irritable and easily-provoked, with a marked tendency to become quickly frustrated and discontented.
- Volatile, hostile reaction to being corrected or criticized, with a dislike of sympathy or consolation. This is linked to competitive, perfectionist tendencies.
- Very inclined to pick a quarrel when feeling unwell, and tends to feel relieved and improved after an outburst.

■ Jittery and unable to switch off after work, often as a result of resorting to stimulants such as drinking large quantities of caffeine in order to keep going during the day.

■ Because of the reliance on stimulants to keep alert, and sedatives in order to relax, addiction may become an additional problem.

■ Generally jittery and anxious about health, work, the future and financial security.

Head Symptoms

■ Classic tension headaches that stem from tightness at the back of the neck.

■ Headaches are worse from exposure to draughty, cold conditions, and much improved by warmth and firm pressure.

■ Sick headaches with constipation, nausea and total lack of appetite.

■ Classic 'morning after' headache with dizziness, disorientation, heavy, painful sensation at the back of the head, and awful sensitivity to noise and strong smells, and persistent nausea.

■ Constrictive, tense head pains that are relieved by sound sleep.

Eye Symptoms

■ Extreme light sensitivity on waking, with watering and irritation of eyes.

■ Smarting, itching, burning eyes.

Ear, Nose And Throat Symptoms

■ Cold symptoms are generally more uncomfortable indoors, and feel better in the fresh, open air.

■ Terrible sensitivity to noise, including the speaker's own voice.

■ Troublesome, irritating itching in the ears.

■ Severe sneezing with raw feeling in throat.

■ Great sensitivity to strong smells, with a nose that is alternately dry and stuffed up or running like a tap.

■ Pains in throat that shoot to the ears when not swallowing.

Chest Symptoms

■ Coughing spasms are relieved by warm drinks and are very sensitive to cold draughts of air.

■ Coughing bouts give rise to severe headaches.

■ Dry, tickling, irritating cough that is worse at night.

Digestive Symptoms

■ A stressful, workaholic lifestyle, and attendant regular intake of convenience foods, strong tea, coffee and alcohol, compound digestive problems.

■ Indigestion, wind and colicky pains are made more intense by eating, or pressure of clothes, and are improved and eased by warmth.

■ Persistent nausea with extreme difficulty in vomiting from *reverse peristalsis* (food seems to remain in the stomach, rather than moving freely and easily upwards in order to be expelled). However, once food can be voided from the stomach, relief is felt instantaneously.

■ Becomes quickly flushed and uncomfortably overheated after eating, with attendant feelings of drowsiness and sleepiness.

■ When stressed and anxious, the stomach feels heavy, queasy, and uneasy, especially after eating.

■ Pains associated with gall-bladder problems are intensified by pressure and movement, and soothed by warmth.

■ Constipation with lots of straining and urging, but *reverse peristalsis* operates at this end of the digestive tract as well (stool seems to slip back into the rectum, rather than being easily expelled).

Urinary Problems

■ Right-sided burning pains and terrible difficulty in passing water.
■ Itching or burning sensations when urinating.
■ Severe discomfort in bladder at night.

Gynaecological Problems

■ Severe pre-menstrual syndrome with marked irritability, anger and violent temper.
■ Chilly and faint with period pains.
■ Morning sickness, persistent nausea, and headaches in pregnancy.
■ Dry, painful retching during labour, with distress and difficulty in bringing up stomach contents.

Sleep

■ Difficulty in switching off and getting to sleep: the mind remains alert and full of ideas.
■ Light, fitful sleep which is disturbed by frightening dreams.
■ Wakes from light, restless sleep feeling anxious and unrefreshed.
■ Feels refreshed and ready to get up in the early hours of the morning, but after falling asleep again feels tired and heavy-headed when it is time to get up.
■ Always feels improved by a cat nap or sound sleep if tired during the day.
■ May become addicted to, or dependent on, sleeping pills in order to sleep.

Flushes And Fever

■ Chilly and irritable, with terrible intolerance and dislike of the slightest draught of cold air.
■ Although flushed and hot in appearance, discomfort arises from not being well covered.

Joint And Muscle Symptoms

■ Stiff, immobile joints and muscles that are especially uncomfortable on initial movement in the morning.

■ Weakness in the joints is made worse by exposure to cold and physical exertion.

■ Cramping pains in the muscles are especially severe at night, with the calves being particularly affected.

■ Spasmodic, sharp, bruised pains in joints and muscles, especially affecting those that extend from the nape of the neck to the base of the spine.

Aggravated By:
■ Exposure to cold draughts.
■ Mornings.
■ Lack of sleep.
■ Eating.
■ Coffee.
■ Cigarettes.
■ Strong smells.
■ Noise.
■ Stress.
■ Touch.
■ Being constipated.

Improved By:
■ Warmth.
■ Rest.
■ Sound sleep.
■ Peace and quiet.
■ Night.
■ Humidity.
■ Regular bowel movements.

Phosphorus (The element white phosphorus)

Often Indicated For:
■ Anaemia
■ Anxiety
■ Blood loss
■ Catarrh
■ Chilblains
■ Croup
■ Diarrhoea
■ Headaches
■ Heartburn
■ Nosebleeds

- Post-natal depression
- Sinusitis
- Sore throats
- Swollen glands
- Vomiting
- Wheezing

Essential Features

■ **Phosphorus** is often required when there is an underlying 'free-floating' anxiety that surfaces by attaching itself to a range of specific fears when illness sets in.

■ Exhaustion sets in rapidly and severely during illness, leading to a fundamentally weakened state that is lacking in stamina. This may be associated with an underlying tendency to anaemia.

■ Energy levels are extremely erratic, with short bursts of energy alternating with exhaustion, apathy and introversion.

■ Burning sensations may occur anywhere in the body. These are linked to poor circulatory function, which results in alternating chilliness and abrupt flushes of heat.

■ Hands, ankles, feet and eyelids become swollen and puffy as a result of a general tendency to fluid retention.

Emotional State

■ Extremely sensitive and reactive to all sorts of stimuli: light, noise, colour, touch, music and perfume.

■ Extremely sensitive to atmospheres and people with a possibly highly-developed sense of psychic awareness.

■ Craves physical affection and reassurance: responds very positively to displays of physical affection.

■ Easily mentally and physically exhausted.

■ Anxious and full of worries and fears. These may include a fear of thunder, spiders, being alone, illness and of the dark.

■ Although extremely extrovert, vivacious and outgoing when energetic, physical and mental exhaustion develops rapidly, leading to apathy and total indifference.

■ Tearfulness quickly comes to the surface when feeling weary and unwell.

■ Extreme sensitivity to the feelings of others with a marked capacity for empathy. As a result, emotional 'burn out' can occur very easily.

■ Generally anxious and low when alone or feeling neglected. Feels perked up by sympathy, attention and general displays of care and affection.

Head Symptoms

■ Headache and weak, nauseated feeling may be induced by going too long without food and before a thunderstorm.

■ Burning, flushed face with a headache.

■ Headache is aggravated by warm, stuffy rooms and lying down.

■ Pains are relieved by exposure to fresh, cool air and eating a little.

■ If there is a tendency to low blood pressure, headaches may be accompanied by disorientation and dizziness when getting up too quickly from a sitting or kneeling position. This may also occur as a result of turning the head too quickly, eating or stooping.

Ear, Nose And Throat Symptoms

■ Dry, stuffed-up nose which makes breathing difficult at night.

■ Yellowy-green, offensive nasal discharge with colds.

■ Colds rapidly affect the throat and chest, with swelling and inflammation of the glands in the neck.

■ Painless hoarseness, or complete loss of voice.

■ Sore throat with great sensitivity to touch and to inhaling cold air.

■ Coughs constantly in an effort to clear the throat.

Chest Symptoms

■ Tight, wheezy chest that is eased by warmth.

■ Dry, irritating cough that is made more intense by changing temperatures and when lying down.

■ Chest feels most comfortable when sitting propped-up in bed.

■ Coughs up yellow-coloured phlegm.

■ Coughing spasms are brought on by abrupt changes of temperature.

Digestive Symptoms

■ Nausea and vomiting are much worse in overheated, stuffy rooms.

■ Burning pains in the stomach with weak, queasy feelings are temporarily relieved by cold drinks, until they become warmed by the stomach.

■ Constant nausea with fullness and burning sensations in the stomach.

■ Burping causes distress, with an attendant unpleasant taste rising into the gullet with each eructation.

■ Gurgling and rumbling occurs in the stomach and the gut.

■ Warm drinks and food are vomited back up.

■ Profuse, painless diarrhoea may be passed involuntarily.

■ Diarrhoea develops during, or may be made worse by, hot weather.

Urinary Symptoms

■ Burning sensations with a frequent need to pass reduced amounts of concentrated urine.

■ Blood-streaked, discoloured urine which may have a fatty-looking deposit floating on the surface.

■ Increased thirst with frequent passage of pale-coloured urine. (If this symptom occurs, tests should be conducted in order to rule out the possibility of diabetes.)

Gynaecological Symptoms

■ Extremely depressed and tearful with pre-menstrual syndrome.

■ Heavy, long-lasting periods.

■ Menopausal distress includes burning hot flushes, anxiety, palpitations, and flooding periods with bright red, clotted flow.

■ May be required before or during labour where panic and anxiety are causing great distress.

Flushes And Fever

■ Anxiety and panic attacks precede hot flushes.

■ Sudden alterations and variations in blood flow lead to chilliness with alternating, sporadic flushes of heat.

■ Despite burning sensations, legs and feet feel icy-cold.

■ Unquenchable thirst for ice-cold drinks when feverish, which are vomited back as soon as they become warmed in the stomach.

Joint And Muscle Symptoms

■ Weakness and stiffness in the arms, neck, back and fingers that is especially marked in the mornings.

■ Sore, painful spine and hip joints that are very sensitive to the lightest touch.

■ Burning pains in the spine in bed at night, while the legs and knees feel very cold.

■ Burning, tingling, itching, numb sensations may affect the arms, fingers, spine or back.

Aggravated By:

■ Too much excitement.

■ Being alone.

■ Early evening.

■ Darkness.

■ Thunderstorms.

■ Lying on the left side.

■ Damp and cold.

■ Crowds.

■ Heights.

Improved By:

■ Massage.

■ Physical expressions of affection and comfort.

■ Reassurance.

- Sound sleep.
- Warmth (except for stomach symptoms).
- Eating little but often

Pulsatilla (Wind flower)

Often Indicated For:
- Catarrh
- Chickenpox
- Chilblains
- Croup
- Depression
- Digestive disorders
- Earache
- German Measles
- Grief
- Hayfever
- Headaches
- Heartburn
- Hot flushes
- Indigestion
- Influenza
- Irregular periods
- Labour
- Mastitis
- Measles
- Morning sickness
- Mumps
- Osteoarthritis
- Painful periods
- Pre-menstrual syndrome
- Sinusitis
- Stress incontinence
- Swollen glands
- Teething
- Thrush
- Varicose veins

Essential Features
- Complaints calling for **Pulsatilla** are generally those that have developed slowly and insidiously over the space of a few days. Therefore, this remedy is seldom required in the initial stages of illness, but often indicated in a later,

established stage (e.g. in measles once the rash has come out, or with catarrhal symptoms that may be persistent).

■ **Pulsatilla** symptoms have a constantly shifting, mutable quality, with a tendency to change character and position very rapidly. This instability has both an emotional and physical effect, with resulting tendencies to severe mood swings in combination with changing physical symptoms.

■ Many problems are linked to the effects of shifting hormone levels, with the result that this is a remedy that is often indicated during puberty, pregnancy, the post-natal periods and the menopause.

■ All **Pulsatilla** symptoms are relieved by gentle movement which stimulates sluggish circulation, and made worse by lying down or resting.

■ **Pulsatilla** has the following unusual features which are characteristic of the remedy: chilliness which is aggravated by contact with warmth and relieved by cool, fresh air; and dry mouth without thirst.

■ Symptoms are often restricted to, or worse on, the right side of the body.

■ Discharges are characteristically thick, bland, and yellowish-green in colour.

Emotional State

■ Emotional distress is eased by consolation, sympathetic company and physical displays of affection.

■ Unstable, shifting, rapidly changing moods that swing from tearfulness to irritability, anxiety, depression or happiness very rapidly.

■ Emotional problems and insecurities are particularly marked before a period or when pregnant.

■ In need of reassurance and consolation when anxious and depressed.

■ Feels much better after a good cry in sympathetic company when depressed.

■ Shy, timid and in need of a lot of attention and encouragement.

■ Indecisive and unable to stick to a decision as a result of poor self-esteem or general lack of confidence.

■ Becomes rapidly low and depressed when feeling ignored, uncared for or unsupported.

■ Anxious and fearful of crowds, open spaces, being alone and losing their reason.

■ Children become characteristically weepy, clingy and very demanding when unwell.

Head Symptoms

■ Headache with upset stomach from eating too many rich, fatty foods, or from spending too long in a badly-ventilated, stuffy environment.

■ Headaches develop or get worse after eating, or come on during the evening.

■ Dizziness may be especially severe when getting up after lying down, or when walking out of doors.

■ Firm pressure, cool flannels or gentle exercise in the fresh air also helps ease head pains.

Eye Symptoms

■ Eye infections with yellow, thick discharge that sticks the lids together overnight.

■ Recurrent styes may affect the lower lid.

■ Irritated, burning, itchy eyes with a constant desire to rub them.

■ Light sensitivity with sharp pains in the eyes.

Ear, Nose And Throat Symptoms

■ Earache may be brought on by exposure to cold air.

■ Ear pain is often accompanied by deafness and/or thick, yellowish-coloured discharge.

■ Heat, pain, redness and swelling of the external ear.

■ Dry, sore throat without thirst.

■ Sore, swollen nose during a cold with loss of smell and taste.

■ Blocked sensation that alternates from side to side. It is improved by fresh air, and gets worse when in overheated or stuffy rooms.

■ Persistent yellowy-green, thick, bland catarrh.

Chest Symptoms

■ Dry cough on waking, which alternates with a loose, productive cough at night.

■ Uncomfortable feeling in chest when lying down, that is relieved by sitting up or moving about.

■ Phlegm is thick and yellowish-green in colour.

Digestive Symptoms

■ Stomach upsets with heavily coated, discoloured tongue that looks white or yellow.

■ Dry mouth with unpleasant taste and lack of thirst.

■ Faintness, chilliness and persistent nausea that are made more distressing in a stuffy or overheated room.

■ Burning indigestion is aggravated by taking warm food or drink, and eased by cool things.

■ Burping with 'repeating' of foods eaten a while before.

■ Craves foods that upset the stomach most. These include: fatty, creamy, rich ingredients such as cheese, pork, butter and cream.

■ Nausea and vomiting follow overexcitement, emotional upset or stress.

■ Violent, burning diarrhoea that is triggered by eating too much fruit or ice cream, and is worse at night.

■ Painful, itchy, protruding haemorrhoids that are aggravated by warmth and soothed by cool. They may be the result of long-standing problems with constipation, with resulting straining in an effort to completely empty the rectum.

Urinary Symptoms

■ Persistent or recurrent cystitis with burning and smarting that is much worse for contact with warmth and better for cool.

- Pain and soreness persists even after passing water.
- Discomfort in bladder is worse when lying on the back, and if there is any delay in being able to pass water.
- Involuntary seepage of urine when sitting, walking, coughing or lying down.

Gynaecological Symptoms

- Late or irregular periods: never knows when the next one might be due.
- Changeable flow which may be heavy or clotted, and then shift to very scant.
- Severe symptoms of pre-menstrual syndrome with tender, swollen breasts and extreme mood swings.
- Recurrent thrush which causes violent itching and irritation. Vaginal discharge is thick and whitish-yellow in appearance.
- Menopausal symptoms include abrupt onset of hot flushes with intolerance of heat, stress incontinence, low back pain with possible prolapse, and very irregular, flooding periods.
- Morning sickness where vomiting lasts all day, or gets worse during the evening and at night.
- Varicose veins, thrush or cystitis may be especially troublesome in pregnancy.
- Slow to start, feeble, changeable or unproductive labour pains often call for **Pulsatilla**.

Sleep

- Sleepy on going to bed but wakes from becoming overheated or too sweaty during the night.
- Unable to get comfortable at night with resulting restlessness. Throws off bed covers, gets too chilly, then pulls them back on again.
- Sleeps with arms extended above the head and feet pushed out of the covers in search of a cool spot.

Flushes And Fever

- Although basically chilly, there is a marked dislike of becoming overheated in an airless, stuffy room.
- Alternating hot and cold flushes with an aversion to being too well covered in bed.
- Palpitations with hot flushes often occur after eating a rich, heavy meal.
- Feels most comfortable near an open window which gives easy access to fresh, cool air.
- Although the mouth is often dry and parched with high temperature, there is no thirst.

Skin

- Terribly itchy skin which is made worse by contact with heat in any form.
- Discomfort is soothed by washing in cool water and contact with cool air.

Joint And Muscle Symptoms
- Changeable, flitting pains that move rapidly from one part of the body to another.
- Legs feel heavy during the day and ache at night.
- Stiffness and immobility of the joints and muscles feels worse on first movement after rest, contact with warmth, and resting in bed. They are made more comfortable by cool compresses, contact with cool air, firm pressure and gentle movement.
- Pains and discomfort in the lower back with possible spinal disorders such as curvature of the spine.

Aggravated By:
- Hot, stuffy rooms.
- Lack of fresh air.
- Being wrapped up warmly.
- Humidity.
- Rest.
- Lying down.
- Evening and at night.
- When pregnant.

Improved By:
- Affection.
- A good cry in sympathetic company.
- Sympathy and attention.
- Cool, fresh air.
- Cool bathing.
- Cold compresses.
- Gentle exercise.
- Firm pressure to painful area.

Rhus tox (Poison ivy)

Often Indicated For:
- Chickenpox
- Chilblains
- Cold sores
- Depression
- Influenza
- Insomnia
- Mumps
- Muscular overexertion
- Nappy rash
- Osteoarthritis

- Sciatica
- Sprains
- Strains
- Swollen glands

Essential Features

- Most commonly indicated for aches and pains which are eased by movement and made much more uncomfortable by resting.
- Pain and stiffness also comes on after exposure to cold, damp conditions.
- Joint and muscle problems are accompanied by sharp, shooting pains and a great deal of stiffness.
- Symptoms generally respond well to warm bathing.
- Discomfort and distress are characteristically more intense at night, with severe depression descending when resting at night.
- Extreme restlessness accompanies most symptoms.
- **Rhus tox** is one of the major remedies indicated for blistery, itchy skin eruptions such as eczema, hives (urticaria), chickenpox or cold sores.

Emotional State

- Extreme mental and physical restlessness that is very distressing at night.
- Depressed, apathetic, withdrawn and lacking interest in everything.
- Anxiety and fear, with sadness and weepiness over things that wouldn't normally cause an upset: bursts into tears for no obvious reason.
- Depression and anxiety are at their most marked in bed at night.
- Irritable and nervous with anxieties about finances, business and domestic affairs, or there may be a general, diffused fear about the future.
- Broods on unsettling or unpleasant events from the past, especially at night when there is little to provide a diversion or distraction.

Head Symptoms

- Headaches follow anger, frustration or becoming chilled.
- Severe headaches that are eased by warmth, and when bending the head backwards.
- Migraine headaches are eased a great deal by walking in the open, fresh air.

Eye Symptoms

- Watery, irritated eyes with stiff sensations in eyeballs.
- Styes with stiff sensation in eyelids.

Ear, Nose And Throat Symptoms

- Sneezing and frequent nosebleeds on waking.
- Redness, heat and swelling of the nose with burning pain when inflamed part is touched.
- Dry, painful, cracked lips and mouth with recurrent cold sores.
- Hoarseness when speaking which improves the more the voice is used.

■ Dry throat with bruised pain when speaking, and shooting pain on swallowing.

Chest Symptoms

■ Raw feeling in air passages with unpleasant, bloody or salty taste in mouth.

■ Severe headache from coughing spasms.

■ Dry, tickly cough that is brought on by exposure to the least draught of cold, damp air.

Digestive Symptoms

■ Inflamed, sore, coated tongue with red triangular tip.

■ Severe, colicky stomach pains are relieved by gentle movement and bending double.

■ Nausea is made worse by lying down.

■ Severe, painless, morning diarrhoea.

■ Exhausted with involuntary passage of diarrhoea.

Sleep

■ Restless, fitful sleep: especially after midnight.

■ Constantly moves about the bed in an effort to get comfortable.

■ Depressed and exhausted on waking from unrefreshing sleep with disturbed dreams.

Flushes And Fever

■ High temperature with sweating and trembling which is aggravated by taking warm drinks.

■ Unquenchable thirst for cold drinks, especially at night.

■ Delirium when feverish, with muttering in sleep when disturbed.

Skin

■ Constant irritation of skin in bed at night, with persistent urge to scratch.

■ Blistery, puffy skin eruptions with intolerable itching and burning.

Joint And Muscle Symptoms

■ Joint and muscle pains are brought on by exposure to damp, cold, draughty conditions.

■ Extreme, distressing restlessness with joint pains that promotes constant movement in an effort to get comfortable.

■ Muscular aches and pains follow a period of overvigorous or overly-long physical activity.

■ Severely, painful, stiff, swollen joints that are eased by continued, gentle movement. They are made more painful by resting, initial movement after keeping still, and any physical activity that is continued for long with resulting exhaustion.

■ Stiff, painful neck that is worse in the morning when first movement occurs after rest.

Aggravated By:

- Cold, damp weather.
- Rest.
- Too much physical effort.
- In bed.
- Standing.
- First movement after rest.
- After night.
- Scratching.

Improved by:

- Continued, gentle movement.
- Warm, dry weather.
- Heat.
- Warm bathing.
- Warm compresses.
- Wrapping up well.

Ruta (Rue)

Often Indicated For:

- Archilles tendon
- Bruises
- Eye strain
- Sciatica
- Sprains
- Tendonitis

Essential Features

- Aching pains in the bones and joints are a major characteristic of this remedy. Pains that respond well to **Ruta** arise from injury to the periosteum (the membranous sheath that covers the bones, providing for the attachment of tendons). Pains of this kind persist long after the date of initial injury and well after superficial bruising has healed.
- Marked restlessness and inability to keep still for any extended period of time.
- Generally chilly, with a need to be as warm as possible.
- Drowsy during the day, but unable to sleep at night, with a frequent need to stretch the limbs.
- Weary and exhausted with joint pains.

Emotional State

- Weepy and depressed, or irritable with joint pains.
- Restlessness and anxiety that is very noticeable in the evening.

Eye Symptoms

■ Pains in the eyes, or eye strain after reading or doing fine work of any kind.

■ Hot, burning eyes with possible blurring of sight which is worse in the evening.

■ Eyes water and smart after rubbing.

Digestive Symptoms

■ Pinching, gnawing pains in the stomach are soothed by taking milky drinks.

■ Stitching, tearing pains in the rectum are more intense when sitting still.

■ Haemorrhoids with possible prolapse, and constant need to pass a soft stool.

Urinary Symptoms

■ Constant discomfort and tearing pains in the bladder.

■ Frequent need to empty the bladder, with difficulty in urinating when it is time to do so.

■ Poor tone of the sphincter muscle at the neck of the bladder leads to stress incontinence during the day, or involuntary passage of urine at night.

Joint And Muscle Symptoms

■ Pains especially affect the wrists, knuckles, knees or ankles.

■ Sense of weakness in the joints that is most intense when rising from a sitting position, or when going up or down steps.

■ Walking is difficult because of bruised pains in the thighs.

■ Discomfort and bruised pains in the spine and lower back that are eased by lying on the back and made more intense when sitting down.

■ Restless legs: moves them constantly in an effort to get comfortable and settled.

Aggravated By:

■ Rest.

■ Touch.

■ Stooping.

■ Lying on the painful part.

■ Walking in the open air.

Improved By:

■ Warmth.

■ Gentle movement indoors.

Sepia (Cuttlefish ink)

Often Indicated For:

■ Back pain

■ Depression

■ Eating disorders

- Headache
- Indigestion
- Irregular periods
- Morning sickness
- Painful periods
- Post-natal depression
- Pre-menstrual syndrome
- Prolapse
- Stress Incontinence
- Thrush
- Varicose veins

Essential Features

- Physical, mental and emotional weariness, exhaustion and depression.
- Pervading sense of indifference and lack of motivation that are linked to extremely low energy levels.
- A general sense of sagging or drooping is a characteristic **Sepia** symptom, wherever it occurs in the body. There may also be a sensation of obstruction by a ball or lump.
- Poor circulation leads to problems with varicose veins, unstable body temperature and haemorrhoids.
- Nausea and dizziness are typically caused by unstable blood sugar levels and, as a result, are aggravated by going for long intervals without food. **Sepia** is often called for when these symptoms occur in pregnancy or pre-menstrually, provided the general symptoms agree.
- Despite a general sense of exhaustion, all emotional and physical symptoms are improved by vigorous exercise, such as walking briskly or running in the fresh air.
- Often indicated for depressive feelings during the menopause, after child-birth, or during severe pre-menstrual syndrome if other guiding symptoms fit.

Emotional State

- Black depression with extreme irritability and severe changes of mood.
- Although weepy, little or no relief is obtained after having a good cry.
- Terribly irritable, emotionally volatile and impatient with family, especially when feeling overwhelmed by domestic or emotional demands.
- Although energized and able to deal competently with day-to-day tasks when well, once ill health sets in, a strong feeling of being unable to cope develops.
- Anxiety and agitation when feeling overburdened. Shouts and screams in frustration, or wants to run away from emotional ties and responsibilities.
- Completely lacking in energy and drive: feels droopy and dragged down by the slightest effort.
- Marked aversion to intercourse, and total indifference to sexual partner.

■ Mentally and emotionally improved after vigorous exercise such as an aerobics class or a brisk walk in the open air.

■ Emotional symptoms are at their height after pregnancy, during the menopause or pre-menstrually.

Head Symptoms

■ Giddiness on waking from poor circulation or low blood pressure.

■ One-sided, severe headaches with throbbing, shooting pains.

■ Migraines or headaches are made worse by light, noise and the atmosphere before a storm. Associated nausea is much worse for coming into contact with the sight or smell of food.

■ Head pains are eased by sound sleep and contact with fresh air.

Eye Symptoms

■ Burning, watering and gritty feelings in the eyes.

■ Visual disturbance such as zig-zags or sparks before the eyes.

■ Visual distortion or temporary loss of vision occurs before a migraine.

Ear, Nose And Throat Symptoms

■ Frequent or recurrent colds with dry, sore, crusty nostrils.

■ Inflamed and swollen tip of the nose with troublesome loss of sense of smell.

Chest Symptoms

■ Coughing bouts lead to nausea, vomiting and retching.

■ Troublesome, hacking cough that is worse on waking or during the night.

■ Pains and uneasiness in the chest feel better for firm pressure to the affected area.

Digestive Symptoms

■ Faintness and nausea rapidly develop as a result of skipping regular meals.

■ Eating temporarily relieves nausea if it is caused by low blood sugar levels.

■ Acidic pains or an unpleasant sensation of constant movement in the stomach.

■ Constipation with small, dry, hard stools which are slow and difficult to pass.

■ A sense of a ball, or lump, or fullness remains in the rectum after a stool has been passed.

■ Severe pain occurs after passing a stool, from bleeding, inflamed haemorrhoids.

Urinary Symptoms

■ Constant desire to pass water day and night, with a marked sense of pressure in the bladder.

■ Strong-smelling, discoloured urine with reddish sediment.

Gynaecological Symptoms

■ Pre-menstrual weariness and complete mental and physical exhaustion.

■ Terrible pre-menstrual syndrome with mood swings, lethargy, irritability and delayed, scanty periods.

■ Awful morning sickness that is made much worse for delaying meals and improved by eating little and often.

■ Prolapse of the womb with a feeling that everything is about to fall out of the pelvic cavity.

■ Symptoms are worse for standing or walking for long periods of time, and are eased by sitting with the legs crossed.

■ Great distress and aversion to intercourse because of painful vaginal dryness. This symptom is most likely to develop after the menopause.

■ Additional menopausal symptoms include violent hot flushes and heavy perspiration after very little physical effort.

■ Vaginal itching with yellowy-greenish discharge.

Flushes And Fever

■ Hot flushes alternate with distressing, heavy sweats.

■ Perspiration occurs after the least physical effort.

■ Although hot flushes may feel overpowering, there is very little redness of the skin.

■ Upward moving flushes of heat, that travel from the legs to the neck and head in a wave-like motion.

Sleep

■ Drowsy by day, but unable to sleep at night – wakeful for hours.

■ Feels totally unrefreshed on waking.

■ Perspiration and flushes are especially severe at night.

Skin

■ Hormonal fluctuations may be closely related to the developing of skin conditions (e.g. acne may develop at puberty, eczema during the menopause, or urticaria (hives) may be worse during ovulation or before a period).

■ Itching, irritated skin feels worse out of doors, and better for warmth. However, it is made worse by becoming warm or overheated in bed.

■ Poor circulation leads to a mottled appearance of the skin, and/or varicose veins.

Joint And Muscle Symptoms

■ Heavy, dragging sensation with lower back pain that is relieved by firm pressure. Back pain may be associated with prolapse of the womb or period pains.

■ Weak, heavy feelings in the legs and knee joints that 'give out' when walking.

■ Knee pains with puffiness and swelling that are worse from descending stairs.

■ Resting makes bruised pains in the joints more intense.

Aggravated By:

■ Emotional demands.

■ Before, during or after a period.

- Skipping meals.
- Damp conditions.
- Resting (joint pains especially).
- Perspiring.
- Touch.
- Mental effort.

Improved By:

- Vigorous exercise such as running, walking or dancing.
- Fresh air.
- Eating little amounts at frequent intervals.
- Warmth.
- After sleep.
- Firm pressure.
- Elevating the legs.

Silica (Flint)

Often Indicated For:

- Abscesses
- Acne
- Boils
- Dizziness
- Eating disorders
- Sinusitis
- Stress incontinence
- Swollen glands
- Ulcers
- Wounds

Essential Features

- Slow, insidiously-developing conditions that come on over an extended period of time.
- Symptoms of emotional and physical illness gradually emerge after experiencing extremely stressful, shocking or distressing life events.
- Extreme tiredness and listlessness, with inability to throw off infections involving the throat and glandular system. Consequently, recurrent swollen glands and inflamed, sore throats are a frequent problem.
- Slow-healing wounds that become infected easily, or leave stubborn scars. When infection sets in, there is a tendency for discharges to be thin, clear or pussy.
- Although hot flushes can occur as a result of unstable circulation, chilliness is characteristic of the **Silica** state.

Emotional State

■ Timid, anxious and extremely lacking in confidence. Because of a strong conviction that any undertaking is likely to result in failure, any situations that are stressful or demanding are avoided.

■ Indecisive from an underlying lack of confidence, with a resulting inability to make a firm decision about anything.

■ May become obsessive or develop phobias. These may include a fear of sharp or pointed objects, leading to a marked fear of injections.

■ Short-tempered and irritable when feeling under pressure.

■ Develops fixed, rigid ideas that are very difficult to shift because of an underlying lack of security or self-confidence.

■ Jumps, flinches and starts at loud noises when feeling nervous and over-wrought.

■ Emotional and physical 'burn out' leads to great problems in thinking clearly and constructively. A hopeless depression may set in as a result of this exhausted, overwrought state.

■ Although meticulous, conscientious and hard-working when well, ill-health results in the opposite state of lack of drive, energy and initiative.

Head Symptoms

■ Hot flushes rise to the head which especially affect the crown and the right side.

■ Recurrent, bursting, severe headaches that start at the base of the skull, spreading over the whole head.

■ Headaches are eased by tight pressure, heat and wrapping up warmly. They are aggravated by exposure to cold, movement, light and noise.

Eye Symptoms

■ Dizziness and visual disturbance with headaches.

■ Dry, gritty eyes which tend to water in the open air.

Ear, Noise And Throat Symptoms

■ Itchy ears when swallowing.

■ Ears are extremely sensitive to cold air and noise.

■ Temporary hardness of hearing disappears when blowing the nose.

■ Persistent colds with sneezing, and alternately dry and running nose.

■ Uncomfortably blocked nose with painful sinuses.

■ Persistent sore throats or tonsillitis with swollen glands.

■ Swollen and tender salivary glands with sore throats and colds.

Chest Symptoms

■ Hoarseness with dry cough that is aggravated by cold drinks or when speaking.

■ Irritating cough and tickling sensation in chest are eased by warm drinks.

■ Coughing bouts are so severe, they leave the patient gasping and exhausted.

Digestive Symptoms
- Nausea with aversion to water which tastes unpleasant, and warm food or drinks.
- Abdominal tenderness and discomfort are relieved by warmth.
- Severe or persistent constipation with extreme difficulty in passing even soft stools. Sticking pains persist for some time after passing a stool.
- Tendency to anal fissure or terribly sensitive haemorrhoids.

Gynaecological Symptoms
- Absent, irregular or painful periods.
- Irregular bleeding or 'spotting' may occur at intervals between periods.
- Discharge from the vagina which is smarting and milky in appearance.

Skin
- Easily infected and poor-healing skin. The smallest scratch or wound rapidly becomes septic and inflamed.
- Slow healing capacity of the skin leads to frequent or recurring abscesses, boils and carbuncles.
- Scars refuse to heal, or remain painful for a very long time.
- Brittle or poor-quality bones that tend to break easily.

Joint And Muscle Symptoms
- Weakness and cramping pains in arms and legs.
- 'Pins and needles' and rapidly-developing numbness are caused by poor or inefficient circulation.
- Back pains are eased by warmth and aggravated by first movement after rest.

Aggravated By:
- Cold air.
- Windy, dry, cold weather.
- Pressure.
- Lying on painful part.
- During periods.

Improved By:
- Summer weather.
- Hot compresses.
- Being wrapped up warmly.
- Rest.

Staphysagria (Stavesacre)

Often Indicated For:
- After-pains in incised wounds (e.g. after Caesarian section)
- Bites

- Cystitis
- Grief
- Joint pains
- Neuralgia
- Post-natal depression
- Prostatitis
- Shingles
- Styes
- Tonsillitis
- Toothache

Essential Features

- Physical symptoms that require treatment with **Staphysagria** characteristically emerge as a result of anger, rage or indignation being suppressed or denied their natural expression.
- Extreme sensitivity on mental, emotional and physical levels, with terrific sensitivity to pains that are stinging, sharp or stitching in nature.
- Often indicated in situations of emotional and/or sexual abuse.
- Problems often follow surgical procedures that are viewed by the patient as an imposition or violation of privacy. This may often happen after invasive tests involving the genital area, or radical surgery relating to these organs (e.g. after a complete hysterectomy, especially if the patient has not been prepared for the procedure).
- Generally sensitive, shivery and chilly.

Emotional State

- Terribly inwardly resentful and angry: tends to brood and smoulder rather than freely expressing emotions.
- Shakes and trembles with the force of suppressed anger, becoming disproportionately irritated and upset by slightest criticism.
- Symptoms of illness emerge following experiences where anger, humiliation, grief or rejection are appropriate responses, but have been suppressed.
- Broods on the past, keeping a 'stiff upper lip' about unfair treatment or injustices.
- Sleep disturbance with persistent or frustrating thoughts leads to apathy and depression during the day.

Head Symptoms

- Headaches with pains in the forehead, and a general sensation of the whole head feeling numb, tight or prickling.
- Dizziness is eased by moving around, and made more intense when sitting or lying down.

Eye Symptoms

- Recurrent styes with itchy margins of eyelids.

Digestive Symptoms
■ Discomfort and irritation in the stomach that is aggravated when smoking.
■ Retching with pressure and burning pains in the stomach.
■ Discomfort in the stomach is brought on by getting tense and irritable, or drinking cold water.
■ Stinging, burning, extremely sensitive haemorrhoids.

Urinary Symptoms
■ 'Honeymoon cystitis' with constant, urgent need to pass water, and distressing burning pains that persist afterwards.
■ Persistent and irritating sensation of a drop of urine making its way along the urethra.
■ Concentrated, dark-coloured urine.
■ Cystitis may be brought on or aggravated by intercourse.

Gynaecological Symptoms
■ Itchy, extra-sensitive vagina with aversion to sexual contact, or increased libido.
■ Suppressed anger or depression after Caesarian delivery, episiotomy, hysterectomy, or any surgical procedure associated with feelings of assault, violation or bitter disappointment (e.g. following a 'high tech' birth when lack of medical intervention had been desired or anticipated).
■ Stinging pains or general sensitivity in scars that remain long after surgery.

Sleep
■ Wakes feeling irritable, bad-tempered and unrefreshed by sleep.
■ Constantly yawns with drowsiness during the day, but finds it extremely difficult to fall into a deep sleep at night.

Skin
■ Persistent stinging pains in slow-healing wounds or scars.
■ Scaly, weepy skin that burns before and after scratching.
■ Itch/scratch/itch cycle, with itching moving to another place once one area has been scratched.
■ Sharp, stinging pains during and after shingles.

Joint And Muscle Symptoms
■ Aching, stiff joints that are aggravated by touch and movement.
■ Joints become misshapen with bony nodules in well-established arthritis.
■ Discomfort and pain in the back is aggravated during the night, and when at rest.
■ Right-sided pain in the shoulder is made more intense by movement.

Aggravated By:
■ Suppressed feelings of anger, indignation or frustration.

- Mental effort.
- Slight touch.
- Intercourse.
- Smoking.
- Early morning.

Improved By:
- Rest.
- Warmth.
- Sound sleep.
- After breakfast.

Sulphur (Brimstone)

NB Although often indicated for itching and irritation of the skin, **Sulphur** should be used very sparingly and with caution because of its very dynamic and deep-acting nature. It is best to avoid giving this remedy frequently over an extended period of time, especially where there is a history of well-established or severe skin problems such as eczema or psoriasis.

Often Indicated For:
- Acne
- Addictions
- Boils
- Bronchitis
- Catarrh
- Cradle cap
- Diarrhoea
- Dizziness
- Eczema
- German measles
- Hot flushes
- Measles
- Nappy Rash
- Sleep disturbance
- Swollen glands
- Thrush
- Wheezing

Essential Features
- Marked discomfort from becoming overheated in stuffy, badly-ventilated rooms, with great relief following contact with cool, fresh air (provided it doesn't overchill).

■ Itchy, burning skin which is much worse for becoming warm in bed or after washing. The feet are especially sensitive to heat, and need to be stuck out of the bed covers in order to feel comfortable.

■ Red, hot skin that becomes flushed very rapidly, with the areas around the mouth, eyelids and wings of the nose looking especially bright red and inflamed.

■ Poor stamina with a tendency for conditions to relapse from a general state of exhaustion and lack of vitality.

■ Unstable or low blood sugar levels, with a marked dip in energy around 11 a.m., and associated dizziness, weakness and pangs of hunger.

■ Discharges are characteristically profuse, discoloured (yellowish-green), and offensive in odour and consistency.

■ Strong aversion to washing because it always aggravates symptoms in general.

Emotional State

■ Poor or deficient, long-term stamina and persistence for tasks or challenges that call for staying power.

■ Touchy, depressed and self-absorbed with a tendency to be extremely short-tempered and irritable.

■ Impatient, with a rapid tendency to sulk when offended.

■ Endlessly speculates and philosophizes: beats around the bush rather than being straightforward.

■ Combination of fastidiousness with untidiness: study is chaotic, while work that is produced is immaculate.

■ Anxious, weepy, introspective and depressed during periods and the menopause.

■ Obsessional thoughts may develop about religious ideas, moral issues, or anxieties about health and disease.

Head Symptoms

■ Dizziness occurs frequently, and may be especially severe when standing for any length of time.

■ Light-headedness may be combined with nausea, weakness and breathlessness.

■ Periodic headaches (e.g. each weekend, or during a holiday). These may occur due to the release of stress during a period of relaxation.

■ Headaches are worse out of doors or when stooping, and better for resting in a moderate, stable temperature.

Eye Symptoms

■ Red edges of the eyelids with a yellowish, crusty discharge.

■ Itchy, red, burning eyes.

Ear, Nose And Throat Symptoms

■ Stuffed-up indoors with fluent nasal discharge when out of doors.

■ Persistent or recurrent colds with thick, offensive, persistent nasal discharge.

- Sore, dry throat with a sensation of a ball or lump that refuses to move when swallowing.

Chest Symptoms

- Tight, constricted feeling in the chest that is worse at night.
- Suffocative coughing bouts are eased by contact with open, fresh air.
- Wheezing bouts alternate with skin problems such as eczema.

Digestive Symptoms

- Ravenous appetite, with sinking sensation in the stomach around mid-morning.
- Queasiness that is made much worse for skipping meals.
- Violent burping with burning indigestion.
- Craves spicy, fatty foods and alcohol which aggravate indigestion, or may show a marked dislike of fat, eggs and milk.
- Painless, early morning diarrhoea with great urgency: rushes to the toilet in order to get there in time.
- Alternating constipation and diarrhoea.
- Diarrhoea results in red, sore, burning or itching anus that may be the cause of great discomfort in bed at night.

Urinary Symptoms

- Distressing burning, smarting pains when passing water.
- Recurrent kidney problems with general state of shivering, cold sweat and muscle aches on urinating.

Gynaecological Symptoms

- Irregular periods with intermittent menstrual flow that stops and starts.
- Periods may be delayed or early, with dark menstrual flow that is alternately heavy and scanty.
- Menopausal hot flushes, shivering and faintness.
- Bearing down sensations with prolapse that are aggravated when standing.
- Vaginal burning and itching that is much worse during the menopause.

Sleep

- Wakes regularly around 3 a.m. unable to get back to sleep.
- Starts violently when on the verge of falling asleep.
- Unrefreshed by sleep, with a constant need to lie in.

Flushes And Fever

- During a hot flush the skin remains generally hot and dry, or it may be swiftly followed by a distressing, clammy, drenching perspiration.
- Although very hot and flushed, there is a marked dislike of both overheated and draughty rooms.

- Head is often uncomfortably hot while the feet are chilly, or feet may feel burning hot.
- Very thirsty for lots of cold drinks, but little sweat is produced.

Skin

- Itchy, inflamed, unhealthy skin that burns, weeps or bleeds after scratching.
- Intense itching that feels much worse for contact with heat in any form, such as warmth of the bed, or bathing in warm water.
- Skin is also very sensitive to contact with wool.

Joint And Muscle Symptoms

- Painful, stiff joints that are especially uncomfortable when rising from a sitting position.
- Easily-developing 'pins and needles' when a limb is kept immobile for any length of time.
- Cramps and muscle pains may be brought on by becoming warm in bed.
- Sensitive, painful spine which is aggravated by the slightest pressure or jarring movement.
- Curvature of the spine as a result of weak, poorly-toned spinal muscles.

Aggravated By:

- Heat.
- Warmth of the bed.
- Cold draughts or chill.
- Standing for prolonged periods of time.
- Washing.
- Eating.
- On walking.
- Mid-morning.

Improved By:

- Dry, warm weather.
- Moderate temperatures.
- Lying on the right side.

Homoeopathic Remedies And Their Abbreviations

Aconitum napellus	Aconite
Aesculus hippocastum	
Allium cepa	
Aloe alumina	
Ammonium muriaticum	Ammonium mur
Antimonium tartaricum	Ant tart
Apis mellifica	Apis
Argentum nitricum	Argentum nit
Arnica montana	Arnica
Arsenicum album	Arsenicum alb
Belladonna	
Bellis perennis	
Borax	
Bryonia alba	Bryonia
Calcarea carbonica	Calc carb
Calcarea phosphorica	Calc phos
Calendula officinalis	Calendula
Cantharis	
Carbo vegetabilis	Carbo veg
Caulophyllum	Caul
Causticum	
Chamomilla	
Cimicifuga racemosa	Cimic
Coccus cacti	
Colocythis	
Corallium rubrum	
Cuprum metallicum	Cuprum
Dioscorea	

Drosera	
Eupatorium perfoliatum	Eupatorium
Euphrasia	
Ferrum phosphoricum	Ferrum phos
Gelsemium sempervirens	Gelsemium
Glonoin	
Gnaphaleum	
Graphites	
Graphiteum	
Hamamelis	
Hepar sulphuris calcareum	Hepar sulph
Hypericum perfoliatum	Hypericum
Ignatia amara	Ignatia
Ipecacuana	Ipecac
Jaborandi	
Kali bichromium	Kali bich
Kali carbonicum	Kali carb
Kreosotum	
Lachesis	
Ledum palustre	Ledum
Lycopodium	
Magnesia phosphorica	Mag phos
Mercurius solubilis	Mercurius
Natrum muriaticum	Nat mur
Nux vomica	
Phosphorus	
Phytolacca decandra	Phytolacca
Podophyllum	
Pulsatilla nigricans	Pulsatilla
Rhus toxicodendron	Rhus tox
Rumex crispus	Rumex
Ruta graveolens	Ruta
Sabadilla	
Sanguinaria	
Sepia	
Silica	
Spongia tosta	Spongia
Staphysagria	
Sulphur	
Symphytum officinale	Symphytum
Urtica urens	Urtica
Veratrum album	Veratrum alb

Useful Addresses

Council for Complementary and Alternative Medicine
179 Gloucester Place
London NW1 6DX
Tel: 0171 724 9103

Natural Medicines Society
Market Chambers
13A Market Place
Heanor
Derbyshire
DE75 7AA
Tel: 01773 710002

British Complementary Medical Association
St Charles' Hospital
Exmoor Street
London W10 6DZ
Tel: 0181 964 1206

The Society of Homoeopaths
2 Artizan Road
Northampton
NN1 4HU
Tel: 01604 21400

The British Homoeopathic Association
27a Devonshire Street
London WC1N 3HZ
Tel: 0171 935 2163

The Homoeopathic Society
Hahnemann House
Powis Place
Great Ormond Street
London WC1N 1RJ
Tel: 0171 837 9469

Ainsworths Homoeopathic Pharmacy
38 New Cavendish Street
London W1M 7LH
Tel: 0171 935 5330 (Daytime) 0171 487 5252 (24-hour answering machine service)

Helios Homoeopathic Pharmacy
97 Camden Road
Tunbridge Wells
Kent TN1 2QP
Tel: 01892 536393 (Daytime) 01892 537254 (24-hour answering machine service)

The Homoeopathic Supply Company
4 Nelson Road
Sherringham
Norfolk NR26 8BU
Tel: 01263 824683

Recommended Reading

General Books on Homoeopathy

Castro, Miranda, *The Complete Homoeopathy Handbook: A Guide to Everyday Health Care*, Macmillan, 1990

Cummings, Dr Stephen, and Ullman, Dana, *Everybody's Guide to Homoeopathic Medicines: Taking Care of Yourself and Your Family With Safe and Effective Remedies*, Gollancz, 1986

Hammond, Dr Christopher, *How to Use Homoeopathy*, Element, 1991

Lockie, Dr Andrew, *The Family Guide to Homoeopathy: The Safe Form of Medicine for the Future*, Elm Tree Books, 1989

MacEoin, Beth, *Homoeopathy: Headway Lifeguides*, Headway, 1992

Panos, Maesimund and Heimlich, Jane, *Homoeopathic Medicine at Home*, Corgi, 1980

Ullman, Dana, *Homoeopathy, Medicine for the Twenty-First Century*, Thorsons, 1989

Vithoulkas, George, *Homoeopathy, Medicine for the New Man*, Thorsons, 1985

Weiner, Michael and Goss, Kathleen, *The Complete Book of Homoeopathy*, Bantam, 1982

For those who are interested in a more detailed explanation of homoeopathic philosophy, theory and history, the following books will be appropriate:

Campbell, Anthony, *The Two Faces of Homoeopathy*, Robert Hale Ltd, 1984

Coulter, Harris, *Divided Legacy: The Conflict Between Homoeopathy and the American Medical Association*, North Atlantic Books, 1982

Coulter, Harris, *Homoeopathic Science and Modern Medicine: The Physics of Healing With Microdoses*, North Atlantic Books, 1980

Nicholls, Phillip, *Homoeopathy and the Medical Profession*, Croom Helm, 1988

Vithoulkas, George, *The Science of Homoeopathy*, Thorsons, 1986

Homoeopathy For Women

Castro, Miranda, *Homoeopathy for Mother and Baby: Pregnancy, Birth, and the Post-Natal Year*, Macmillan, 1992

Handley, Rima, *Homoeopathy for Women*, Thorsons, 1993

Lockie, Dr Andrew, and Geddes, Dr Nicola, *The Woman's Guide to Homoeopathy: The Natural Way to a Healthier Life for Women*, Hamish Hamilton, 1992

MacEoin, Beth, *Homoeopathy For Women: A Guide to Vital Health*, Headway, 1995

Moskowitz, Dr Richard, *Homoeopathic Medicines for Pregnancy and Child-birth*, North Atlantic Books, 1992

General Health Guides For Women

Bradford, Nikki, *The Well Woman's Self-Help Directory*, Sidgwick and Jackson, 1990

Kahn, Ada, and Linda Hughey Holt, *Menopause: The Best Years of Your Life*, Bloomsbury, 1993

Kenton, Leslie, *Passage to Power: Natural Menopause Revolution*, Ebury, 1995

Llewellyn-Jones, Derek, *Everywoman: A Gynaecological Guide for Life*, Penguin, 1993

MacEoin, Beth, *Healthy by Nature: A Woman's Guide to Positive Health and Vitality in a Stressful World*, Thorsons, 1994

Phillips, Angela and Rakusen, Jill, *The New Our Bodies Ourselves: A Health Book for and by Women*, Penguin, 1989

Scott, Julian and Susan, *Natural Medicine for Women: Drug-Free Healthcare for Women of All Ages*, Gaia, 1991

Stoppard, Dr Miriam, *Every Woman's Lifeguide: How to Achieve and Maintain Fitness, Health and Happiness in Today's World*, Optima, 1988

Stoppard, Dr Miriam, *Menopause: The Complete Practical Guide to Managing Your Life and Maintaining Physical and Emotional Well-Being*, Dorling Kindersley, 1994

Westcott, Patsy, *Alternative Health Care For Women: A Compendium of Natural Approaches to Women's Health and Well Being*, Grapevine, 1987

Homoeopathy For Children

Castro, Miranda, *Homoeopathy For Mother and Baby: Pregnancy, Birth, and the Post-Natal Year*, Macmillan, 1992

Herscu, Paul, *The Homoeopathic Treatment of Children: Pediatric Constitutional Types*, North Atlantic Books, 1991

MacEoin, Beth, *Homoeopathy for Babies and Children: A Parents' Guide*, Headway, 1994

Morgan, Lyle W., *Homoeopathy and Your Child*, Healing Arts Press, 1992

Ullman, Dana, *Homoeopathic Medicine For Children and Infants*, Piatkus, 1994

The Issue of Vaccination

Neustaeder, Randall, *The Immunization Decision: A Guide For Parents*, North Atlantic Books, 1990

Chaitow, Leon, *Vaccination and Immunization: Dangers, Delusions and Alternatives*, C.W. Daniel, 1987

Kenton, Leslie, *Nature's Child: Guide, Nourish and Protect Your Child the Gentle Way*, Ebury Press, 1993

Articles

'The Immunization Debate', *Childright*, January/February 1992

Stress and Relaxation

Benson, Herbert, *Beyond the Relaxation Response*, Collins, 1985

Benson, Herbert, *The Relaxation Response*, Collins, 1976

Chaitow, Leon, *Your Complete Stress-Proofing Programme*, Thorsons, 1986

Horn, Sandra, *Relaxation: Modern Techniques for Stress Management*, Thorsons, 1986

Kenton, Leslie, *Ten Day De-stress Plan: Make Stress Work for You*, Ebury, 1994

Krista, Alix, *The Book of Stress Survival: How to Relax and Live Positively*, Ebury, 1986

Souter, Dr Keith, *Homoeopathy: Heart and Soul: Treatment for Emotional Problems*, C.W. Daniel, 1993

Homoeopathy and Fitness

Subotnick, Steven, *Sports and Exercise Injuries: Conventional, Homoeopathic and Alternative Treatments*, North Atlantic Books, 1991

Index

abbreviations 336-7
abdominal pains 90, 114-17, 218
Achilles tendonitis 92-4
Aconite *see* Aconitum napelus
Aconitum napelus 236-9
   for anxiety 198
   chickenpox 112
   colds 50
   croup 118
   earache 121
   German measles 125
   grief 205
   influenza 78
   insomnia 209
   labour pains 175
   measles 127
   mumps 131
   shock 44
   sore throats 85
   teething 138
acute illness 10-11
addictions 189, 194
addresses 338-9
adenoids 120
aerobic exercises 54
Aesculus hippocastanum, for
   haemorrhoids 215
Agnus castus 239-40
alcoholism 194
allergens 47-8
Allium cepa
   for colds 51
   hayfever 67
Aloe, for haemorrhoids 215
Alumina and aluminium
   for constipation 54, 55, 74
   haemorrhoids 214
Ammonium muriaticum, for
   sciatica 232
Anacardium orientale 241-2
Ant tart *see* Antimonium tartaricum
antacids 74
Antimonium tartaricum
   for chickenpox 112
   whooping cough 142
anxiety 60, 87, 157, 194-8
   see also depression; insomnia
Apis mellifica 242-5
   for bites/stings 26
   cystitis 148

hayfever 66
measles 128
mumps 132
nappy rash 135
osteoarthritis 225
puncture wounds 42
shock 45
sore throats 85
appendicitis, vomiting and 87
Argentum nitricum 245-7
   for anxiety 197
   diarrhoea 62
   hiatus hernia 218
Arnica montana 247-9
   for Achilles tendonitis 93
   blood loss 29
   burns 34
   cream 24
   cuts/bruises 36
   fractures 39
   grief 205
   insomnia 209
   muscle aches 95
   muscle sprains 98
   osteoarthritis 225
   post-delivery 178
   shock 44
   tendonitis 104
   varicose veins 235
   whooping cough 142
aromatherapy oils 20, 95, 184,
   196, 208
Arsenic *see* Arsenicum album
Arsenicum album 250-3
   for addictions 194
   anxiety 197
   chickenpox 112
   colds 51
   coughs 57
   cystitis 147
   depression 202
   diarrhoea 61
   hayfever 66
   hiatus hernia 217
   indigestion 75
   influenza 79
   measles 129
   morning sickness 170
   nappy rash 135
   period pains 164

pregnancy 173
thrush 152
varicose veins 234
asthma 46-8
   see also eczema; hayfever

babies *see* children and babies
Belladonna 253-6
   for blood loss 30
   chickenpox 112
   colds 51
   colic 115
   cystitis 148
   earache 121
   German measles 125
   influenza 78
   mastitis 180
   measles 127
   mumps 131
   nappy rash 136
   period pains 164
   sore throats 85
   sun/heat stroke 101
   teething 138
Bellis perennis
   for Achilles tendonitis 93
   cuts/bruises 37
   post-delivery 178
   tendonitis 104
bereavement 204-6
   see also anxiety; depression;
   insomnia
bites/stings 25-8
black snakeroot *see* Cimicifuga
   racemosa
bladders, cystitis and 145, 146, 147
blood loss 28-31
books 21, 340-2
Borax, for thrush 152
breast-feeding 114, 180
brimstone *see* Sulphur
British Homoeopathic Association
   21, 338
bruises/cuts 35-7
Bryonia alba 257-60
   for colic 116
   constipation 55
   coughs 57
   fractures 39
   haemorrhoids 214

headaches 71
hiatus hernia 217
indigestion 75
influenza 79
insomnia 210
mastitis 181
measles 128
mumps 131
muscle aches 96
muscle sprains 98
osteoarthritis 224
burns/scalds 31-5

Calc carb *see* Calcarea carbonica
Calc phos *see* Calcarea
  phosphorica
Calcarea carbonica 260-3
  for nappy rash 136
  PMS 159
  teething 139
  thrush 153
Calcarea phosphorica
  for fractures 40
  osteoarthritis 226
  teething 139
calcium carbonate *see* Calcarea
  carbonica
calcium sulphide *see* Hepar
  sulphuris calcareum
Calendula officinalis 263
  cream/tincture 23, 24, 134, 233
  for post-delivery 178
Candida albicans 149, 150, 151
Cantharis 264-5
  for bites/stings 27
  burns 34
  cystitis 148
  nappy rash 135
Carbo vegetabilis 266-8
  for blood loss 30
  diarrhoea 61
  hiatus hernia 218
  indigestion 74
  shock 45
  sun/heat stroke 102
  varicose veins 235
  whooping cough 141
Caulophyllum, for labour pains 176
Causticum 268-71
  for burns 34
chamomile *see* Chamomilla
Chamomilla 271-4
  for colic 115
  earache 122
  labour pains 177
  period pains 165
  teething 138
chaste tree *see* Agnus castus
chest pains 59
chickenpox 110-13
childbirth, pre/post 174-9
children and babies
  behaviour 106
  infectious diseases 108-13, 124-
    33, 140-3
  sore throats 87
children and babies, signs/
    symptoms in 108

China officinalis 274-5
chiropractor 224
chronic illness 11
Cimicifuga racemosa 276-8
  for depression 202
  period pains 165
  PMS 161
  post-natal depression 185
clubmoss *see* Lycopodium
Coccus cacti, for whooping cough
    141
coeliac disease 60
colds 49-52
colic 114-17
Colocynthis
  for colic 115
  period pains 165
  sciatica 231
constipation 52-6
contraception 147, 160, 162
Corallium rubrum, for whooping
    cough 142
coughs 56-9
creams/tinctures 24, 26
  see also specific names
Crohn's disease 60
croup 117-20
Cuprum metallicum, for sun/heat
    stroke 102
cuts/bruises 35-7
cuttlefish ink *see* Sepia
cycling 94, 95, 163, 192
cystitis 145-9

deadly nightshade *see* Belladonna
dehydration 60, 63, 88, 90, 100
depression 182-6, 199-203
  see also anxiety; insomnia
diabetes, thrush and 150
diarrhoea 60-3
  see also nausea; vomiting
Dioscorea
  for colic 116
  sciatica 231
discharge, vaginal 150, 152, 153,
    154
diuretics 53, 66, 163
dosage, remedies 6-7, 14-15
dowager's hump 226
Drosera
  for coughs 58
  croup 118
  whooping cough 142
drug dependency 189-94

earache 120-3
eating disorders 52, 88, 199, 227
eczema 63-5
  see also asthma; hayfever
endorphins 157, 192
Eupatorium perfoliatum
  for fractures 39
  influenza 79
Euphrasia
  for colds 51
  hayfever 67
  measles 128
eustachian tubes 120

evening primrose oil 65, 151, 158,
    163
exercise 94-5, 163, 192, 195, 200,
    213, 227
eye pains 90

Ferrum phosphoricum
  for colds 51
  earache 122
  German measles 125
first aid kits 23-5
first aid techniques 26, 28-9, 32-3,
    35, 41, 43-4
flint *see* Silica
food poisoning 88
fractures 38-40

garlic 50, 57, 78, 81, 147
Gelsemium sempervirens 278-80
  for anxiety 197
  diarrhoea 62
  headaches 70
  influenza 79
  labour pains 177
  measles 128
  sciatica 230
genital thrush 149-54
German measles 124-6
Glonoin
  for hot flushes 221
  sun/heat stroke 101
Gnaphalium, for sciatica 231
golfer's elbow 103
GPs (doctors) 17-18, 20
Graphites
  for constipation 56
  mastitis 182
  nappy rash 136
grief 204-6
gynaecological problems 154-65

haemorrhoids 212-15
Hamamelis
  haemorrhoids 214
  varicose veins 234
hangovers 68, 70
hayfever 65-8
  see also asthma; eczema
headaches 68-72, 102
heartburn, in pregnancy 171-4
heat exhaustion 99-103
heel pains 92, 94
Hepar sulphuris calcareum 280-2
  for coughs 59
  croup 119
  earache 122
  sinusitis 82
  sore throats 86
herb teas 60, 69, 156, 196, 200
hiatus hernia 215-18
holism/holistic treatment 4-6,
    7-8
homoeopaths 21-2
honey bee *see* Apis mellifica
hot flushes 219-22
HRT (Hormone Replacement
    Therapy) 227
humidifiers 57, 84

Hypercal cream/tincture 23, 24,
    84, 110, 111, 134
Hypericum perfoliatum 282-3
    for bites/stings 27
    cuts/bruises 36
    post-delivery 178
    puncture wounds 42
    sciatica 230

Ignatia amara 283-5
    for grief 206
    indigestion 76
    insomnia 210
    post-natal depression 185
    sore throats 86
impetigo 64
indigestion 72-6, 171-4
infectious diseases 108-13, 124-33
influenza 76-81
insomnia 206-10
    see also anxiety; depression
Ipecacuanha 286-7
    for blood loss 30
    morning sickness 169
    period pains 165
    vomiting 89
    whooping cough 141
Irritable Bowel Syndrome 54, 60

Jaborandi, for mumps 132
jogging 94, 95, 163

Kali bichromium 288-90
    for coughs 58
    croup 119
    German measles 125
    sinusitis 82
Kali carbonicum 290-3
    for labour pains 176
    PMS 159
    sciatica 231
    thrush 153
    whooping cough 142
Kreosotum
    for teething 138
    thrush 154

labour pains 175-7
Lachesis 293-6
    for addictions 193
    croup 119
    depression 201
    earache 123
    headaches 70
    hot flushes 221
    mumps 131
    period pains 164
    PMS 159
    sore throats 87
    varicose veins 235
laryngitis 84, 86
laxatives 53, 54
Ledum palustre 296-8
    for bites/stings 27
    cuts/bruises 36
    muscle sprains 99
    osteoarthritis 225
    puncture wounds 41

tendonitis 104
Lycopodium 298-301
    for addictions 193
    anxiety 198
    colic 116
    constipation 55
    hiatus hernia 218
    indigestion 74
    PMS 159
    pregnancy 173
    sore throats 87

Mag phos see Magnesia
    phosphorica
Magnesia phosphorica
    for colic 116
    sciatica 231
marigold see Calendula officinalis
marking nut see Anacardium
    orientale
mastitis 179, 182
Materia Medica 7
measles 126-9
meditation 189
Mercurius solubilis 301-4
    for chickenpox 113
    earache 122
    influenza 80
    mastitis 181
    mumps 133
    sinusitis 83
    sore throats 86
    thrush 153
migraines 68
monkshood see Aconitum napelus
morning sickness 166-71
mountain daisy see Arnica montana
mumps 130-2
muscles, over-exercise of 94-6

nappy rash 133-6
Nat mur see Natrum muriaticum
Natrum muriaticum 304-7
    for colds 52
    depression 202
    grief 206
    hayfever 67
    headaches 70
    morning sickness 169
    PMS 159
    post-natal depression 186
    thrush 152
nausea 72, 76
    see also diarrhoea; vomiting
night sweats 220
Nux vomica 307-11
    for addictions 193
    anxiety 197
    colds 52
    colic 115
    constipation 55
    cystitis 149
    haemorrhoids 214
    hayfever 68
    headaches 70
    hiatus hernia 217
    indigestion 75
    insomnia 209

labour pains 176
morning sickness 171
period pains 164
PMS 158
pregnancy 173
vomiting 90

oesophagus 215
oils, aromatherapy 95, 196, 201,
    208
older people 211-35
oophoritis 130
orchitis 130
osteoarthritis 222-6
osteopaths 224
osteoporosis 54, 226-9

painkillers 69, 72
    see also TENS machines
pains
    abdominal 90, 114-7, 218
    chest 59
    eye 90
    heel 92, 94
    labour 175-7
    period 161-6
period pains 161-6
Peruvian bark see China officinalis
pharmacies, homoeopathic 213
pharyngitis 84
Phosphorus 311-15
    for anxiety 198
    blood loss 30
    coughs 58
    croup 118
    diarrhoea 62
    headaches 71
    pregnancy 174
    sinusitis 83
    sore throats 85
    vomiting 90
phytolacca decandra
    Achilles tendonitis 93
    mastitis 181
    mumps 132
Phytolacca decandram, sore
    throats 86
pilates 91
PMS (Pre-Menstrual Syndrome)
    144, 145, 154-61
Podophyllum, for diarrhoea 62
poison ivy see Rhus toxicodendron
poison nut see Nux vomica
post-natal depression 182-6
potassium bichromate see Kali
    bichromium
potassium carbonate see Kali
    carbonicum
potassium hydrate see Causticum
Pre-Menstrual Syndrome see PMS
    (Pre-Menstrual Syndrome)
pregnancy
    and constipation 52, 56
    diarrhoea 63
    German measles 126
    heartburn 171-4
    morning sickness 166-71
    problems 144

thrush 150
varicose veins 232
prostoglandin 162
psoriasis 63-4, 81
Pulsatilla nigricans 315-19
    for chickenpox 113
    colic 117
    coughs 59
    cystitis 149
    depression 202
    earache 123
    German measles 126
    grief 205
    hayfever 67
    headaches 71
    hiatus hernia 217
    hot flushes 221
    indigestion 75
    influenza 80
    labour pains 176
    mastitis 182
    measles 128
    morning sickness 170
    mumps 133
    osteoarthritis 225
    period pains 166
    PMS 159
    pregnancy 174
    sinusitis 82
    teething 139
    thrush 153
    varicose veins 234
    vomiting 90
puncture wounds 40-3

quicksilver see Mercurius solubilis

rashes
    chickenpox 110-13
    German measles 124
    measles 127
    nappy 133-6
relaxation 54, 188-9
remedies 336-7
    administration 15-16
    buying 18
    dosage 6-7, 14-15
    names see specific
    response to 16-17
    storing 19-20
remedy tables, use of 13-14
Reye's syndrome 111
rheumatic fever 87
Rhus toxicodendron 319-22
    for Achilles tendonitis 94
    chickenpox 113
    depression 203
    influenza 80
    insomnia 210
    mumps 132
    muscle aches 96
    muscle sprains 98
    nappy rash 135
    osteoarthritis 224
    sciatica 230
    tendonitis 104
ruue see Ruta graveolens
Rumex see Rumex crispus

Rumex crispus, for coughs 59
Ruta graveolens 322-3
    for Achilles tendonitis 93
    cuts/bruises 37
    muscle sprains 98
    tendonitis 104

Sabadilla, for hayfever 67
St Ignatius' bean see Ignatia amara
St John's wort see Hypericum
        perfoliatum
salt, common see Natrum
        muriaticum
Sanguinaria, for hot flushes 222
scalds/burns 31-5
sciatica 229-32
senile dementia 54
Sepia 323-7
    for depression 203
    headaches 71
    indigestion 76
    morning sickness 169
    period pains 166
    PMS 158
    post-natal depression 184
    thrush 152
sex 147, 150
shock 40, 43-5, 103
Silica 327-9
    for puncture wounds 42
    sinusitis 83
silver nitrate see Argentum
        nitricum
sinusitis 81-3
Society of Homoeopaths 21, 338
sore throats 83-7
Spanish fly see Cantharis
Spongia tosta
    for coughs 58
    croup 118
sports 91-105, 163, 192, 201
sprains 96-9
Staphysagria 329-32
    for bites/stings 27
    cuts/bruises 37
    cystitis 148
    grief 206
    post-delivery 179
    post-natal depression 185
stavesacre see Staphysagria
stings/bites 25-8
strains 96-9
stress 157, 188-9
stridor 117
sugars, cystitis and 146-7
Sulphur 332-5
    for addictions 194
    diarrhoea 63
    German measles 126
    headaches 72
    hot flushes 222
    measles 129
    nappy rash 136
    thrush 154
sun/heat stroke 99-103
Surukuku snake venom see
        Lachesis
Symphytum officinale

for cuts/bruises 36
    fractures 39
'symptom pictures' 8-9, 12-13

tables, use of 13-14
t'ai chi 91, 195
teething 137-40
tendonitis 103-5
tennis elbow 103-5
tenosynovitis 92
TENS (Transcutaneous Electrical
        Nerve Stimulation) machines
        162-3
tension headaches 68, 69
tetanus 37-8, 42
thrush, genital 149-54
tinctures, see creams/tinctures
tonsillitis 83, 87, 120

ulcerative colitis 60
Urtica urens
    for bites/stings 27
    burns 33
    cream/tincture 23, 110, 111
urticaria 64

vaccination 109-10
vaginal discharge, thrush and 150,
        152, 153, 154
varicose veins 232-5
vegetable charcoal see Carbo
        vegetabilis
Veratrum album
    for diarrhoea 61
    morning sickness 170
    sun/heat stroke 102
    vomiting 89
vitamin B supplement
    for depression 200
    PMS 157, 163
    thrush 151
vitamin C supplement
    for colds 49-50
    coughs 57
    cystitis 147
    influenza 77
    PMS 158, 163
    sinusitis 81
    sore throats 84
    thrush 151
vomiting 87-90
    see also diarrhoea; nausea

walking 94, 95, 157, 163
warts 64
wheezing 59, 68
white bryony see Bryonia alba
whooping cough 140-3
wild rosemary see Ledum palustre
wind flower see Pulsatilla
witch hazel 213, 214
wounds 28-31, 40-3

yellow jasmine see Gelsemium
        sempervirens
yoga 91, 95, 157, 195